T0260828

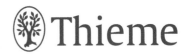

Top 3 Differentials in Gastrointestinal Imaging

A Case Review

Rocky C. Saenz, DO, FAOCR
Vice Chairman, Department of Radiology
Program Director of Diagnostic Radiology Residency
Director of MRI and Musculoskeletal Imaging
Beaumont Hospital, Farmington Hills Campus
Farmington Hills, Michigan
Clinical Assistant Professor
Michigan State University College of Osteopathic Medicine
Lansing, Michigan

Series Editor:

William T. O'Brien, Sr., DO, FAOCR
Director, Pediatric Neuroradiology Fellowship
Cincinnati Children's Hospital Medical Center
Associate Professor of Radiology
University of Cincinnati College of Medicine
Cincinnati, Ohio

206 illustrations

Thieme
New York • Stuttgart • Delhi • Rio de Janeiro

Executive Editor: William Lamsback
Managing Editor: Apoorva Goel
Director, Editorial Services: Mary Jo Casey
Production Editor: Shivika
International Production Director: Andreas Schabert
Editorial Director: Sue Hodgson
International Marketing Director: Fiona Henderson
International Sales Director: Louisa Turrell
Director, Institutional Sales: Adam Bernacki
Senior Vice President and Chief Operating Officer:
   Sarah Vanderbilt
President: Brian D. Scanlan

Library of Congress Cataloging-in-Publication Data
is available from the publisher.

©2019 Thieme Medical Publishers, Inc.

Thieme Medical Publishers New York
333 Seventh Avenue
New York, New York 10001 USA
+1 800 782 3488
customerservice@thieme.com

Thieme Publishers Stuttgart
Rüdigerstrasse 14, 70469 Stuttgart, Germany
+49 [0]711 8931 421, customerservice@thieme.de

Thieme Publishers Delhi
A-12, Second Floor, Sector-2, Noida-201301
Uttar Pradesh, India
+91 120 45 566 00, customerservice@thieme.in

Thieme Publishers Rio de Janeiro,
Thieme Publicações Ltda.
Edifício Rodolpho de Paoli, 25º andar
Av. Nilo Peçanha, 50 – Sala 2508,
Rio de Janeiro 20020-906 Brasil
+55 21 3172-2297

Cover design: Thieme Publishing Group
Typesetting by DiTech Process Solutions, India

Printed in USA by King Printing Company, Inc.   5 4 3 2 1

ISBN 978-1-62623-358-4

Also available as an e-book:
eISBN 978-1-62623-359-1

Important note: Medicine is an ever-changing science undergoing continual development. Research and clinical experience are continually expanding our knowledge, in particular our knowledge of proper treatment and drug therapy. Insofar as this book mentions any dosage or application, readers may rest assured that the authors, editors, and publishers have made every effort to ensure that such references are in accordance with **the state of knowledge at the time of production of the book.**

Nevertheless, this does not involve, imply, or express any guarantee or responsibility on the part of the publishers in respect to any dosage instructions and forms of applications stated in the book. **Every user is requested to examine carefully** the manufacturers' leaflets accompanying each drug and to check, if necessary in consultation with a physician or specialist, whether the dosage schedules mentioned therein or the contraindications stated by the manufacturers differ from the statements made in the present book. Such examination is particularly important with drugs that are either rarely used or have been newly released on the market. Every dosage schedule or every form of application used is entirely at the user's own risk and responsibility. The authors and publishers request every user to report to the publishers any discrepancies or inaccuracies noticed. If errors in this work are found after publication, errata will be posted at www.thieme.com on the product description page.

Some of the product names, patents, and registered designs referred to in this book are in fact registered trademarks or proprietary names even though specific reference to this fact is not always made in the text. Therefore, the appearance of a name without designation as proprietary is not to be construed as a representation by the publisher that it is in the public domain.

The views expressed in this book are those of the author and contributors, and do not reflect the official policy or position of the United States Government, the Department of Defense, Department of the Army or the Department of the Air Force

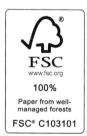

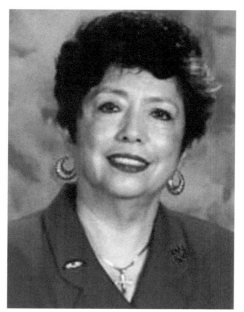

1939–2016

I dedicate this work to my mother, Angelita Hernandez Saenz. You were the greatest mother giving all your love and countless selfless acts to your children and grandchildren. The first college-educated in your family and achieving an advanced degree are just obvious reasons you are my personal inspiration. It is because of your guidance throughout my life that I have been able to accomplish all my goals, both professionally and personally. Your grandchildren's future success is only possible because of the endless sacrifices you endured and your dedication toward education. The thousands of students you taught, during your career, are lucky to have been in the presence of a great woman like you.

I will love you forever!

Your son,

Rocky C. Saenz

Contents

Series Foreword

The original "Top 3" concept was something engrained in us during our residency training in the military. From day 1, our program emphasized the importance of having gamut-based differentials as part of our daily readout sessions, as well as during didactic and clinical case-based conferences. The bulk of residency training was then centered around learning the key clinical and imaging manifestations of each entity on the list of differentials to be able to distinguish one from another, when possible. To avoid providing clinicians with a laundry list of differentials that would be of little value, we were encouraged to consider the "Top 3" differentials and any other important considerations based on the specific clinical scenario or imaging finding(s) presented. I found that concept and approach to radiology so useful that I continue to utilize it to this day.

One thing I have learned throughout my radiology career, especially as a residency program director, is that not every individual learns or processes information in the same manner. Some individuals can read through a traditional textbook that is organized by pathology (i.e., developmental abnormalities, infectious processes, neoplasms, etc.) and readily recognize that the developmental abnormality in Chapter 1 is in the same differential for the infectious process in Chapter 2 and a few neoplasms in Chapter 3. Others, like me, best learn from gamut-based resources where content is organized based on the key imaging findings, similar to how we practice radiology. If you are part of the latter group, then the "Top 3" approach may be the right fit for you. The intent of the series is to provide a comprehensive case-based alternative to traditional subspecialty textbooks where the focus remains on differential diagnoses. After all, when the dust settles and the core and certifying exams are nothing but distant (and hopefully pleasant) memories, this is what radiology is all about.

The Gastrointestinal Imaging (GI) Top 3 book is edited by Dr. Rocky C. Saenz, who is an academic radiologist and residency program director with the Michigan State University consortium. I have known Dr. Saenz for nearly 10 years and have worked closely with him on numerous academic projects, including annual board review courses that he pioneered in Detroit, Michigan, and at the American Osteopathic College of Radiology annual meetings. His experience and academic acumen, along with his presentation and teaching style, make him an ideal editor for this subspecialty Top 3 book.

Top 3 Differentials in Gastrointestinal Imaging is organized into five parts: hepatobiliary, pancreas and spleen, GI tract, mesentery and vascular, and abdominal wall and soft tissues. The carefully selected cases provide illustrative examples across all imaging modalities, providing a high-yield and well-rounded GI review. As with the original Top 3 book, the emphasis is on differential-based cases with the addition of Roentgen Classics where appropriate.

It is my sincere hope that you find this subspecialty Top 3 book both enjoyable and educational.

William T. O'Brien, Sr., DO, FAOCR

Preface

This book is for both residents (radiology, surgery, and gastrointestinal fellows) and practicing physicians. I feel strongly that it will provide you the knowledge you need to learn gastrointestinal radiology. We have followed the "Top 3" format and present unknown cases followed by a brief discussion on the most common pathology. For simplicity, the book is organized into five parts: hepatobiliary, pancreas and spleen, gastrointestinal tract, mesentery and vascular, and abdominal wall and soft tissues.

Our goal is to create a quick reference book for the physicians (resident and attending). This book emphasizes on the diagnosis of frequent pathologies and covers multiple modalities (X-ray, ultrasound, MRI, barium fluoroscopy, and CT). The book will be great for board study or in daily practice.

Rocky C. Saenz, DO, FAOCR

Acknowledgments

I would like to thank Dr. William O'Brien for including me in his "Top 3" radiology series. Dr. O'Brien's concept of "Top 3 Differentials" is a great approach to learning radiology. I hope you, the reader, enjoy this gastrointestinal edition that follows the same format as the original book. Next, I would like to thank the Department of Radiology at Beaumont Hospital, Farmington Hills (formerly known as Botsford Hospital), for agreeing to contribute and help me put together this project. This includes my fellow staff radiologists, Reehan Ali, Elias Antypas, Kathy Borovicka, Sarika Joshi, Kristin Kamienecki, Tim McKnight, Andy Mizzi, and Mickey Schwartz as well as my devoted residents, Gregory Puthoff, Chelsea Jeranko, Dan Knapp, Jules Cameron, Julia Hobson, Sara Boyd, Jake Figner, VJ Williams, Alex Martin, Zophia Martinez, Mike Legacy, and Raj Aravapalli for their hard work and dedication in contributing cases. I would also like to thank Sharon Kreuer and Stacy Ries for finding the time away from motherhood and private practice to contribute toward this book. Thank you again to all of you; I would not have been able to complete this project without your collaboration.

Lastly and most importantly I would like to extend my gratitude toward my family. I thank my brother, Roland Saenz, who has provided me emotional support. I thank my wife Blanca and sons, Rocky, Russell, Ronin, and Rex, for their understanding and patience, watching me spend countless hours on my laptop computer to complete this book. I could not and would not be able to complete this academic project or any other without their love and support.

Rocky C. Saenz, DO, FAOCR

Contributors

Reehan M. Ali, DO
Clinical Assistant Professor
Michigan State University College of
  Osteopathic Medicine
Lansing, Michigan
Director of CT and Thoracic Imaging
Beaumont Hospital
Farmington Hills Campus
Farmington Hills, Michigan

Elias Antypas, MD, PhD
Clinical Assistant Professor
Michigan State University College of
  Osteopathic Medicine
Lansing, Michigan
Director of Interventional Radiology
Beaumont Hospital
Farmington Hills Campus
Farmington Hills, Michigan

Rajeev Aravapalli, DO
Radiology Resident
Beaumont Hospital
Farmington Hills Campus
Farmington Hills, Michigan

Kathy M. Borovicka, MD
Clinical Assistant Professor
Michigan State University College of
  Osteopathic Medicine
Lansing, Michigan
Staff Radiologist
Beaumont Hospital
Farmington Hills Campus
Farmington Hills, Michigan

Sara K. Boyd, DO
Radiology Resident
Beaumont Hospital
Farmington Hills Campus
Farmington Hills, Michigan

Julia D. Cameron-Morrison, DO
Radiology Resident
Beaumont Hospital
Farmington Hills Campus
Farmington Hills, Michigan

Cam Chau, MD
Department of Diagnostic Imaging
UC Davis Medical Center
Sacramento, California

Paul B. DiDomenico, MD
Clinical Instructor of Radiology
Department of Radiology and Biomedical Engineering
Yale University School of Medicine
VA Connecticut Health Care System
New Haven, Connecticut

Jake Figner, DO
Radiology Resident
Beaumont Hospital
Farmington Hills Campus
Farmington Hills, Michigan

Julia J. Hobson, DO
Radiology Resident
Beaumont Hospital
Farmington Hills Campus
Farmington Hills, Michigan

Chelsea M. Jeranko, DO
Radiology Resident
Beaumont Hospital
Farmington Hills Campus
Farmington Hills, Michigan

Robert A. Jesinger, MD, MSE
Colonel
United States Air Force
Academic Chair
Diagnostic Radiology Residency Program
David Grant USAF Medical Center
Travis Air Force Base
Associate Clinical Professor of Radiology
UC Davis School of Medicine
Sacramento, California

Sarika N. Joshi, MD
Clinical Assistant Professor
Michigan State University College of
  Osteopathic Medicine
Lansing, Michigan
Director of Gastrointestinal Imaging
Beaumont Hospital
Farmington Hills Campus
Farmington Hills, Michigan

Kristin Kamienecki, DO
Clinical Assistant Professor
Michigan State University College of
  Osteopathic Medicine
Lansing, Michigan
Director of Ultrasound
Beaumont Hospital
Farmington Hills Campus
Farmington Hills, Michigan

Daniel E. Knapp, DO
Radiology Resident
Beaumont Hospital
Farmington Hills Campus
Farmington Hills, Michigan

Sharon Kreuer, DO
Clinical Assistant Professor of Radiology
University of Pittsburgh Medical Center
Community Division
Monroeville, Pennsylvania

Grant E. Lattin, Jr., MD
Lieutenant Colonel
United States Air Force
Program Director
Diagnostic Radiology Residency and
  Body Imaging Fellowship
National Capital Consortium
Walter Reed National Military Medical Center
Associate Professor
Uniformed Service University of the Health Sciences
Bethesda, Maryland

Michael Legacy, DO
Radiology Resident
Beaumont Hospital
Farmington Hills Campus
Farmington Hills, Michigan

Brian J. Lewis, DO
Major
United States Air Force
Department of Radiology
10th Medical Group
United States Air Force Academy
Colorado Springs, Colorado

Shaun Loh, MD, MBA
Department of Diagnostic Imaging
UC Davis Medical Center
Sacramento, California

Alex R. Martin, DO
Radiology Resident
Beaumont Hospital
Farmington Hills Campus
Farmington Hills, Michigan

Zophia Martinez, DO
Radiology Resident
Beaumont Hospital
Farmington Hills Campus
Farmington Hills, Michigan

Timothy McKnight, DO
Clinical Assistant Professor
Michigan State University College of
  Osteopathic Medicine
Lansing, Michigan
Assistant Program Director of Radiology Residency
Beaumont Hospital
Director of Nuclear Medicine and Radiation Safety
Farmington Hills Campus
Farmington Hills, Michigan

Andrew Mizzi, DO
Clinical Assistant Professor
Michigan State University College of
  Osteopathic Medicine
Lansing, Michigan
Director of Mammography
Beaumont Hospital
Farmington Hills Campus
Farmington Hills, Michigan

William T. O'Brien, Sr., DO, FAOCR
Director, Pediatric Neuroradiology Fellowship
Cincinnati Children's Hospital Medical Center
Associate Professor of Radiology
University of Cincinnati College of Medicine
Cincinnati, Ohio

Eleanor L. Ormsby, MD, MPH
Department of Diagnostic Imaging
UC Davis Medical Center
Sacramento, California

Gregory D. Puthoff, DO
Radiology Resident
Beaumont Hospital
Farmington Hills Campus
Farmington Hills, Michigan

Stacy J. Ries, DO
Clinical Faculty
Michigan State University
Lansing, Michigan
Clinical Faculty
Oakland University
Rochester
X-Ray Associates of Port Huron
Port Huron, Michigan

Rocky C. Saenz, DO, FAOCR
Vice Chairman, Department of Radiology
Program Director of Diagnostic Radiology Residency
Director of MRI and Musculoskeletal Imaging
Beaumont Hospital, Farmington Hills Campus
Farmington Hills, Michigan
Clinical Assistant Professor
Michigan State University College of
  Osteopathic Medicine
Lansing, Michigan

Michael L. Schwartz, MD
Clinical Assistant Professor
Michigan State University College of
  Osteopathic Medicine
Lansing, Michigan
Chairman
Beaumont Hospital
Farmington Hills Campus
Farmington Hills, Michigan

Rebecca Stein-Wexler, MD
Professor of Pediatric Radiology
Director, Radiology Residency Program
UC Davis Medical Center and Children's Hospital
Sacramento, California

Vernon F. Williams, Jr., DO
Radiology Resident
Beaumont Hospital
Farmington Hills Campus
Farmington Hills, Michigan

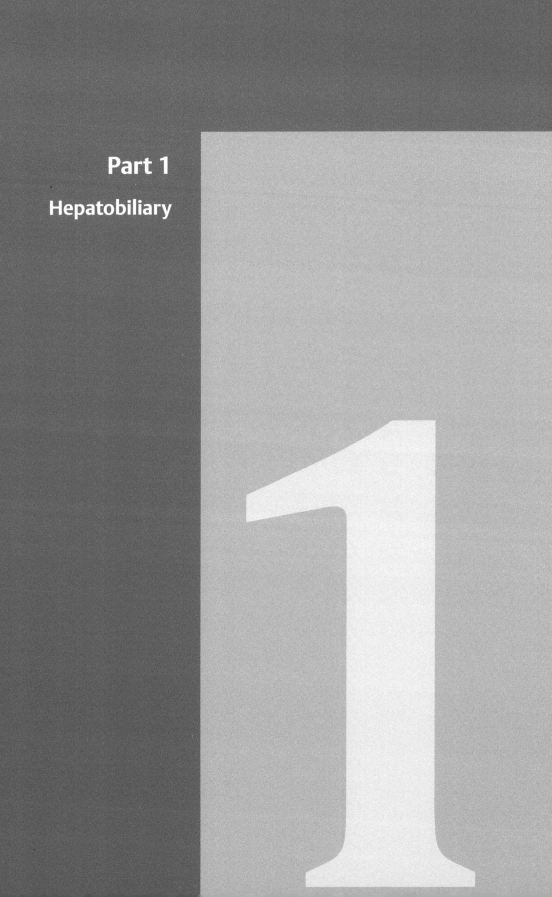

Part 1

Hepatobiliary

Case 1

Rocky C. Saenz

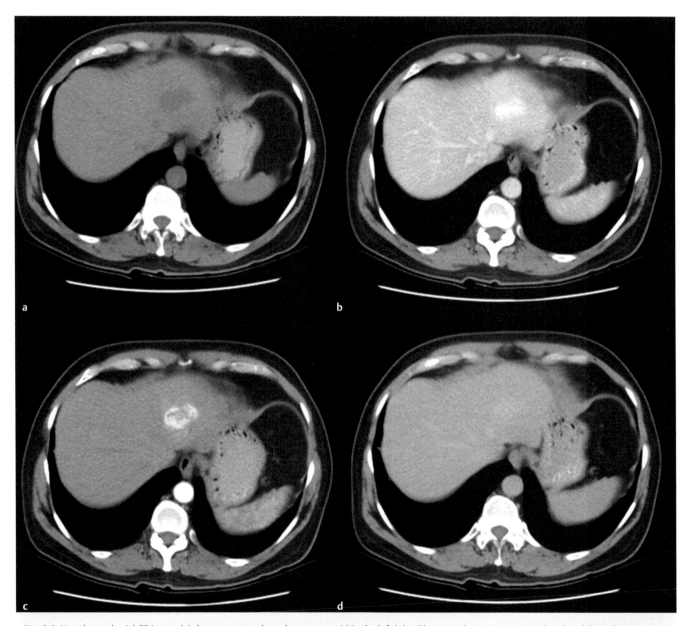

Fig. 1.1 Unenhanced axial CT image (a) demonstrates a hypodense mass within the left lobe. The mass demonstrates peripheral nodular enhancement on arterial phase imaging with a central hypodense scar (b). On venous phase imaging (c), the mass is hyperdense to surrounding hepatic parenchyma. On delayed imaging (d), the lesion is isodense to the surrounding hepatic parenchyma.

■ Clinical History

A 26-year-old woman with intermittent discomfort (▶Fig. 1.1).

■ Key Finding

Liver mass with peripheral nodular enhancement.

■ Top 3 Differential Diagnoses

- **Hemangioma:** Hemangiomas are the most common benign lesion with incidence reported as high as 20% in the general population. The classic imaging findings are initial progressive peripheral nodular enhancement in the arterial phase which on delayed imaging becomes isodense to the surrounding liver parenchyma. On MRI, hemangiomas are hyperintense on T2 (light bulb sign) and hypointense on T1-weighted imaging with similar enhancement patterns as seen with CT. On ultrasound, most hemangiomas are well circumscribed hyperechoic lesions.
- **Focal nodular hyperplasia (FNH):** FNH is an uncommon hepatic lesion with a 5% incidence in the general population. The lesion is composed of hepatocytes and classically contains a central low-density scar. On MRI, FNH is intermediate to low signal on T2 with a bright central scar. Since FNH is composed of hepatocytes, it demonstrates enhancement on delayed intracellular imaging (with gadoxetate disodium), which is helpful in distinguishing FNH from other hepatic lesions.
- **Hepatic adenoma:** Hepatic adenomas are benign lesions predominantly seen in women (90%). Most often they are solitary but may occasionally be multiple, especially in patients with glycogen storage disease. There is an association with oral contraceptive use. Hepatic adenomas have a variable contrast enhancement pattern. Adenomas are typically hypervascular; internal hemorrhage can lead to heterogeneity. The minority of cases may have macroscopic fat and calcifications.

■ Additional Diagnostic Considerations

- **Hepatocellular carcinoma (HCC):** HCC is the most common visceral malignancy in the world. The most common etiology is cirrhosis. The lesions are typically hypodense and demonstrate increased arterial phase enhancement due to blood supply from the hepatic artery. Portal or hepatic vein invasion is common. MRI can be helpful in these instances since HCC typically displays increased T2 signal intensity. Clinically, HCC is associated with elevated alpha-fetoprotein (poor prognosis with average survival time of 6 months).
- **Metastases:** Metastases are usually multiple but may present as a solitary lesion. Tumors that classically metastasize to liver commonly include lung, breast, melanoma, colon, and pancreas. On contrasted-enhanced imaging, metastases have a variable appearance.

■ Diagnosis

Hemangioma.

✓ Pearls

- Hemangiomas demonstrate peripheral, nodular, enhancement, which becomes isodense to liver.
- A hepatic lesion with portal or hepatic vein invasion is HCC until proven otherwise.
- Hepatic adenomas are associated with oral contraceptives.

Suggested Readings

Federle MP, Jeffrey RB, Woodward PJ, Borhani A. Diagnostic Imaging: Abdomen. 2nd ed. Philadelphia, PA: Lippincott Williams & Wilkins; 2009

Kamel IR, Lawler LP, Fishman EK. Comprehensive analysis of hypervascular liver lesions using 16-MDCT and advanced image processing. AJR Am J Roentgenol. 2004; 183(2):443–452

Saenz RC. MRI of benign liver lesions and metastatic disease characterization with gadoxetate disodium. J Am Osteopath Coll Radiol. 2012; 1(4):2–9

Case 2

Zophia Martinez

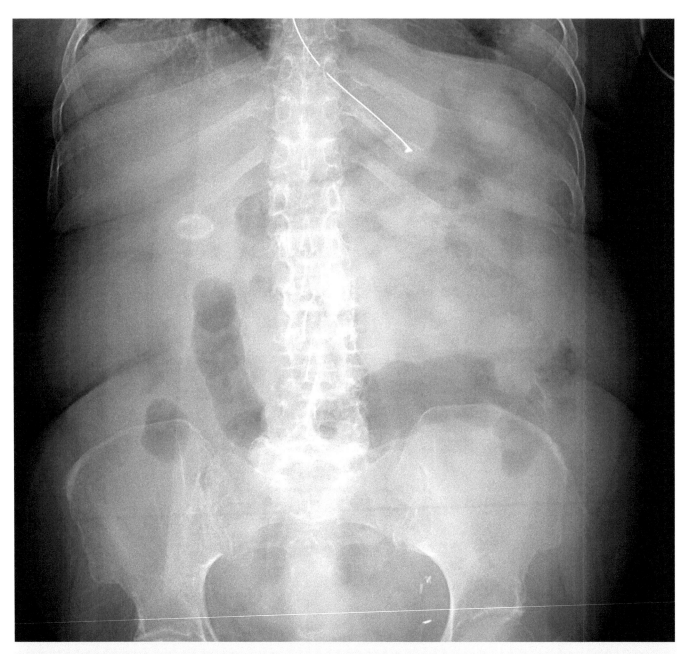

Fig. 2.1 Frontal radiograph of the abdomen demonstrates a round, peripherally dense calcification in the right upper quadrant. An enteric tube is seen overlying the stomach.

■ Clinical History

A 57-year-old female with occasional postprandial pain (▶Fig. 2.1).

■ Key Finding

Calcific density in the right upper quadrant.

■ Top 3 Differential Diagnoses

- **Gallbladder calcification:** Gallstones are a common cause of right upper quadrant calcification, despite the fact that only a minority contain enough calcium making them visible on X-ray. The "Mercedes-Benz" sign is an additional radiographic indicator of cholelithiasis caused by nitrogen gas collecting in degenerating gallstones. Porcelain gallbladder is an additional consideration as it represents gallbladder wall calcification. Recent studies have shown a much weaker association between porcelain gallbladder and gallbladder carcinoma than traditionally thought.
- **Renal calcification:** Numerous etiologies are possible for renal calcification, with nephrolithiasis being the most common. Most renal calculi are predominantly composed of calcium and demonstrate uniform opacity. Clustered, diffuse, mottled, or thin rim-like renal calcification can be seen in medullary and cortical nephrocalcinosis. Additionally, approximately 10% of renal cell carcinomas (RCCs) contain calcification, typically in an amorphous pattern.
- **Hepatic calcification:** The etiologies of liver calcification are numerous. The most common etiology is calcified granuloma, which can form as a result of numerous infections, most commonly histoplasmosis. These often appear as multiple punctate, solid calcifications. Punctate calcification involving the spleen and/or lungs in addition to the liver is highly suggestive of granulomatous disease. Certain malignant neoplasms can also calcify, especially metastasis from mucinous adenocarcinomas of the colon, breast, stomach, or ovary. These calcifications tend to be faint and amorphous rather than dense.

■ Additional Diagnostic Considerations

Adrenal calcification: The most common cause of adrenal calcification is prior adrenal hemorrhage, which is more common in neonates than in adults and can appear as amorphous paraspinal calcification. Calcifications are typically seen greater or equal to 1 year after hemorrhage in adults and within 1 to 2 weeks in neonates.

■ Diagnosis

Cholelithiasis.

✓ Pearls

- Cholelithiasis is the most common cause of right upper quadrant calcifications.
- Nephrolithiasis is the most common cause of renal calcification.
- Subcentimeter calcifications involving the liver, spleen, and/or lungs are highly suggestive of old healed granulomatous disease.

Suggested Readings

Bortoff GA, Chen MYM, Ott DJ, Wolfman NT, Routh WD. Gallbladder stones: imaging and intervention. Radiographics. 2000; 20(3):751–766

Dyer RB, Chen MY, Zagoria RJ. Abnormal calcifications in the urinary tract. Radiographics. 1998; 18(6):1405–1424

Stoupis C, Taylor HM, Paley MR, et al. The Rocky liver: radiologic-pathologic correlation of calcified hepatic masses. Radiographics. 1998; 18(3):675–685, quiz 726

Case 3

Rocky C. Saenz

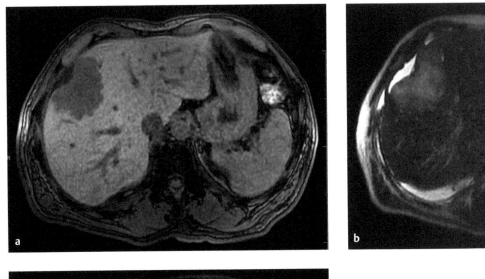
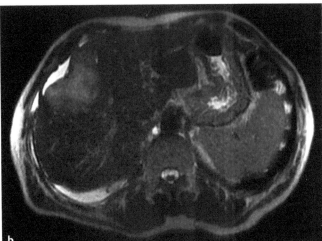
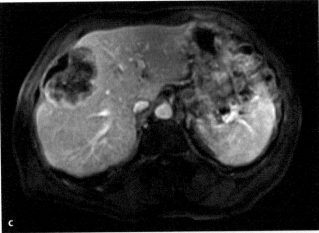

Fig. 3.1 MRI axial images. T1 precontrast fat saturation image **(a)** shows a low signal lesion with capsular retraction in the right lobe. The T2 image demonstrates the lesion to be of intermediate signal **(b)**. Contrast enhanced axial T1 fat saturation image shows the lesion with an irregular enhancement pattern **(c)**. A small amount of free fluid is seen in the right upper quadrant.

■ Clinical History

A 66-year-old female with a lung nodule and axillary lump (►Fig. 3.1).

■ Key Finding

Hepatic lesion with capsular retraction.

■ Top 3 Differential Diagnoses

• **Metastases:** Metastasis is the most common tumor and malignancy of the liver. The most common source of metastatic disease is melanoma, lung, breast, pancreas, and colon carcinomas. Hepatic metastases on dynamic cross-sectional imaging most commonly show enhancement on the early arterial phase. Imaging findings depend on the primary tumor type, but lesions are often poorly circumscribed with variable enhancement and are usually multiple. Remember, the liver is the most common organ site for metastatic disease.

• **Hepatocellular carcinoma (HCC):** HCC is the most common primary hepatic malignancy. The key imaging features include its characteristic dynamic enhancement pattern (early arterial phase enhancement with washout on delayed imaging)

and a tumor capsule. The capsule is best seen on the portal venous and delayed images. MRI has a high accuracy of identifying an HCC capsule. Clinical correlation with serum alpha-fetoprotein levels may be helpful and should be elevated.

• **Cholangiocarcinoma:** Cholangiocarcinoma is a rare cancer of the bile ducts. Cholangiocarcinomas are typically infiltrative lesions with segmental peripheral intrahepatic bile duct dilation. These tumors are the second most common primary hepatic malignancy. On dynamic CT, the majority of cases does not demonstrate any significant arterial enhancement and show delayed maximum enhancement (beyond 10 minutes), which is a key distinguishing feature. The lesion commonly is seen in the left lobe of the liver. Cholangiocarcinoma has a poor prognosis and less than 20% are resectable.

■ Additional Diagnostic Considerations

Hepatic lymphoma: Hepatic lymphoma may be primary or secondary. Secondary hepatic lymphoma is seen in greater than 50% of all lymphoma patients. Most lesions are lobulated

in appearance and are multiple in number. Non-Hodgkin's lymphoma (NHL) is more common to have hepatic involvement than Hodgkin.

■ Diagnosis

Metastasis from breast carcinoma.

✓ Pearls

• A hepatic lesion with capsular retraction should be considered malignant until proven otherwise.

• HCC will achieve maximum enhancement in the arterial phase, and cholangiocarcinoma has maximum enhancement on delayed imaging.

• Cholangiocarcinoma is the only liver lesion that is more common in the left lobe.

Suggested Readings

Federle MP, Jeffrey RB, Woodward PJ, Borhani A. Diagnostic Imaging: Abdomen. 2nd ed. Philadelphia, PA: Lippincott Williams & Wilkins; 2009

Saenz RC. MRI of benign liver lesions and metastatic disease characterization with gadoxetate disodium. J Am Osteopath Coll Radiol. 2012; 1(4):2–9

Tang A, Bashir MR, Corwin MT, et al. LI-RADS Evidence Working Group. Evidence supporting LI-RADS major features for CT- and MR imaging-based diagnosis of hepatocellular carcinoma: a systematic review. Radiology. 2018; 286(1):29–48

Case 4

Sara K. Boyd

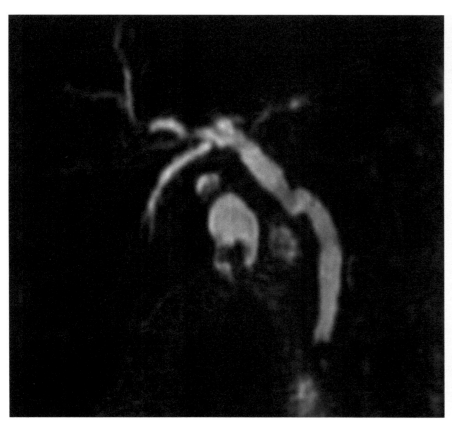

Fig. 4.1 Single MRCP T2-weighted coronal image shows a dilated common bile duct with a round low signal focus proximally at the level of the pancreatic head. (Image courtesy of Rocky C. Saenz.)

■ Clinical History

A 54-year-old male with acute right upper quadrant pain and elevated total bilirubin (▶ Fig. 4.1).

■ Key Finding

Common bile duct dilation.

■ Top 3 Differential Diagnoses

• **Choledocholithiasis:** Obstructing biliary stones are a common cause of a dilated common bile duct and occur in about 10% of patients with gallstones. Magnetic resonance cholangiopancreatography (MRCP) is very sensitive for their detection and stones will appear as one or more low-signal filling defects with angular margins and surrounding high-signal bile with associated ductal dilation. The central or segmental bile ducts may be involved in isolation or there can be dilation of the whole biliary tree. Chronic choledocholithiasis can result in biliary strictures, which will appear as smooth symmetric short segment narrowing of the duct either superior or inferior to the calculi on MRCP. Patients are at risk of developing cholangitis and cholestasis.

• **Strictures:** Biliary strictures are classified as either benign or malignant. The features of benign strictures (causes include iatrogenic, pancreatitis, and inflammatory conditions) are smooth margins, symmetric tapering, and are typically short segment with or without duct dilation on MRCP. In contrast, malignant strictures (caused by tumor) are longer in length, asymmetric, and demonstrate abnormal irregular luminal shouldering.

• **Neoplasm:** Tumors such as cholangiocarcinoma, pancreatic adenocarcinoma, gallbladder malignancies, and metastasis may invade the biliary system. These tumors can result in focal narrowing of the common bile duct and poststenotic dilation. Malignant strictures involving the common bile duct create an abrupt caliber change with intraluminal shouldering and eccentric asymmetry, which is often present at the transition point between the dilated obstructed duct and the smaller caliber decompressed duct. Extrinsic compression from malignant masses, lymphadenopathy, or dilated collateral vasculature may also produce poststenotic ductal dilation.

■ Additional Diagnostic Considerations

• **Choledochol cyst:** A type 1 choledochol cyst is defined by dilation of the common bile duct. This can be seen in isolation or with concomitant dilation of the common hepatic duct. The common bile duct may be focally enlarged distally or can be enlarged in a fusiform morphology. These lesions will demonstrate bile-type signal on MRCP and MR studies.

• **Papillary stenosis:** Defined as obstruction of bile flow at the sphincter of Oddi without the presence of a mass or inflammation at the ampulla, papillary stenosis appears as common bile duct dilation on MRCP. The most common cause is dysfunction of the sphincter of Oddi and patients typically present clinically with jaundice and pancreatitis. Papillary size less than 12 mm suggests an underlying benign cause. Endoscopic retrograde cholangiopancreatography (ERCP) is useful in determining the cause.

■ Diagnosis

Choledocholithiasis.

✓ Pearls

• Choledocholithiasis appears as a filling defect with a dilated common bile duct.

• Benign strictures are typically short with smooth tapering, and malignant strictures are characteristically long with irregular luminal shouldering and asymmetry.

• Neoplasm may present with poststenotic common bile duct dilation as the mass narrows the duct from direct invasion or from extrinsic compression from tumor, lymphadenopathy, or enlarged collateral vessels.

Suggested Readings

Nikolaidis P, Hammond NA, Day K, et al. Imaging features of benign and malignant ampullary and periampullary lesions. Radiographics. 2014; 34(3):624–641

O'Connor OJ, O'Neill S, Maher MM. Imaging of biliary tract disease. AJR Am J Roentgenol. 2011; 197(4):W551–8

Yeh BM, Liu PS, Soto JA, Corvera CA, Hussain HK. MR imaging and CT of the biliary tract. Radiographics. 2009; 29(6):1669–1688

Case 5

Rocky C. Saenz

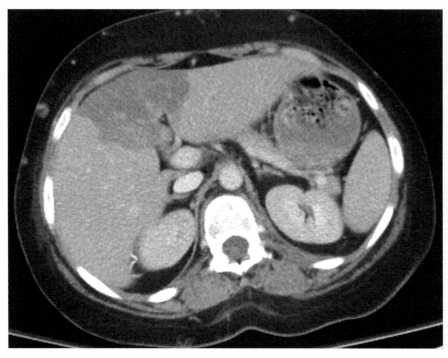

Fig. 5.1 CT with intravenous contrast of the abdomen shows the liver with a geographic area of low attenuation involving both the right and left lobe.

■ **Clinical History**

A 27-year-old female with a generalized pain (▶Fig. 5.1).

■ Key Finding

Geographic liver lesion.

■ Top 3 Differential Diagnoses

- **Steatosis:** Hepatic steatosis also known as fatty liver is due to the accumulation of triglycerides in the hepatocytes. The etiology may be from alcoholic or non-alcoholic liver disease (nonalcoholic steatohepatitis, NASH). Steatosis has many appearances including: diffuse, diffuse with sparring, focal, multifocal, and geographic. The focal form is less common. A key imaging feature is noting normal vessels coursing through the lesion. On CT, the diagnosis can be made by noting Housfield Units (HU) less than 40 on non-contrast imaging or HU 20 less than splenic parenchyma on portal venous phase.
- **Metastases:** Metastasis is the most common lesion of the liver. The most common appearance of hepatic metastases on CT is a low-density lesion with respect to the liver parenchyma.

Imaging findings depend upon the primary tumor type, but lesions are often poorly circumscribed with variable enhancement and typically multiple. Metastasis is more than 10 times more common than primary liver malignancies. The liver is the most common organ site for metastatic disease.
- **Hepatic infarction:** Hepatic infarcts are not common due to the dual blood supply of the liver. Etiologies include postsurgical ligation, vasculitis, blunt trauma, hypercoagulable states, and rare infections. Hepatic artery occlusion is more common than portal vein thrombosis. The most reliable finding is wedge shaped nonenhancement on all phases of a dynamic study. Angiography may be necessary to confirm hepatic artery occlusion. Treatment includes revascularization and transplantation.

■ Additional Diagnostic Considerations

- **Hepatic lymphoma:** Hepatic lymphoma is known as the great mimicker. Although most often it is lobulated and multiple, it could also appear geographic in appearance. Non-Hodgkin's lymphoma (NHL) is more common to have hepatic involvement than Hodgkin.
- **Laceration:** On CT, a laceration is usually a linear and of low attenuation on postcontrast images. Advanced lacerations are

large and may appear geographic in shape and are associated with hemoperitoneum. Imaging needs to be done in dual phase manner with delayed imaging in order to exclude vascular extravasation. Grading of injuries is done utilizing AAST (American Association for Surgical Trauma) scale. Treatment for patients with vascular extravasation who are unstable needs surgical intervention.

■ Diagnosis

Focal fatty infiltration.

✓ Pearls

- The key to diagnose focal fatty infiltration is noting normal vessels coursing through the lesion.

- Advanced AAST grades V to VI liver injuries are usually surgical.
- Consider infarct in a postsurgical patient.

Suggested Readings

Coast, et al. Fat-containing liver lesions on imaging: detection and differential diagnosis. Am J Roentgen. 2018; 210:1–10

Federle MP, Jeffrey RB, Woodward PJ, Borhani A, et al. Diagnostic Imaging: Abdomen. 2nd ed. Philadelphia, PA: Lippincott, Williams & Wilkins; 2009

Saenz RC. MRI of benign liver lesions and metastatic disease characterization with gadoxetate disodium. J Am Osteopath Coll Radiol. 2012; 1(4):2–9

Case 6

Rajeev Aravapalli

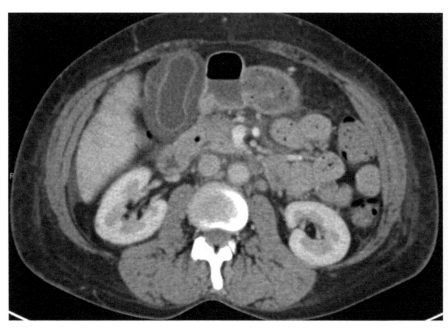

Fig. 6.1 CT image of the abdomen with IV contrast shows gallbladder wall thickening. Fluid is seen adjacent to the liver laterally but not layering in the gallbladder fossa or Morrison's pouch. (Image courtesy of Rocky C. Saenz.)

■ Clinical History

A 41-year-old female with right upper quadrant pain (▶ Fig. 6.1).

■ Key Finding

Gallbladder wall thickening.

■ Top 3 Differential Diagnoses

- **Acute cholecystitis:** Most frequent inflammatory condition of the gallbladder. Cholecystitis is suspected on CT when a thick-walled gallbladder and fat stranding are seen. However, this is not pathognomonic and should be confirmed on ultrasound. Additional signs should include obstructing gallstone, hydropic dilatation of the gallbladder, pericholecystic fluid, and positive sonographic Murphy sign (most reliable).
- **Chronic cholecystitis:** It is caused by gallbladder stones that create transient obstruction which leads to prolonged inflammation and fibrosis. This fibrosis may lead to a contracted gallbladder, and is almost always seen with cholelithiasis. Imaging findings include gallstones in thick-walled gallbladder with no pericholecystic fluid and lack of wall hyperemia.
- **Gallbladder carcinoma:** More than 90% are adenocarcinomas with a 5-year survival rate of less than 5%. This entity can appear as a mass replacing the gallbladder, an intraluminal polypoid mass, or wall thickening that is focal or diffuse. Most gallbladder carcinomas present after 65. CT and MR are useful in defining extent of disease, adenopathy, and evaluating for metastasis.

■ Additional Diagnostic Considerations

- **Adenomyomatosis:** Idiopathic, benign condition that has excessive proliferation of surface epithelium within dilated Rokitansky–Aschoff sinuses deep into the muscular wall. The most common findings are nonspecific wall thickening (focal, segmental, or diffuse), sludge, and calculi. The most common form is focally in the fundus. CT is less specific than ultrasound for detection, but it may show cystic-appearing thickening of the gallbladder wall or enhancing epithelium within intramural diverticula surrounded by relatively unenhanced hypertrophied gallbladder muscularis.
- **Systemic disease:** Heart, renal, and liver failure may cause gallbladder wall thickening in the absence of inflammation. This may be related to elevated portal venous pressure, low intravascular osmotic pressure, hypoalbuminemia, and sepsis. Wall thickening may be pronounced (> 10 mm).

■ Diagnosis

Acute cholecystitis.

✓ Pearls

- Gallbladder wall thickening greater than 3 mm is abnormal.
- On CT when acute cholecystitis is suspected it should be confirmed on ultrasound.
- The most common sites of metastasis for gallbladder carcinoma are the liver and peritoneum.

Suggested Readings

Federle MP, Jeffrey RB, Woodward PJ, Borhani A. Diagnostic Imaging: Abdomen. 2nd ed. Philadelphia, PA: Lippincott Williams & Wilkins; 2009

Runner GJ, Corwin MT, Siewert B, Eisenberg RL. Gallbladder wall thickening. AJR Am J Roentgenol. 2014; 202(1):W1–W12

van Breda Vriesman AC, Engelbrecht MR, Smithuis RH, Puylaert JB. Diffuse gallbladder wall thickening: differential diagnosis. AJR Am J Roentgenol. 2007; 188(2):495–501

Case 7

Rocky C. Saenz

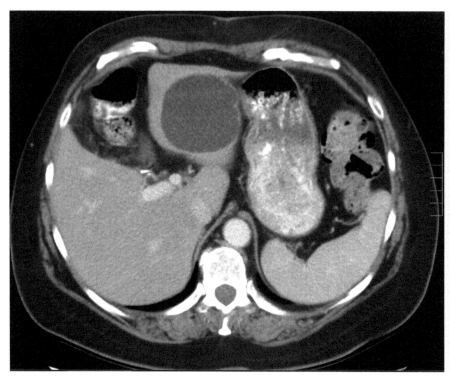

Fig. 7.1 Contrast enhanced axial CT image through the upper abdomen demonstrates a low-density lesion in the left lobe.

■ **Clinical History**

A 25-year-old female with a generalized pain (▶Fig. 7.1).

■ Key Finding

Solitary, nonenhancing liver lesion.

■ Top 3 Differential Diagnoses

• **Hepatic cyst:** Hepatic cysts are thought to be congenital lesions arising from developmental defects of the biliary ducts. They are well circumscribed with very thin or imperceptible walls. These are benign lesions and are more commonly seen in women. When cysts are innumerable, these may be associated with autosomal dominant polycystic kidney disease (ADPKD) or tuberous sclerosis. Simple cysts do not enhance.

• **Hepatic abscesses:** Hepatic abscesses are uncommon and can be categorized into pyogenic (80%), amebic (10%), and fungal (10%). Pyogenic hepatic abscesses, being the most common, are found in the setting of diverticulitis and sepsis. Amebic abscesses are prone to rupture. Imaging findings include thick-walled, hypoattenuating liver masses with internal septations, peripheral lesion enhancement, and gas in up to 20% of cases. Pyogenic abscesses are commonly multilocular. Untreated, liver abscesses have a high mortality rate.

• **Biliary hamartoma:** Biliary hamartomas are uncommon, benign, congenital malformations of the biliary tract. These are classically multiple (may be solitary), fluid attenuated, and measure less than 1.5 cm. There is no gender bias and these are asymptomatic, not requiring any treatment. The lesions typically do not enhance but if associated with solid components may enhance or show thin wall enhancement. These are also known as von Meyenburg complexes.

■ Additional Diagnostic Considerations

• **Biliary cystadenoma:** Biliary cystadenomas are uncommon, multilocular, well-defined cystic masses arising from the bile ducts which are premalignant. They typically occur in middle-aged women who complain of chronic abdominal pain. The cyst wall may enhance. Malignant transformation to cystadenocarcinoma can occur.

• **Metastases:** Metastasis is the most common lesion of the liver. The most common appearance of hepatic metastases on CT is a low-density lesion with respect to the liver parenchyma. Imaging findings depend on the primary tumor type, but lesions are often poorly circumscribed with variable enhancement and typically multiple. Metastasis is more than 10 times more common than primary liver malignancies. The liver is the most common organ site for metastatic disease.

■ Diagnosis

Hepatic cyst.

✓ Pearls

• The key to diagnose hepatic cysts is confirming nonenhancement.

• Hepatic cysts follow fluid on all MRI sequences.
• Consider abscess with septic patients with a multilocular foci.

Suggested Readings

Federle MP, Jeffrey RB, Woodward PJ, Borhani A. Diagnostic Imaging: Abdomen. 2nd ed. Philadelphia, PA: Lippincott Williams & Wilkins; 2009

Mortelé KJ, Ros PR. Cystic focal liver lesions in the adult: differential CT and MR imaging features. Radiographics. 2001; 21(4):895–910

Saenz RC. MRI of benign liver lesions and metastatic disease characterization with gadoxetate disodium. J Am Osteopath Coll Radiol. 2012; 1(4):2–9

Case 8

Rajeev Aravapalli

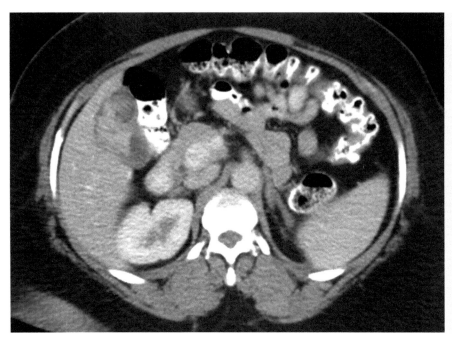

Fig. 8.1 CT axial image with intravenous and oral contrast shows an enhancing focus in the gallbladder which is non-dependent. (Image courtesy of Rocky C. Saenz.)

■ Clinical History

A 70-year-old female with right upper quadrant pain (▶ Fig. 8.1).

■ Key Finding

Gallbladder mass.

■ Top 3 Differential Diagnoses

- **Cholelithiasis:** Gallstones commonly present with right upper quadrant discomfort after a fatty meal in women in their 40s. It is the most commonly encountered gallbladder mass. Ultrasound is the best modality for detecting gallstones. Calcified gallstones appear hyperattenuated on CT, while pure cholesterol stones are hypoattenuating on CT. Isodense stones may be missed on CT. Treatment of choletlithiasis may be conservative if asymptomatic. Surgical removal of the gallbladder may be necessary if symptomatic.
- **Gallbladder polyp:** These are nonmobile masses protruding from the gallbladder wall that may simulate focal wall thickening. These can be polypoid or sessile. The majority of polyps less than 10 mm are benign (>90%). CT is useful for staging larger polyps where there is an increased risk of malignancy. Polyps greater than 10 mm warrant resection. These are classified into adenoma, adenocarcinoma, cholesterol polyps, and inflammatory polyps.
- **Gallbladder carcinoma:** There are several different imaging appearances. It can appear as a mass completely replacing the gallbladder which is most common. There can be focal or diffuse gallbladder wall thickening. Additionally, it can present as an intraluminal polypoid mass. Typically hypodense on venous phase. Calcified gallstones or porcelain gallbladder may be present.

■ Additional Diagnostic Considerations

- **Adenomyomatosis:** Results in diffuse or focal thickening of the muscular wall of the gallbladder. There will be cystic non-enhancing spaces within gallbladder wall reflecting intramural diverticula. Deposition of cholesterol crystals into mucosal diverticula called Rokitansky–Aschoff sinuses. This a benign finding that is incidentally discovered. Contrast-enhanced CT is limited in the evaluation of adenomyomatosis.
- **Tumefactive sludge:** Usually a result of biliary stasis from prolonged fasting or hyperalimentation. Most biliary sludge presents as a layering in the dependent gallbladder. Tumefactive sludge presents as an intraluminal polypoid mass that can mimic a tumor (> 25 HU). It should not enhance; however, vicarious excretion of iodinated contrast may confuse evaluation.

■ Diagnosis

Gallbladder adenocarcinoma.

✓ Pearls

- Gallstones may contain nitrogen gas centrally which is called the "Mercedes-Benz" sign.
- Size is most important predictor of malignancy with gallbladder polyps.
- Increased risk of gallbladder carcinoma in patients with porcelain gallbladder.

Suggested Readings

Federle MP, Jeffrey RB, Woodward PJ, Borhani A. Diagnostic Imaging: Abdomen. 2nd ed. Philadelphia, PA: Lippincott Williams & Wilkins; 2009

Furlan A, Ferris JV, Hosseinzadeh K, Borhani AA. Gallbladder carcinoma update: multimodality imaging evaluation, staging, and treatment options. AJR Am J Roentgenol. 2008; 191(5):1440–1447

McKnight T, Patel A. Gallbladder masses: multimodality approach to differential diagnosis. J Am Osteopath Coll Radiol. 2012; 1(4):22–31

Case 9

Rocky C. Saenz

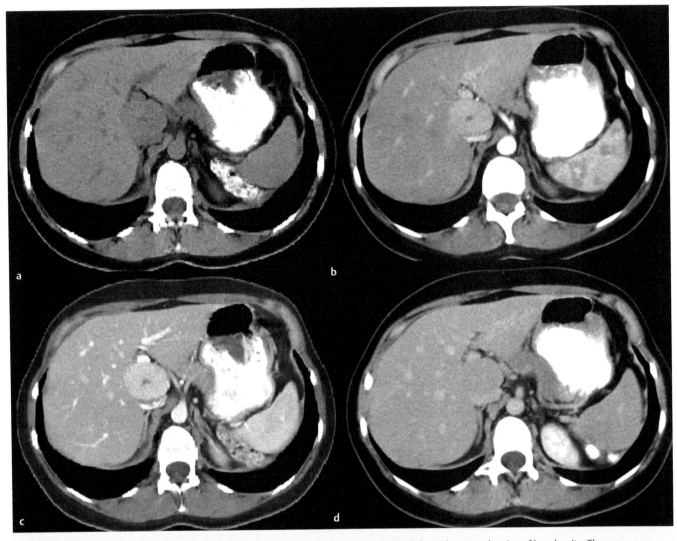

Fig. 9.1 Unenhanced axial CT image (a) demonstrates a hypodense mass within the caudate lobe with a central region of low density. The mass demonstrates homogeneous increased enhancement on arterial phase imaging with a central hypodense scar (b). On venous phase imaging (c), the mass is hyperdense to surrounding hepatic parenchyma with maintenance of the central hypodense scar. On delayed imaging (d), the central scar fills-in and the entire lesion is now isodense and imperceptible to the surrounding hepatic parenchyma.

■ Clinical History

A 34-year-old woman with vague abdominal discomfort
(▶ Fig. 9.1).

■ Key Finding

Liver mass with a central scar.

■ Top 3 Differential Diagnoses

• **Hemangioma:** Hemangiomas are the most common benign hepatic lesion. The classic imaging findings are initial discontinuous peripheral nodular enhancement in the arterial phase with delayed central filling. Smaller hemangiomas may demonstrate flash-filling during the arterial phase, while larger lesions may have central regions of fibrosis or cystic changes. On MRI, hemangiomas are hyperintense on T2 (light bulb sign) and hypointense on T1-weighted imaging with similar enhancement patterns as seen with CT. On ultrasound, most hemangiomas are well circumscribed hyperechoic lesions.

• **Focal nodular hyperplasia (FNH):** FNH is an uncommon hepatic lesion that typically presents in young females (75%). The lesion is composed of hepatocytes and classically contains a central low-density scar. On arterial phase imaging, there is enhancement of the lesion with a low-density central scar, which fills in on delayed imaging. The central scar is hyperintense on T2-weighted MR imaging. Since FNH is composed of hepatocytes, it may demonstrate uptake of sulfur colloid (other hepatic lesions demonstrate cold defects) on scintigraphy, although this examination has been somewhat supplanted by MRI. Hepatocyte specific MR contrast agents with delayed imaging are less than 95% specific in distinguishing FNH from other hepatic lesions.

• **Hepatocellular carcinoma (HCC):** HCC is the most common primary hepatic malignancy with an increased incidence in patients with chronic liver disease. Patients may present with a single lesion, multiple lesions, or diffuse hepatic involvement. The lesions are typically hypodense and demonstrate increased arterial phase enhancement due to blood supply from the hepatic artery. Portal or hepatic vein invasion is common. Diagnosis can be difficult in cirrhosis with regenerating nodules. MRI can be helpful in these instances since HCC typically displays increased T2 signal intensity. Clinically, HCC is associated with elevated alpha-fetoprotein.

■ Additional Diagnostic Considerations

• **Hepatic adenoma:** Hepatic adenomas are benign lesions predominantly seen in women (90%). Most often they are solitary but may occasionally be multiple, especially in patients with glycogen storage disease. Hepatic adenomas have an increased frequency and risk of rupture with the use of oral contraceptives. Adenomas are typically hypervascular; internal hemorrhage can lead to heterogeneity.

• **Hypervascular metastases:** Hypervascular metastases are usually multiple but may occasionally present as a solitary mass. Tumors that classically result in hypervascular metastases include melanoma, renal cell carcinoma (RCC), choriocarcinoma, thyroid, carcinoid, pancreatic islet cell tumors, and sarcomas.

■ Diagnosis

FNH.

✓ Pearls

• FNH demonstrates variable enhancement with the scar being isoattenuated on delayed phase imaging.
• A hypervascular hepatic lesion within a cirrhotic liver is HCC until proven otherwise.

• Hepatic adenomas are associated with oral contraceptives and are prone to hemorrhage.

Suggested Readings

Federle MP, Jeffrey RB, Woodward PJ, Borhani A. Diagnostic Imaging: Abdomen. 2nd ed. Philadelphia, PA: Lippincott Williams & Wilkins; 2009

Kamel IR, Lawler LP, Fishman EK. Comprehensive analysis of hypervascular liver lesions using 16-MDCT and advanced image processing. AJR Am J Roentgenol. 2004; 183(2):443–452

Saenz RC. MRI of benign liver lesions and metastatic disease characterization with gadoxetate disodium. J Am Osteopath Coll Radiol. 2012; 1(4):2–9

Case 10

Chelsea M. Jeranko

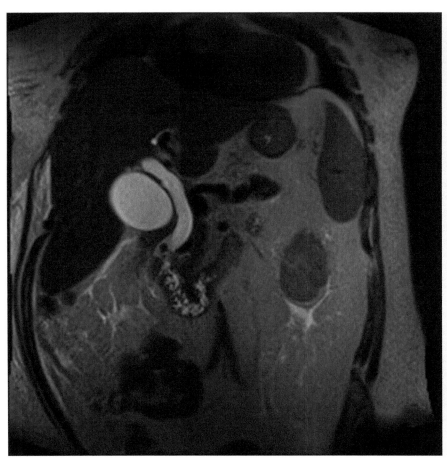

Fig. 10.1 Coronal T2-weighted image of the abdomen demonstrates a low T2 signal round focus in the common bile duct. The common bile duct is also dilated.

■ **Clinical History**

A 54-year-old female with right upper quadrant pain (▶ Fig. 10.1).

■ Key Finding

Round focus in common bile duct.

■ Top 3 Differential Diagnoses

- **Choledocholithiasis:** Choledocholithiasis is one of the most common indications for magnetic resonance cholangiopancreatography (MRCP) of the biliary system, which has a high sensitivity and specificity for their detection. The vast majority of common bile duct stones originate from the gallbladder. Both cholesterol and pigmented stones manifest as low signal on T2-weighted images, however their T1 characteristics can vary. Nondilated biliary ducts can be seen in up to one-third of patients with biliary stones. Therefore, a nondilated biliary tract should still be scrutinized for filling defects, as intermittent obstruction can occur.
- **Ascending cholangitis:** The classical clinical presentation of ascending cholangitis includes fever, jaundice, and right upper quadrant pain (Charcot's triad). Ascending cholangitis occurs in the setting of biliary obstruction, most commonly from choledocholithiasis/hepatolithiasis. There is resultant bile stasis with subsequent infection, typically ascending from the duodenum. Irregular, dilated bile ducts with wall enhancement and biliary obstruction are characteristic. Occasionally, low signal intensity biliary calculi can be seen on T2-weighted images.
- **Recurrent pyogenic cholangitis:** Recurrent pyogenic cholangitis is endemic in Southeast Asia and has a strong association with parasitic infections of the bile ducts. The disease is characterized by recurrent attacks of bacterial cholangitis with associated biliary calculi (pigmented stones). Dilated bile ducts with intrahepatic biliary strictures and intraductal calculi are characteristic. Atrophy of the affected hepatic segment is commonly present.

■ Additional Diagnostic Considerations

Cholangiocarcinoma: Cholangiocarcinoma can be classified based on the anatomic location. Hilar (Klatskin tumor) is the most common and classically involves the biliary confluence. Extrahepatic cholangiocarcinoma involves the common hepatic or common bile duct and peripheral cholangiocarcinoma arises from intrahepatic bile ducts. The tumors characteristically demonstrate slow, progressively increasing enhancement that persists on delayed images. Proximal biliary ductal dilatation and abrupt biliary stricture/occlusion can be seen on MRCP.

■ Diagnosis

Choledocholithiasis.

✓ Pearls

- Stones are characterized on T2 images as low signal intensity foci within the bile duct.
- Ascending cholangitis occurs in the setting of biliary obstruction, most commonly from gallstones.
- Suspect recurrent pyogenic cholangitis in the setting of bile duct dilatation/stones in Southeast Asian patients.

Suggested Readings

Catalano OA, Sahani DV, Forcione DG, et al. Biliary infections: spectrum of imaging findings and management. Radiographics. 2009; 29(7):2059–2080
Leyendecker JR, Brown JJ, Merkle EM. Practical Guide to Abdominal and Pelvic MRI, 2nd ed. Philadelphia, PA: Lippincott Williams & Wilkins; 2011
Yeh BM, Liu PS, Soto JA, Corvera CA, Hussain HK. MR imaging and CT of the biliary tract. Radiographics. 2009; 29(6):1669–1688

Case 11

Michael Legacy

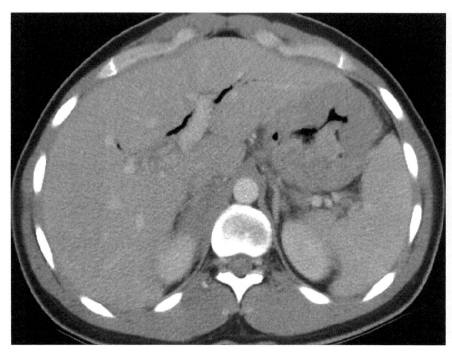

Fig. 11.1 CT axial image with intravenous and oral contrast shows central hepatic air consistent with pneumobilia. In addition, there is concentric gastric wall thickening related to gastritis. (Image courtesy of Rocky C. Saenz.)

■ Clinical History

A 26-year-old male with abdominal pain (▶Fig. 11.1).

■ Key Finding

Pneumobilia.

■ Top 3 Differential Diagnoses

- **Sphincter of Oddi dysfunction:** Choledocholithiasis and patulous sphincter of Oddi are the most common causes of a dysfunctional sphincter of Oddi. Passage of gallstones through the sphincter of Oddi may cause incompetence of the sphincter and result in passage of bowel gas into the bile ducts. A patulous sphincter of Oddi is primarily seen in the elderly and typically the pneumobilia will be minimal.
- **Iatrogenic/postsurgical:** Patients typically have a history of enteric or biliary intervention such as endoscopic retrograde cholangiopancreatography (ERCP) biliary-enteric anastomosis, or sphincterotomy. Biliary sphincterotomy and patent biliary stents are common surgical causes of pneumobilia. Incising the sphincter of Oddi during an ERCP for removal of gallstones, and/or placement of a stent enables bowel gas to pass through the stent or the postsurgical sphincter into the bile ducts.
- **Infection/inflammation:** Emphysematous cholecystitis, most commonly in diabetic and the elderly, may reflux air into the bile ducts. Look for surrounding inflammatory changes.

■ Additional Diagnostic Considerations

Fistula: Gallstone ileus may cause the gallstone to erode through inflamed bile duct or gallbladder wall into the small bowel creating a cholecystoduodenal fistula. Extensive inflammatory changes are usually present.

■ Diagnosis

Pneumobilia post-sphincterotomy.

✓ Pearls

- Pneumobilia can reflux into the gallbladder and mimic emphysematous cholecystitis.
- Portal venous gas is along the periphery of the liver.
- Occluded biliary stents do not allow passage of bowel gas into the bile ducts.

Suggested Readings

Catalano OA, Sahani DV, Forcione DG, et al. Biliary infections: spectrum of imaging findings and management. Radiographics. 2009; 29(7):2059–2080

Federle MP, Jeffrey RB, Woodward PJ, Borhani A. Diagnostic Imaging: Abdomen. 2nd ed. Philadelphia, PA: Lippincott Williams & Wilkins; 2009

Patel NB, Oto A, Thomas S. Multidetector CT of emergent biliary pathologic conditions. Radiographics. 2013; 33(7):1867–1888

Shah PA, Cunningham SC, Morgan TA, Daly BD. Hepatic gas: widening spectrum of causes detected at CT and US in the interventional era. Radiographics. 2011; 31(5):1403–1413

Case 12

Rajeev Aravapalli

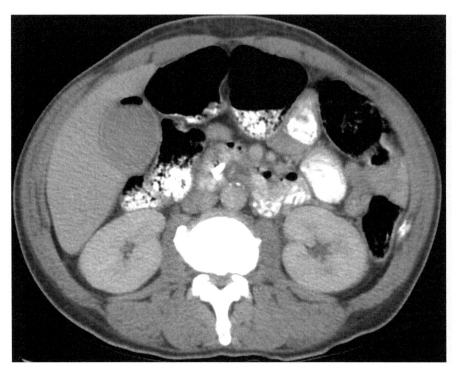

Fig. 12.1 CT axial image of the abdomen with intravenous and oral contrast demonstrates an air-fluid level in the gallbladder without any wall thickening. (Image courtesy of Rocky C. Saenz.)

■ Clinical History

A 44-year-old female with generalized abdominal pain (▶Fig. 12.1).

■ Key Finding

Gallbladder intraluminal air.

■ Top 3 Differential Diagnoses

- **Emphysematous cholecystitis:** Emphysematous cholecystitis is a rare form of acute cholecystitis due to secondary infection by gas-forming organisms. The pathogenesis is thought to be secondary to vascular compromise of cystic artery. This is considered a surgical emergency. There is a high risk of gangrene, perforation, and sepsis if untreated. An urgent cholecystectomy is the definitive treatment. A cholecystostomy may be needed to bridge to cholecystectomy in high-risk poor surgical candidates. Emphysematous cholecystitis most commonly occurs in elderly or diabetic patients.
- **Sphincter of Oddi dysfunction:** Incompetence of the sphincter of Oddi may result in passage of bowel gas into the bile ducts and into the gallbladder. This incompetence is caused by choledocholithiasis, senescent change, or a patulous sphincter. The sphincter may also be dysfunctional secondary to prior instrumentation (esophagogastroduodenoscopy, sphincteroplasty, or papillotomy).
- **Cholelithiasis:** These may present with gas filled fissures. About 50% of gallstones have fissures, however less than half have gas. This triradiate pattern of nitrogen gas is called the "Mercedes-Benz sign." This can be mistaken for emphysematous cholecystitis. The presence of air-filled gallstones does not imply infection.

■ Additional Diagnostic Considerations

- **Gangrenous cholecystitis:** The most common complication of acute cholecystitis affecting 15% of patients. It occurs as a result of ischemia with necrosis of the gallbladder wall. CT signs include gallbladder wall or lumen gas, focal irregularity or defect in the gallbladder wall, intraluminal membranes, absence of mural enhancement, and pericholecystic abscess.
- **Fistula:** There may be an abnormal connection between the bowel and the gallbladder. This connection allows air from the bowel to enter into the gallbladder. The cholecystocolonic fistula is uncommon, occurring in around 0.1% of patients with biliary disease. The cholecystoduodenal fistula is the most common type involving the gallbladder. A complication of cholecystocolonic fistula is perforation of the colon with resultant fecal peritonitis which can progress to sepsis or death.

■ Diagnosis

Sphincter of Oddi dysfunction secondary to a patulous sphincter.

✓ Pearls

- *Clostridium perfringens* is the most common gas forming organism in emphysematous cholecystitis.
- CT is the best modality for identifying intramural or intraluminal gas.
- Portal venous gas may mimic biliary gas.

Suggested Readings

Federle MP, Jeffrey RB, Woodward PJ, Borhani A. Diagnostic Imaging: Abdomen. 2nd ed. Philadelphia, PA: Lippincott Williams & Wilkins; 2009

Grayson DE, Abbott RM, Levy AD, Sherman PM. Emphysematous infections of the abdomen and pelvis: a pictorial review. Radiographics. 2002; 22(3):543–561

Smith EA, Dillman JR, Elsayes KM, Menias CO, Bude RO. Cross-sectional imaging of acute and chronic gallbladder inflammatory disease. AJR Am J Roentgenol. 2009; 192(1):188–196

Case 13

Rocky C. Saenz

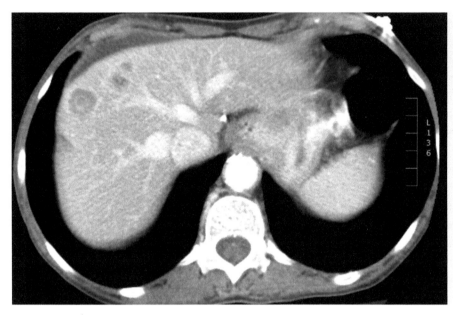

Fig. 13.1 CT axial image with intravenous contrast through the upper liver and spleen demonstrates a target enhancing lesion in the right lobe. There are at least three other subcentimeter liver lesions. Free fluid is seen in the right upper quadrant.

■ Clinical History

A 45-year-old female with a breast lump (▶ Fig. 13.1).

■ Key Finding

Target liver lesion.

■ Top 3 Differential Diagnoses

- **Metastases:** Metastasis is the most common tumor and malignancy of the liver. The most common source of metastatic disease is melanoma, lung, breast, pancreas, and colon carcinomas. Metastatic lesions can have peripheral rim- or target-like enhancement. Imaging findings depend on the primary tumor type, but lesions are often poorly circumscribed with variable enhancement and typically multiple. Metastasis .is more than 10 times more common than primary liver malignancies. The liver is the most common organ site for metastatic disease.
- **Hepatocellular carcinoma (HCC):** HCC is the most common primary hepatic malignancy. Patients may present with multiple lesions. The lesions typically demonstrate increased arterial phase enhancement due to blood supply from the hepatic artery with washout of contrast on delayed imaging. MRI can be helpful in these instances since HCC typically displays increased T2 signal intensity. Clinically, HCC is associated with elevated alpha-fetoprotein.
- **Hepatic lymphoma:** Hepatic lymphoma may be primary or secondary. Secondary hepatic lymphoma is seen in more than 50% of all lymphoma patients. Most lesions are lobulated in appearance and are multiple in number. Non-Hodgkin's lymphoma (NHL) is more common to have hepatic involvement than Hodgkin.

■ Additional Diagnostic Considerations

Hepatic abscesses: Hepatic abscesses are uncommon and can be categorized into pyogenic (80%), amebic (10%), and fungal (10%). Pyogenic hepatic abscesses are the most common and found in the setting of diverticulitis and sepsis. Amebic abscesses are prone to rupture. Imaging findings include thick-walled, hypoattenuating liver masses with internal septations, peripheral lesion enhancement, and air in up to 20% of cases. Untreated, liver abscesses have a high mortality rate.

■ Diagnosis

Metastasis from breast carcinoma.

✓ Pearls

- A hepatic lesion with a target enhancement should be considered metastatic until proven otherwise.
- A hepatic metastatic target lesion is classically from breast or gastrointestinal adenocarcinoma.
- HCC will have an elevated serum alpha-fetoprotein.

Suggested Readings

Federle MP, Jeffrey RB, Woodward PJ, Borhani A. Diagnostic Imaging: Abdomen. 2nd ed. Philadelphia, PA: Lippincott Williams & Wilkins; 2009

Mortelé KJ, Ros PR. Cystic focal liver lesions in the adult: differential CT and MR imaging features. Radiographics. 2001; 21(4):895–910

Saenz RC. MRI of benign liver lesions and metastatic disease characterization with gadoxetate disodium. J Am Osteopath Coll Radiol. 2012; 1(4):2–9

Case 14

Rocky C. Saenz

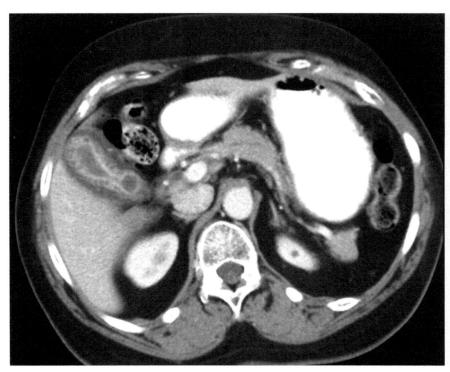

Fig. 14.1 CT image of the upper abdomen shows gallbladder wall thickening with multiple intramural cystic foci.

■ **Clinical History**

A 43-year-old female with right upper quadrant pain (▶ Fig. 14.1).

■ Key Finding

Gallbladder wall thickening with cystic changes.

■ Top 3 Differential Diagnoses

- **Adenomyomatosis:** It is also known as adenomyomatous hyperplasia or diverticulosis of the gallbladder. Adenomyomatosis is a benign condition with cholesterol deposition within dilated Rokitansky–Aschoff sinuses with associated wall thickening. The most common form is focally in the fundus. CT is less specific than ultrasound for detection, but it may show cystic-appearing thickening of the gallbladder wall or enhancing epithelium within intramural diverticula surrounded by relatively unenhanced hypertrophied gallbladder muscularis. On MRI, the intramural diverticula may be seen as high T2 signal foci in line mimicking a "pearl necklace."
- **Acute cholecystitis:** Most frequent inflammatory condition of the gallbladder. Cholecystitis is suspected on CT when a thick-walled gallbladder and fat stranding are seen. However, this is not pathognomonic and should be confirmed on ultrasound or nuclear hepatobiliary scan. On ultrasound, the most reliable sign is a positive sonographic Murphy sign (pain when the sonographer pushes on the gallbladder while imaging).
- **Chronic cholecystitis:** It is caused by gallbladder stones that create transient obstruction which leads to prolonged inflammation and fibrosis. This fibrosis may lead to a contracted gallbladder, and is almost always seen with cholelithiasis. Imaging findings include gallstones in thick-walled gallbladder with no pericholecystic fluid and lack of wall hyperemia.

■ Additional Diagnostic Considerations

Gallbladder carcinoma: The majority are adenocarcinomas with the second most common being squamous cell. This entity can appear as a mass replacing the gallbladder, an intraluminal polypoid mass, or wall thickening that is focal or diffuse. Most gallbladder carcinomas present after 65. CT and MR are useful in defining extent of disease, adenopathy, and evaluating for metastasis.

■ Diagnosis

Adenomyomatosis.

✓ Pearls

- Adenomyomatosis is a benign condition.
- Adenomyomatosis is seen in up to 25% of cholecystectomy specimens.
- On CT when acute cholecystitis is suspected it should be confirmed with ultrasound or nuclear.

Suggested Readings

Federle MP, Jeffrey RB, Woodward PJ, Borhani A. Diagnostic Imaging: Abdomen. 2nd ed. Philadelphia, PA: Lippincott Williams & Wilkins; 2009

McKnight T, Patel A. Gallbladder masses: multimodality approach to differential diagnosis. J Am Osteopath Coll Radiol. 2012; 1(4):22–31

Runner GJ, Corwin MT, Siewert B, Eisenberg RL. Gallbladder wall thickening. AJR Am J Roentgenol. 2014; 202(1):W1–W12

Case 15

Robert A. Jesinger

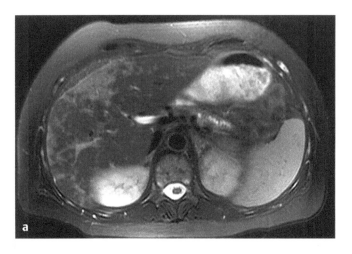

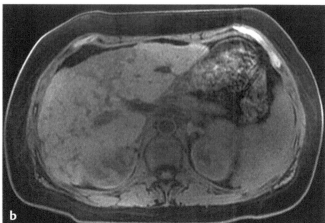

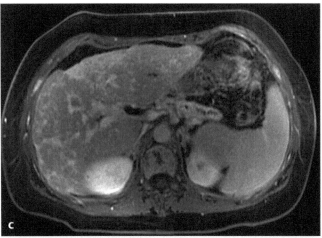

Fig. 15.1 Axial T2-weighted MR image with fat suppression **(a)** demonstrates a nodular liver contour with capsular retraction and numerous confluent wedge-shaped foci of increased signal intensity peripherally. These regions are low in signal intensity on T1-weighted fat suppressed image **(b)** and demonstrate heterogeneous enhancement postgadolinium **(c)**.

■ **Clinical History**

A 67-year-old woman with chronic liver enzyme elevation and a history of breast cancer (▶ Fig. 15.1).

■ Key Finding

Nodular liver contour.

■ Top 3 Differential Diagnoses

- **Cirrhosis:** Cirrhosis is a chronic liver disease characterized by hepatic fibrosis and regenerative hepatic nodules. Common causes include alcohol (micronodular cirrhosis), chronic viral hepatitis (macronodular cirrhosis), autoimmune hepatitis, and chronic metabolic conditions (primary biliary cirrhosis, primary hemochromatosis, Wilson's disease, alpha-1 antitrypsin deficiency). Imaging findings include nodular liver surface contour, distorted hepatic architecture with atrophy, and stigmata of portal hypertension (enlarged main portal vein with slow flow, flow reversal or occlusion; varices, splenomegaly, gallbladder/bowel wall thickening, and ascites). MRI of liver nodules helps distinguish regenerative nodules (low T2 signal) from neoplastic nodules (high T2 signal). The use of gadoxetate disodium can help in distinguishing or characterizing hepatic lesions due to hepatocyte phase of imaging.
- **Treated metastases:** Chemotherapy treatment of liver metastases (commonly from breast, lung, and colorectal cancer) can result in scarring of hepatic tumor implants. Liver parenchyma, between these areas of scarring, can be normal or regenerative. The overall imaging appearance simulates macronodular cirrhosis, and hence is referred to as "pseudocirrhosis." Correlation with appropriate history is helpful.
- **Budd–Chiari syndrome:** Chronic hepatic venous occlusive disease can result in a nodular liver contour, usually as a consequence of regenerative nodules. In chronic Budd–Chiari syndrome, these nodules are usually small, multiple, and hypervascular, and the number of nodules is often underestimated on CT. Large regenerative hypervascular nodules may be seen and are usually hyperintense on T1 MRI sequences. There is no evidence that large regenerative nodules degenerate into malignancy. A central scar in nodules greater than 1 cm can be seen. Caudate hypertrophy occurs as a result of its separate venous drainage into the inferior vena cava (IVC), which may simulate a dominant nodule.

■ Additional Diagnostic Considerations

- **Schistosoma japonicum:** Schistosoma japonicum, a major cause of hepatic schistosomiasis, is highly associated with hepatic fibrosis. Calcified eggs along the portal tracts produce the pathognomonic "turtleback" calcification. The size and shape of the liver can be preserved, but fibrosis and portal tract calcification often result in a nodular liver contour.
- **Confluent hepatic fibrosis:** Confluent hepatic fibrosis may occur in the setting of chronic liver disease. The most common appearance is a wedge-shaped hypodense region on CT which extends from the hilum. The anterior segment of the right hepatic lobe and medial segment of the left hepatic lobe are the most common sites of involvement. There is overlying capsular retraction and little or no enhancement.

■ Diagnosis

Treated breast metastases (pseudocirrhosis).

✓ Pearls

- MRI helps distinguish regenerative (low T2 signal) from neoplastic (high T2 signal) liver nodules.
- Pseudocirrhosis is most commonly seen with treated breast, lung, and colorectal metastases.
- The "turtleback" appearance of the liver is most commonly associated with schistosomiasis.

Suggested Readings

Brancatelli G, Federle MP, Grazioli L, Golfieri R, Lencioni R. Benign regenerative nodules in Budd-Chiari syndrome and other vascular disorders of the liver: radiologic-pathologic and clinical correlation. Radiographics. 2002; 22(4):847–862

Dodd GD, III, Baron RL, Oliver JH, III, Federle MP. Spectrum of imaging findings of the liver in end-stage cirrhosis: part I, gross morphology and diffuse abnormalities. AJR Am J Roentgenol. 1999; 173(4):1031–1036

Saenz RC. MRI of benign liver lesions and metastatic disease characterization with gadoxetate disodium. J Am Osteopath Coll Radiol. 2012; 1(4):2–9

Case 16

Sara K. Boyd

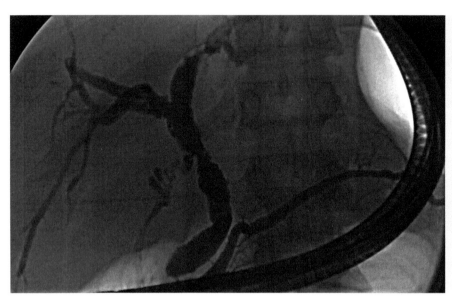

Fig. 16.1 Single ERCP image demonstrates a focal narrowing and dilation of the left primary biliary radicle and narrowing of common bile duct with proximal and distal dilatation (beaded appearance). The pancreatic duct is prominent. (Image courtesy of Rocky C. Saenz.)

■ **Clinical History**

A 26-year-old male with right upper quadrant pain and acquired immunodeficiency syndrome (AIDS) (▶Fig. 16.1).

■ Key Finding

Common bile duct beaded appearance.

■ Top 3 Differential Diagnoses

- **Primary sclerosing cholangitis:** This is an idiopathic progressive chronic disease of the liver and intra- and extrahepatic biliary ducts that has characteristic multiple short segment strictures throughout the biliary system with normal to mildly enlarged intervening ducts. This produces an overall "beaded" appearance on magnetic resonance cholangiopancreatography (MRCP) and endoscopic retrograde cholangiopancreatography (ERCP) and can involve the common bile duct. Fibrotic strictures are often at duct bifurcations and are out of proportion to adjacent upstream duct enlargement. Other cholangiographic findings include webs, diverticula, and stones. Advanced disease will demonstrate peripheral duct obliteration, producing a characteristic "pruned tree" appearance.
- **AIDS cholangiopathy:** A form of secondary cholangitis, this entity results from chronic biliary inflammation and infection from opportunistic infections in AIDS patients with CD4 counts less than 100 cells/mm³. Cytomegalovirus (CMV) and *Cryptosporidium parvum* are the most common infectious agents. MRCP will demonstrate multiple inta- and extrahepatic biliary strictures with intervening ductal dilation. Additional radiologic findings include a distal common bile duct stricture, acalculous cholecystitis, and cholangitis.
- **Posttransplantation strictures:** Common bile duct strictures secondary to liver transplantation are either anastomotic or nonanastomotic. Anastomotic strictures are secondary to iatrogenic ischemia with resultant scarring. MRCP will demonstrate a short-segment narrowing at site of anastomoses, which are often extrahepatic, with or without proximal ductal dilation. Nonanastomotic strictures are due to non-iatrogenic ischemia, such as hepatic arterial thrombosis and are often multiple discontinuous intrahepatic long segment strictures on MRCP.

■ Additional Diagnostic Considerations

- **Ascending cholangitis:** Cholangitis, a purely clinical diagnosis is caused by a bacterial infection within an obstructed biliary system, which may result from strictures, choledocholithiasis, or papillary stenosis. A classic Charcot's triad of clinical symptoms may be present: fever, jaundice, and abdominal pain. MRCP and/or ERCP are useful as an adjunct examination for determining the underlying etiology of the obstruction.
- **Oriental cholangiohepatitis:** This intraductal parasitic infection by *Clonorchis sinensis* or *Ascaris lumbricoides* is endemic to Southeast Asia. The parasites provoke injury and inflammation to the biliary ducts which progress to multiple sites of strictures and post-stenotic dilation. MRCP can demonstrate a "beaded" appearance, ductal stones, disproportionate extrahepatic ductal dilation that is not a result of stricture or stone, and a right-angle branching pattern of the ducts.

■ Diagnosis

AIDS cholangitis.

✓ Pearls

- Primary sclerosing cholangitis is the most common cause of the "beaded" appearance of the intra- and extrahepatic biliary ducts. Advanced disease has a characteristic "pruned tree" appearance.
- Posttransplantation biliary strictures are either anastomotic or nonanastomotic and relate to ischemia.
- AIDS-related cholangitis will have a "beaded" appearance in patients with CD4 counts less than 100 cells/mm³.

Suggested Readings

Ito K, Mitchell DG, Outwater EK, Blasbalg R. Primary sclerosing cholangitis: MR imaging features. AJR Am J Roentgenol. 1999; 172(6):1527–1533

Katabathina VS, Dasyam AK, Dasyam N, Hosseinzadeh K. Adult bile duct strictures: role of MR imaging and MR cholangiopancreatography in characterization. Radiographics. 2014; 34(3):565–586

Vitellas KM, Keogan MT, Freed KS, et al. Radiologic manifestations of sclerosing cholangitis with emphasis on MR cholangiopancreatography. Radiographics. 2000; 20(4):959–975, quiz 1108–1109, 1112

Case 17

Rocky C. Saenz

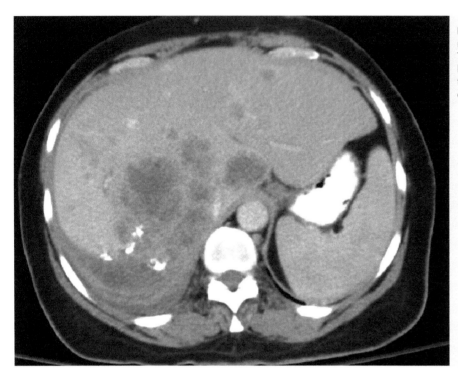

Fig. 17.1 Enhanced axial CT image demonstrates multiple hypodense lesions throughout the liver. The majority of the lesions are within the right lobe with calcifications. Small amount of free fluid in the abdomen and a small right pleural effusion.

■ **Clinical History**

A 54-year-old woman with right upper quadrant pain (▶Fig. 17.1).

■ Key Finding

Cystic liver lesion with calcification.

■ Top 3 Differential Diagnoses

- **Metastases:** Metastasis is the most common liver lesions. The most common source of metastatic lesions with calcifications is colon, ovary, breast, and gastric carcinomas. Metastatic disease to the liver is indicative of late stage cancer. Imaging findings depend on the primary tumor type, but lesions are often poorly circumscribed with variable enhancement and typically multiple. The liver is the most common organ site for metastatic disease.
- **Hepatic abscess:** Fungal infections are uncommon etiology of hepatic abscess accounting for approximately 10%. Pyogenic hepatic abscesses are much more common. These fungal infections usually occur in immunocompromised neutropenic patients. The most common cause is *Candida albicans*. On CT, low density is seen with areas of calcifications. After administration of contrast, a central or eccentric dot of enhancement is seen (likely representing the hyphae). Prognosis is favorable with prompt antifungal treatment.
- **Hydatid cyst:** The most common cause is *Echinococcus granulosus* with *Echinococcus multilocularis* (*alveolaris*) being less common. These cysts can be uni- or mutilocular, well-defined cysts. These cysts commonly have curvilinear ring like calcification. Commonly seen are daughter cysts (smaller adjacent cysts) which also may have calcification. A known complication of these cysts is rupture into the peritoneal cavity causing peritonitis and an anaphylactic reaction.

■ Additional Diagnostic Considerations

Autosomal dominant polycystic liver disease (ADPLD): ADPLD is a hereditary disorder with resulting multiple parenchymal cysts. The cysts are usually more than 20 in number and may have peripheral calcifications related to the prior hemorrhage. None of these cysts enhance. These are benign lesions and are more commonly seen in women. ADPLD is a distinct entity from autosomal dominant polycystic kidney disease (ADPKD). About half of polycystic kidney patients have liver involvement. Approximately 70% of ADPLD also have ADPKD.

■ Diagnosis

Metastasis from colon carcinoma.

✓ Pearls

- In immunocompromised patients the diagnosis of exclusion is an abscess.
- Multiple hepatic and renal cysts are seen consider ADPLD or ADPKD.
- In a foreign-born patient with a cystic calcified lesion consider hydatid disease.

Suggested Readings

Erden A, Ormeci N, Fitoz S, Erden I, Tanju S, Genç Y. Intrabiliary rupture of hepatic hydatid cysts: diagnostic accuracy of MR cholangiopancreatography. AJR Am J Roentgenol. 2007; 189(2):W84–9

Federle MP, Jeffrey RB, Woodward PJ, Borhani A. Diagnostic Imaging: Abdomen. 2nd ed. Philadelphia, PA: Lippincott Williams & Wilkins; 2009
Saenz RC. MRI of benign liver lesions and metastatic disease characterization with gadoxetate disodium. J Am Osteopath Coll Radiol. 2012; 1(4):2–9

Case 18

Eleanor L. Ormsby

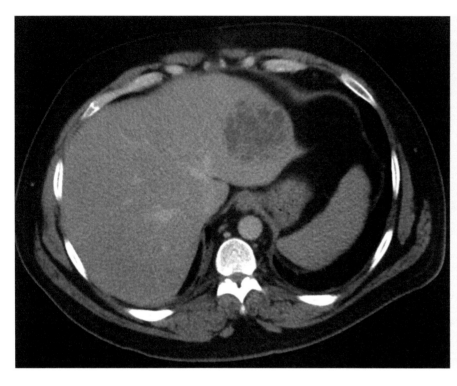

Fig. 18.1 Axial contrast enhanced CT image demonstrates an ill-defined 5 cm hypodense multilocular mass in the left lobe of the liver. The lesion has peripheral rim and septal enhancement. On delayed imaging (not shown), there was no contrast filling in of the mass. (Image courtesy of Rocky C. Saenz.)

■ Clinical History

A 43-year-old male with history of epigastric pain (▶ Fig. 18.1).

■ Key Finding

Solitary hypodense, hypovascular liver mass.

■ Top 3 Differential Diagnoses

- **Hepatic cyst:** Hepatic cysts are thought to be congenital lesions arising from developmental defects of the biliary ducts. They are well circumscribed with very thin or imperceptible walls. They rarely cause symptoms and typically do not result in abnormal liver function tests. Simple cysts do not enhance.
- **Solitary metastasis:** The most common appearance of hepatic metastases on CT is a low-density lesion with respect to the liver parenchyma. There may be a degree of peripheral rim enhancement. Calcifications may be seen in mucinous adenocarcinomas of the colon, stomach, or ovary. Hypovascular metastatic masses are best seen on portal venous phase images. Smaller lesions may fill-in on delayed images.

- **Hepatic abscess:** Hepatic abscesses are most commonly pyogenic usually from ascending cholangitis, hematogenous spread, or direct extension from adjacent sites of infection. They may also occur as a complication after surgery or traumatic events involving the liver. Hepatic abscesses are hypodense with peripheral enhancement. Pyogenic abscesses are commonly multilocular. Amebic abscesses appear similar to pyogenic abscesses but tend to be unilocular. They are common worldwide and have a tendency to rupture. Echinococcal infection (hydatid cyst) can be very large with rim-like calcification. Daughter cysts within the larger cyst are pathognomonic. Mycotic abscesses are typically multiple and small.

■ Additional Diagnostic Considerations

- **Peripheral cholangiocarcinoma:** Intrahepatic cholangiocarcinomas are hypodense on arterial and portal venous phase imaging and characteristically demonstrate delayed (> 10 minutes) peripheral to central enhancement. Overlying capsular retraction is due to fibrosis. The masses tend to be infiltrative with irregular borders. Biliary ductal dilatation is common peripheral to the tumor.

- **Biliary cystadenoma:** Biliary cystadenomas are uncommon, multilocular, well-defined cystic masses arising from the bile ducts. They typically occur in middle-aged women who complain of chronic abdominal pain. The cyst wall may enhance. Malignant transformation to cystadenocarcinoma can occur.

■ Diagnosis

Hepatic abscess (pyogenic).

✓ Pearls

- Delayed imaging with intravenous contrast is helpful in differentiating hepatic cysts from hypodense metastases.
- Amebic abscesses in the liver are fairly common worldwide and have a tendency to rupture.

- Delayed imaging (> 10 minutes) is helpful in the diagnosis of cholangiocarcinoma.

Suggested Readings

Engelbrecht MR, Katz SS, van Gulik TM, Laméris JS, van Delden OM. Imaging of perihilar cholangiocarcinoma. AJR Am J Roentgenol. 2015; 204(4): 782–791

Qian LJ, Zhu J, Zhuang ZG, Xia Q, Liu Q, Xu JR. Spectrum of multilocular cystic hepatic lesions: CT and MR imaging findings with pathologic correlation. Radiographics. 2013; 33(5):1419–1433

Case 19

Rocky C. Saenz

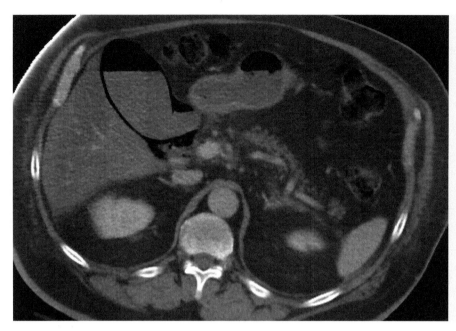

Fig. 19.1 CT image of the upper abdomen shows the gallbladder wall with intramural air circumferentially and an intraluminal air-fluid level. Also, fat stranding is seen adjacent to the neck with air partially seen in cystic duct and common hepatic duct. (Image courtesy of Sharon Kreuer.)

■ Clinical History

A 73-year-old diabetic male with fever and right upper quadrant pain (►Fig. 19.1).

■ **Key Finding**

Gallbladder wall air.

■ **Top 3 Differential Diagnoses**

- **Emphysematous cholecystitis:** Emphysematous cholecystitis is a rare form of acute cholecystitis complicated by secondary infection from a gas-forming organism. The most common organisms include *Escherichia coli* and *Clostridium*. On CT, the best imaging findings include intramural air or intraluminal air. If both intramural and intraluminal air are present, it usually represents advanced disease. If perforation occurs, then pneumoperitoneum may be seen. Septic shock and peritonitis are seen with perforation. An urgent cholecystectomy is the definitive treatment. Emphysematous cholecystitis most commonly occurs in elderly men or diabetic patients.
- **Hepatic abscess:** Hepatic abscesses are usually pyogenic and commonly multilocular secondary to hematogenous spread.

These infections when located in segment V or segment IVb can be associated with direct extension to the gallbladder. Therefore, hepatic abscesses with gallbladder involvement may cause intramural air. Hepatic abscesses are hypodense with peripheral enhancement. Air is seen within the minority of abscesses.
- **Gangrenous cholecystitis:** The most common complication of acute cholecystitis affecting 15% of patients. It occurs as a result of ischemia with necrosis of the gallbladder wall from decreased flow of the cystic artery. CT signs include gallbladder wall or lumen gas, focal irregularity or defect in the gallbladder wall, intraluminal membranes, absence of mural enhancement, and pericholecystic abscess.

■ **Additional Diagnostic Considerations**

Fistula: A fistula can occur between the bowel and the gallbladder. This connection would allow air from the bowel to enter into the gallbladder. A cholecystocolonic fistula is rare. The cho- lecystoduodenal fistula is the most common type. These fistulas would not typically result in intramural air.

■ **Diagnosis**

Emphysematous cholecystitis.

✓ **Pearls**

- Emphysematous cholecystitis is the diagnosis of exclusion with intramural air.
- If gallbladder intramural air is suspected on X-ray or ultrasound; noncontrast CT can be confirmatory.

- Hepatic abscess is only a considered for the etiology of gallbladder intramural air when a discrete hypodense lesion is seen near the gallbladder.

Suggested Readings

Federle MP, Jeffrey RB, Woodward PJ, Borhani A. Diagnostic Imaging: Abdomen. 2nd ed. Philadelphia, PA: Lippincott Williams & Wilkins; 2009
Grayson DE, Abbott RM, Levy AD, Sherman PM. Emphysematous infections of the abdomen and pelvis: a pictorial review. Radiographics. 2002; 22(3):543–561

Smith EA, Dillman JR, Elsayes KM, Menias CO, Bude RO. Cross-sectional imaging of acute and chronic gallbladder inflammatory disease. AJR Am J Roentgenol. 2009; 192(1):188–196

Case 20

Rocky C. Saenz

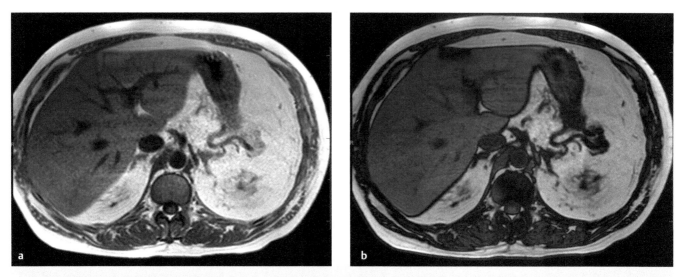

Fig. 20.1 In-phase and out-of-phase imaging of the upper abdomen shows focal high signal on the in-phase **(a)** with corresponding low signal (signal dropout) in segment IVa of the liver **(b)**.

■ Clinical History

A 25-year-old female with a generalized pain (▶Fig. 20.1).

■ Key Finding

Liver lesions with signal drop-out on out of phase.

■ Top 3 Differential Diagnoses

- **Steatosis:** Hepatic steatosis also known as fatty liver is due to the accumulation of triglycerides in the hepatocytes. The etiology may be from alcoholic or nonalcoholic liver disease (nonalcoholic steatohepatitis, NASH). NASH is commonly seen in with hyperlipidemia and diabetes. Steatosis has many appearances including: diffuse, diffuse with sparring, focal, multifocal and geographic. The diffuse form is the most common. A key imaging feature is noting normal vessels coursing through the lesion. On MRI, dual-phase gradient-recalled echo T1-weighted is most reliable to detect loss of signal (hypointense appearance) to surrounding liver on the opposed-phase (out of phase). Steatosis is usually asymptomatic but often associated with mildly increased liver function tests.
- **Hepatocellular carcinoma (HCC):** HCC is the most common primary hepatic malignancy. HCC has been known to have intratumoral fat. Fat is most reliably detected on dual-phase gradient-recalled MRI. The key to diagnosis is using dynamic cross-sectional imaging and noting early (arterial phase) enhancement with washout on delayed imaging. Another typical feature is a tumor capsule. Clinically, HCC is associated with elevated alpha-fetoprotein.
- **Hepatic adenoma:** Hepatic adenomas are benign lesions predominantly seen in women (90%). These lesions are usually seen in women on birth control, athletes on anabolic steroids and patients with metabolic diseases. Hepatic adenomas have an increased risk of rupture when larger than 5 cm. At least four subtypes have been identified with the inflammatory subtype being the most common and typically arise in steatotic livers. Intravoxel fat has been seen in 11 to 20% of the inflammatory subtype. On MRI chemical shift imaging, microscopic fat demonstrates complete dropout on out-of-phase imaging versus macroscopic fat which demonstrates a dark border (India ink staining pattern). Lesions usually are well-circumscribed with variable enhancement but can be heterogeneous due to prior internal hemorrhage.

■ Additional Diagnostic Considerations

- **Metastases:** Metastasis is the most common lesion of the liver and uncommonly may contain fat. The most common primary tumor to have fat is liposarcomas and malignant germ cell tumors. Clear cell renal cell carcinomas (RCCs) are also known to have fat but lesions are often poorly circumscribed with variable enhancement and typically multiple.
- **Angiomyolipoma:** Angiomyolipomas are classified as perivascular epithelioid cell neoplasms (PEComas) which are mesenchymal tumors. The liver is the second most common organ for angiomyolipomas after the kidney. As with renal angiomyolipoma, hepatic lesions may have measurable fat on CT (HU−20). Hepatic angiomyolipomas are also associated with tuberous sclerosis in 6 to 10% of cases, but to a lesser extent the association of renal angiomyolipoma to tuberous sclerosis. Unfortunately, hepatic angiomyolipoma have avid arterial enhancement with delayed washout which mimics HCC. Therefore, many of these lesions are resected.

■ Diagnosis

Focal steatosis.

✓ Pearls

- Focal fatty, geographic liver lesion is likely steatosis.
- On MRI, macroscopic fat does not drop out on chemical shift imaging.
- If serum alpha-fetoprotein level is positive HCC must be excluded.

Suggested Readings

Coast, et al. Fat-containing liver lesions on imaging: detection and differential diagnosis. Am J Roentgen. 2018; 210:1–10

Saenz RC. MRI of benign liver lesions and metastatic disease characterization with gadoxetate disodium. J Am Osteopath Coll Radiol. 2012; 1(4):2–9

Case 21

Rocky C. Saenz

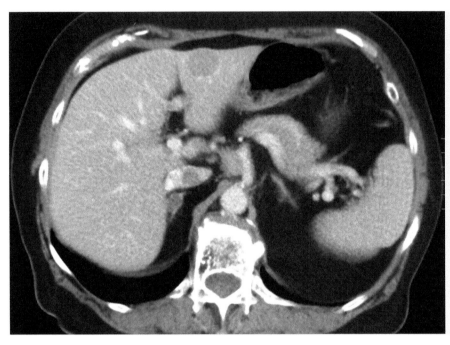

Fig. 21.1 Contrast enhanced axial CT image through the upper abdomen demonstrates a single hypodense lesion in the left lobe of the liver. A right adrenal gland nodule is noted. A filling defect is seen in the inferior vena cava (IVC).

■ Clinical History

A 61-year-old male with weight loss (▶Fig. 21.1).

■ Key Finding

Solid liver lesion.

■ Top 3 Differential Diagnoses

- **Metastases:** Metastasis is the most common tumor and malignancy of the liver. The most common source of metastatic disease is melanoma, lung, breast, pancreas, and colon carcinomas. Metastatic disease to the liver is indicative of late stage cancer. Imaging findings depend on the primary tumor type, but lesions are often poorly circumscribed with variable enhancement and typically multiple. Metastasis is more than 10 times more common than primary liver malignancies. The liver is the most common organ site for metastatic disease.
- **Hemangioma:** Hemangiomas are the most common benign tumor of the liver. The classic dynamic imaging findings are initial discontinuous peripheral nodular enhancement in the arterial phase with delayed central filling. These lesions are more common in females and typically asymptomatic.

Symptomatic lesions are usually large (> 10 cm termed giant hemangiomas) and rarely may be associated with platelet sequestration, resulting in thrombocytopenia, known as Kasabach–Merritt syndrome.
- **Focal nodular hyperplasia (FNH):** FNH is the second most common benign tumor of the liver. It is typically presents in young females (75%). The lesion is composed of hepatocytes and classically solitary with a central scar. On arterial phase imaging, there is variable enhancement of the lesion with a low-density central scar, which fills in on delayed imaging. The central scar is hyperintense on T2-weighted MR imaging. Hepatocyte specific MR contrast agents with delayed imaging are more than 95% specific in distinguishing FNH from other hepatic lesions.

■ Additional Diagnostic Considerations

- **Hepatocellular carcinoma (HCC):** HCC is the most common primary hepatic malignancy. Patients may present with a single lesion, multiple lesions, or diffuse hepatic involvement. The lesions typically demonstrate increased arterial phase enhancement due to blood supply from the hepatic artery with washout of contrast on delayed imaging. MRI can be helpful in these instances since HCC typically displays increased T2 signal intensity. Clinically, HCC is associated with elevated alpha-fetoprotein.
- **Hepatic adenoma:** Hepatic adenomas are benign lesions predominantly seen in women (90%). Most often they are solitary but may occasionally be multiple, especially in patients with glycogen storage disease. Hepatic adenomas have an increased frequency and risk of rupture with the use of oral contraceptives. Adenomas are typically hypervascular; internal hemorrhage can lead to heterogeneity.

■ Diagnosis

Metastasis secondary to colon carcinoma.

✓ Pearls

- Metastasis is the diagnosis of exclusion when there is history of primary carcinoma.
- A hypervascular hepatic lesion within a cirrhotic liver is HCC until proven otherwise.
- Hemangiomas demonstrate progressive, peripheral, nodular enhancement.

Suggested Readings

Federle MP, Jeffrey RB, Woodward PJ, Borhani A. Diagnostic Imaging: Abdomen. 2nd ed. Philadelphia, PA: Lippincott Williams & Wilkins; 2009
Kumashiro Y, Kasahara M, Nomoto K, et al. Living donor liver transplantation for giant hepatic hemangioma with Kasabach–Merritt syndrome with a posterior segment graft. Liver Transpl. 2002; 8(8):721–724
Saenz RC. MRI of benign liver lesions and metastatic disease characterization with gadoxetate disodium. J Am Osteopath Coll Radiol. 2012; 1(4):2–9

Case 22

Rocky C. Saenz

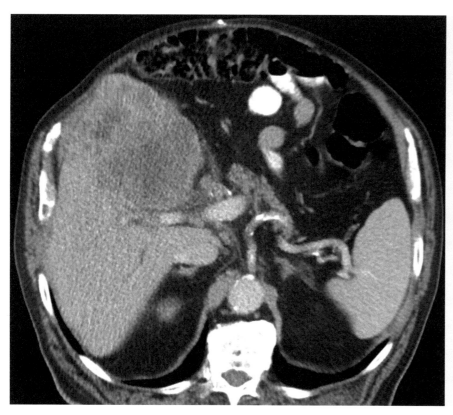

Fig. 22.1 CT axial image with intravenous and oral contrast of the upper abdomen shows a poorly defined enhancing gallbladder mass invading the liver.

■ Clinical History

A 76-year-old male with right upper quadrant pain (▶Fig. 22.1).

■ Key Finding

Gallbladder mass with liver invasion.

■ Top 3 Differential Diagnoses

- **Gallbladder adenocarcinoma:** Adenocarcinomas represents 90% of gallbladder primary malignancies. This entity can appear as a mass replacing the gallbladder with invasion of the adjacent liver. Most gallbladder carcinomas present after 65. The majority of cases have gallstones. A porcelain gallbladder may also be present. Direct invasion can also be seen with the duodenum, stomach, bile ducts, pancreas, and right kidney. Intraperitoneal spread can also be seen with omental studding, ascites, and peritoneal implants. Stage V disease is liver involvement or distant metastasis.
- **Lymphoma:** Gallbladder lymphoma is predominately non-Hodgkin's lymphoma (NHL) with secondary gallbladder involvement. On CT it can present as focal or diffuse wall thickening usually greater than 1 cm or as an intramural mass. Also, significant adenopathy is typically present.
- **Metastasis:** Metastasis presenting as a gallbladder mass is rare and accounts for 2% of gallbladder malignancies. It typically presents as a mucosal surface mass. The most common source of metastasis is melanoma. Malignant melanoma accounts for 50% of metastasis to the gallbladder. Other sources for metastasis to the gallbladder include hepatocellular carcinoma (HCC) and renal cell carcinoma (RCC).

■ Additional Diagnostic Considerations

Gastric gastrointestinal stromal tumors (GISTs): GISTs are the most common mesenchymal origin neoplasm. The majority of these lesions occur in the stomach. It expresses tyrosine kinase growth factor receptor that distinguishes it from leiomyomas, leiomyosarcoma, schwannoma, and neurofibroma. On CT it presents as a large exophytic, hypervascular mass. One may see calcifications in some cases (5–10%). Lymphadenopathy is not seen. GIST is associated with neurofibromatosis type I.

■ Diagnosis

Advanced gallbladder adenocarcinoma.

✓ Pearls

- Gallbladder mass with invasion of the liver should be considered gallbladder adenocarcinoma.
- Gastric gastrointestinal stromal tumors (GISTs) are large masses without adenopathy.
- Gallbladder metastasis is rare and should only be considered with disseminated metastatic disease.

Suggested Readings

Federle MP, Jeffrey RB, Woodward PJ, Borhani A. Diagnostic Imaging: Abdomen. 2nd ed. Philadelphia, PA: Lippincott Williams & Wilkins; 2009

Furlan A, Ferris JV, Hosseinzadeh K, Borhani AA. Gallbladder carcinoma update: multimodality imaging evaluation, staging, and treatment options. AJR Am J Roentgenol. 2008; 191(5):1440–1447

McKnight T, Patel A. Gallbladder masses: multimodality approach to differential diagnosis. J Am Osteopath Coll Radiol. 2012; 1(4):22–31

Case 23

Robert A. Jesinger

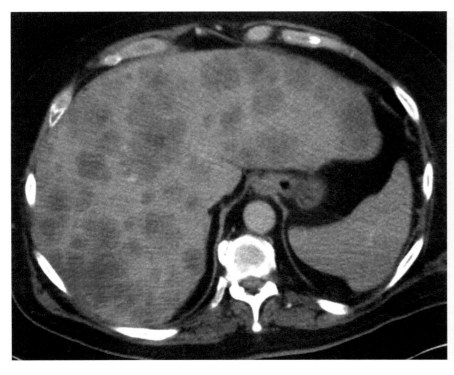

Fig. 23.1 Contrast enhanced axial CT image of the liver demonstrates multiple hypoattenuating hepatic lesions with regions of internal enhancement. (Image courtesy of Rocky C. Saenz.)

■ **Clinical History**

A 58-year-old male with weakness and weight loss (▶Fig. 23.1).

■ Key Finding

Multiple hypoattenuating hepatic lesions.

■ Top 3 Differential Diagnoses

- **Hepatic cysts:** Small isolated hepatic cysts are commonly seen on routine abdominal CT and ultrasound. Hepatic cysts are well-circumscribed, homogeneous masses of near water attenuation value (–20 to +20 HU) that show no enhancement after intravenous contrast administration. When multiple hepatic cysts are seen, polycystic kidney and/or liver disease, biliary hamartomas, and Caroli disease should be considered. Caroli disease is characterized by dilated biliary ducts surrounding an enhancing portal vein and hepatic artery, which is referred to as the central dot sign. When a large solitary liver cyst is noted, hepatic cystadenoma, biloma, and/or hydatid cyst should be considered. Usually hepatic cysts are not associated with biliary obstruction, neither is spontaneous cyst rupture common.
- **Metastatic disease:** Liver metastases rank second to lymph node metastases in cancer patients. Virtually any primary malignant neoplasm can produce liver metastases, but the most common primary tumor sites include the colon, lung, breast, stomach, and pancreas. In children, the most common primary tumors producing hypoattenuating liver metastases include neuroblastoma, Wilms tumor, and leukemia. Most metastatic lesions enhance after intravenous contrast administration, but their visual conspicuity usually results from normally enhancing adjacent liver parenchyma. Surgical resection of isolated metastatic liver lesions has been found to increase survival time in certain cancers (e.g., colon cancer).
- **Multiple hepatic abscesses:** Hepatic abscesses are relatively rare, but when encountered, typically fall into three categories: pyogenic (80%), amebic (10%), and fungal (10%). Historically, pyogenic hepatic abscesses were found in the setting of appendicitis, but currently, diverticulitis and sepsis are more common causes. Amebic abscesses are prone to rupture. Imaging findings include thick-walled, hypoattenuating liver masses with internal septations, peripheral lesion enhancement, and gas in up to 20% of cases. Untreated, liver abscesses have a high mortality rate. However, image-guided catheter drainage has improved mortality rates significantly.

■ Additional Diagnostic Considerations

Cholangiocarcinoma: A rare cancer of the bile ducts, cholangiocarcinomas typically present as multiple hypoattenuating infiltrative lesions, paralleling the bile ducts and causing biliary obstruction. Risk factors include primary sclerosing cholangitis, parasitic liver flukes (e.g., *C. sinensis*), choledochal anomalies, and prior thoratrast exposure. Delayed enhancement (beyond 10 minutes) is a key distinguishing feature. Most patients present late, when curative surgical resection is contraindicated.

■ Diagnosis

Metastatic disease (pancreatic adenocarcinoma).

✓ Pearls

- Hepatic cysts are well-circumscribed, homogeneous masses of near water attenuation.
- Multiple irregularly shaped hypoattenuating lesions in the liver are concerning for metastases.
- Delayed enhancement (beyond 10 minutes) is important in diagnosing hepatic cholangiocarcinomas.

Suggested Readings

Federle MP, Jeffrey RB, Woodward PJ, Borhani A. Diagnostic Imaging: Abdomen. 2nd ed. Philadelphia, PA: Lippincott Williams & Wilkins; 2009

Mortelé KJ, Ros PR. Cystic focal liver lesions in the adult: differential CT and MR imaging features. Radiographics. 2001; 21(4):895–910

Saenz RC. MRI of benign liver lesions and metastatic disease characterization with gadoxetate disodium. J Am Osteopath Coll Radiol. 2012; 1(4):2–9

Case 24

Sara K. Boyd

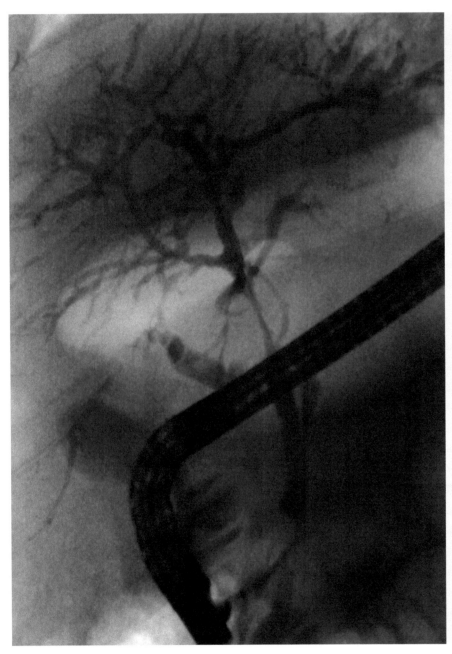

Fig. 24.1 Single endoscopic retrograde cholangiopancreatography (ERCP) image demonstrates a focal common bile duct stricture at the level of the pancreatic head. (Image courtesy of Rocky C. Saenz.)

■ **Clinical History**

A 45-year-old woman with jaundice (▶ Fig. 24.1).

■ Key Finding

Common bile duct stricture.

■ Top 3 Differential Diagnoses

- **Cholangiocarcinoma:** Cholangiocarcinoma can present as a heterogeneously enhancing mass or infiltrative hepatic lesion and the degree of peripheral duct involvement is best evaluated on cross-sectional contrasted MRI–MRCP. Lesions that demonstrate intraductal growth or periductal spread appear as nonspecific single or multifocal sites of narrowing on magnetic resonance cholangiopancreatography (MRCP). Malignant strictures have distinct characteristics compared to benign strictures, including asymmetry, length greater than 1.2 cm, greater than 3 mm of ductal wall thickening, an ill-defined margin, and intraluminal shouldering.
- **Iatrogenic:** Among several iatrogenic causes of common bile duct stricture, the most common is prior hepatobiliary surgery (cholecystectomy or orthotopic liver transplant). Postcholecystectomy biliary strictures are often at the junction of the cystic duct with the common hepatic duct and proximal common bile duct. MRCP will demonstrate a short segment smooth stricture with concurrent intrahepatic ductal dilation. Ductal strictures secondary to liver transplantation are either anastomotic or nonanastomotic. MRCP will demonstrate a short segment stricture at site of anastomosis with or without proximal ductal dilation in the former or multiple discontinuous intrahepatic long segment strictures in the latter.
- **Pancreatitis:** Chronic pancreatitis causes stricture of the intrapancreatic portion of the common bile duct in up to about half of affected patients. Fibrotic changes induced by repeated inflammation of the pancreatic parenchyma narrow the duct and appear as a smooth stricture (1.5–5.5 cm in length) of the distal common bile duct with gradual tapering on MRCP. Although less common, the duct may be abruptly narrowed. Concomitant pseudocysts may obstruct the biliary ducts. Clinical presentation varies from asymptomatic to jaundice in approximately half of patients. Most patients do not require intervention while few with persistent symptoms undergo endoscopic dilation with or without stent placement.

■ Additional Diagnostic Considerations

- **Choledocholithiasis:** Chronic choledocholithiasis induces inflammation which progresses to scar formation and stricture of the common bile duct. On MRCP, choledocholithiasis will appear as one or more low-signal filling defects with angular margins and surrounding high-signal bile. Strictures, if present, will appear as smooth symmetric short segment narrowing of the duct either superior or inferior to the calculi on MRCP. Patients are at risk of developing cholangitis and cholestasis.
- **Immunoglobulin G4-related sclerosing cholangitis:** An immune-mediated systemic disease that affects the biliary ducts, immunoglobulin G4-related Sclerosing Cholangitis has several recognized patterns of strictures. The most common abnormality is a stricture of the distal common bile duct, present in about three-fourth of patients. Diffuse intra- and extrahepatic biliary strictures in isolation or in conjunction with distal common bile duct involvement are less common.

■ Diagnosis

Common bile duct stricture secondary to pancreatitis.

✓ Pearls

- Malignant strictures will have intraluminal shouldering, asymmetry, and ductal wall thickening.
- Postcholecystectomy common bile duct strictures are smooth and short and most often involve the proximal common bile duct.
- Smooth strictures with tapering of the distal common bile duct are commonly present in chronic pancreatitis.

Suggested Readings

Katabathina VS, Dasyam AK, Dasyam N, Hosseinzadeh K. Adult bile duct strictures: role of MR imaging and MR cholangiopancreatography in characterization. Radiographics. 2014; 34(3):565–586

O'Connor OJ, O'Neill S, Maher MM. Imaging of biliary tract disease. AJR Am J Roentgenol. 2011; 197(4):W551:W558

Shanbhogue AK, Tirumani SH, Prasad SR, Fasih N, McInnes M. Benign biliary strictures: a current comprehensive clinical and imaging review. AJR Am J Roentgenol. 2011; 197(2):W295:W306

Case 25

Rocky C. Saenz

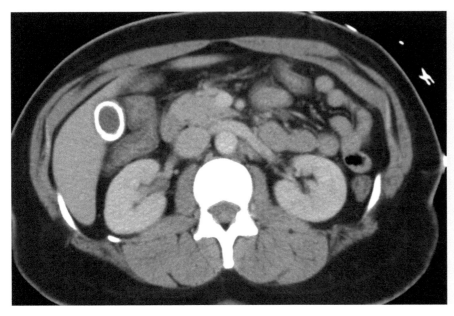

Fig. 25.1 CT axial image with intravenous contrast of the upper abdomen shows gallbladder wall calcification.

■ Clinical History

A 57-year-old male with right upper quadrant pain (▶Fig. 25.1).

■ Key Finding

Gallbladder wall calcification.

■ Top 3 Differential Diagnoses

- **Porcelain gallbladder:** When the gallbladder is calcified it is termed "porcelain." Porcelain gallbladder can be suspected on X-ray when circular right upper quadrant calcifications are seen in the expected location of the gallbladder and may need to be confirmed on CT (no contrast is needed). On CT, the gallbladder wall may involve a portion or the entire wall. Porcelain gallbladder has an association with carcinoma as gallbladder carcinoma is seen in 30% of porcelain cases. Therefore, the treatment of choice is cholecystectomy.
- **Gallbladder carcinoma:** The majority are adenocarcinomas with the second most common being squamous cell. This entity has a variable appearance and may appear as a mass replacing the gallbladder, an intraluminal polypoid mass, or wall thickening that is focal or diffuse. These appearances may be associated with wall calcification. The mean age for gallbladder carcinoma is 72.
- **Cholelithiasis:** When gallstones are enlarged they may fill the entire lumen mimicking a porcelain gallbladder. Gallstones are common seen in 10% of the US population and are more common in women. Risk factors include diabetes, medications, obesity, and ileal disease. Cholelithiasis is seen in 95% of cholecystitis cases and the majority of gallbladder carcinoma cases. The majority of gallstones are not calcified as 80% are cholesterol stones. Therefore, CT and X-ray are not reliable to exclude the diagnosis. So, ultrasound is the gold standard for gallstone evaluation.

■ Diagnosis

Porcelain gallbladder.

✓ Pearls

- Porcelain gallbladder should be treated surgically due to its association with carcinoma.
- Porcelain gallbladder if imaged on ultrasound may be confused with emphysematous cholecystitis and can be differentiated on CT.
- If only a portion of the gallbladder wall is calcified it is still considered a porcelain gallbladder.

Suggested Readings

Federle MP, Jeffrey RB, Woodward PJ, Borhani A. Diagnostic Imaging: Abdomen. 2nd ed. Philadelphia, PA: Lippincott Williams & Wilkins; 2009

Grand D, Horton KM, Fishman EK. CT of the gallbladder: spectrum of disease. AJR Am J Roentgenol. 2004; 183(1):163–170

McKnight T, Patel A. Gallbladder masses: multimodality approach to differential diagnosis. J Am Osteopath Coll Radiol. 2012; 1(4):22–31

Case 26

Rocky C. Saenz

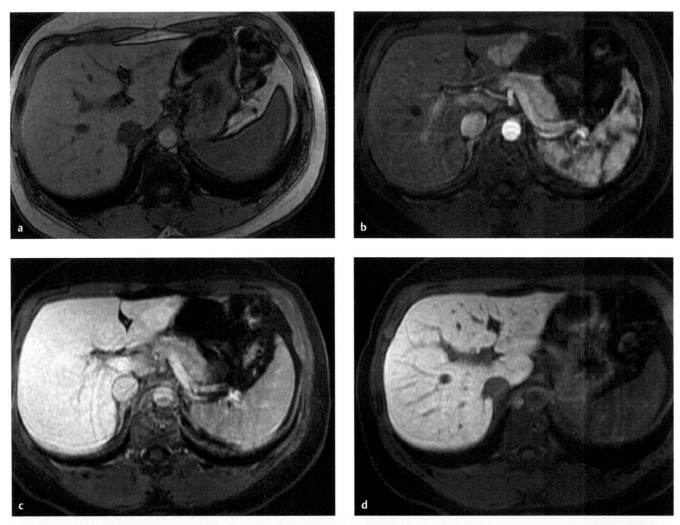

Fig. 26.1 MRI dynamic study utilizing intracellular hepatocyte imaging, noncontrast T1 out-of-phase image **(a)** shows a barely perceptible T1 low signal mass in segment II of the liver left lobe. The mass demonstrates brisk enhancement on the arterial phase **(b)** and retains contrast on the equilibrium phase appearing just brighter than the liver **(c)**. On hepatocyte phase imaging at 20 minutes **(d)**, the lesion is isointense to liver parenchyma and is not visible. (Image with permission from Rocky C. Saenz and J Am Osteopath Coll Radiol, 2012.)

■ **Clinical History**

A 39-year-old woman with non-specific abdominal pain
(►Fig. 26.1).

■ Key Finding

Liver mass isointense to liver parenchyma on hepatocyte imaging.

■ Top 3 Differential Diagnoses

- **Focal nodular hyperplasia (FNH):** FNH is the second most common benign tumor of the liver and is more common in females. The lesion is composed of hepatocytes and classically solitary with a central scar. On MRI, T1 imaging it has low signal and on T2 it has intermediate signal compared to the liver. On dynamic imaging, the arterial phase is usually hyperintense with marked enhancement. During the portal venous phase, the lesions are hyperintense to isointense. On the 20 minute delay hepatocyte/intracellular phase, FNH retains contrast appearing isointense to hyperintense.
- **Hepatocellular carcinoma (HCC):** HCC is the most common primary hepatic malignancy. Patients may present with a single lesion, multiple lesions, or diffuse involvement. On MRI, T1 imaging it is low signal and on T2 it is hyperintense signal compared to the liver. On dynamic imaging, the arterial phase imaging classically demonstrates hyperintense enhancement. The portal venous phase shows the lesion washing out with a hypointense appearance. On the 20 minute delay hepatocyte/ intracellular phase, the lesion typically does not enhance unless the HCC is well circumscribed. Since these well circumscribed HCCs may have remaining functioning hepatocytes which can enhance on the intracellular images but are usually heterogeneous.
- **Hepatic adenoma:** Hepatic adenomas are benign lesions predominantly seen in women of reproductive age. These lesions are composed of hepatocytes arranged in cords separated by dilated sinusoids but do not contain bile ducts unlike FNH. On MRI, T1 imaging it is hypointense and on T2 it is hyperintense signal compared to the liver. The minority of hepatic adenoma on T1 images show hyperintensity due to macroscopic fat. On dynamic imaging, hepatic adenoma enhancement pattern is variable, but typically on arterial phase imaging hyperintense enhancement is seen. The portal venous phase the lesions is hyperintense to isointense. On the 20 minute delay hepatocyte/intracellular phase, hepatic adenomas are hypointense.

■ Additional Diagnostic Considerations

Metastases: Metastasis is the most common tumor and malignancy of the liver. Metastasis is more than 10 times more common than primary liver malignancies. Metastatic disease to the liver is indicative of late stage cancer. Imaging findings depend upon the primary tumor type, but lesions are often poorly circumscribed with variable enhancement on dynamic studies. Since metastasis have primarily an arterial blood supply, the majority enhance on the arterial phase with washout on delayed phase. On the 20 minute delay hepatocyte/intracellular phase, metastasis does not enhance and are hypointense.

■ Diagnosis

FNH.

✓ Pearls

- Classically FNH will be isointense to liver on hepatocyte delayed imaging (gadoxetate disodium).
- Remember all lesions with hepatocytes enhance on hepatocyte imaging. Therefore, a well differentiated HCC can enhance on the delayed hepatocyte phase.
- Hepatic adenomas may have high T1 signal.

Suggested Readings

Kamel IR, Lawler LP, Fishman EK. Comprehensive analysis of hypervascular liver lesions using 16-MDCT and advanced image processing. AJR Am J Roentgenol. 2004; 183(2):443–452

Saenz RC. MRI of benign liver lesions and metastatic disease characterization with gadoxetate disodium. J Am Osteopath Coll Radiol. 2012; 1(4):2–9

Case 27

Rocky C. Saenz

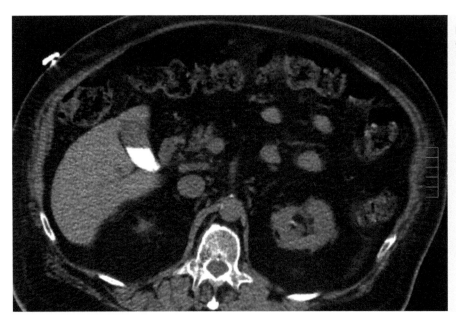

Fig. 27.1 CT image of the abdomen without contrast demonstrates the gallbladder with a high-density fluid–fluid level.

■ **Clinical History**

A 57-year-old male with right upper quadrant pain (▶ Fig. 27.1).

■ Key Finding

Gallbladder high-density fluid–fluid level.

■ Top 3 Differential Diagnoses

- **Milk of calcium:** When the gallbladder has high-density layering dependently it is termed "milk of calcium." The high density is calcium carbonate precipitate. On CT, the high attenuation usually has Hounsfield measurements greater than 150. This is typically an incidental finding.
- **Vicarious excretion:** When the gallbladder fills with contrast due to excretion of parenterally injected contrast medium by organs other than kidneys. Vicarious excretion is inversely related to Glomerular Filtration Rate and may be indicative of diminished renal function. Accumulation of contrast into the gallbladder can be seen in normal patients.
- **Biliary sludge:** Sludge is indicative of highly viscous bile with high bilirubin content. It is typically the result of biliary stasis from prolonged fasting or hyperalimentation. Most biliary sludge presents as a layering in the dependent gallbladder.

■ Additional Diagnostic Considerations

- **Hemobilia:** Hemobilia is uncommon but may be seen with significant gallbladder injury. Gallbladder injury arises from compressive and shearing forces seen typically after motor vehicle accidents. On CT, hemorrhage presents as intraluminal dependent high-density fluid. Delayed imaging is helpful to solidify the diagnosis as it will show increasing amount of dependent high density.
- **Cholelithiasis:** When gallstones are multiple and small in size they may layer dependently in the lumen and may mimic milk of calcium. Cholelithiasis is seen in 95% of cholecystitis cases. The majority of gallstones are not calcified as 80% are cholesterol stones. Therefore, CT and X-ray are not reliable to exclude gallstones. So, ultrasound is the gold standard for gallstone evaluation. On ultrasound, choleliths are hyperechoic with posterior acoustic shadowing.

■ Diagnosis

Milk of calcium.

✓ Pearls

- Ultrasound is the most accurate for cholelithiasis and cholecystitis.
- Vicarious excretion may be a normal finding.
- When considering hemobilia on CT remember to get delayed imaging.

Suggested Readings

Federle MP, Jeffrey RB, Woodward PJ, Borhani A. Diagnostic Imaging: Abdomen. 2nd ed. Philadelphia, PA: Lippincott Williams & Wilkins; 2009

McKnight T, Patel A. Gallbladder masses: multimodality approach to differential diagnosis. J Am Osteopath Coll Radiol. 2012; 1(4):22–31

Wittenberg A, Minotti AJ. CT diagnosis of traumatic gallbladder injury. AJR Am J Roentgenol. 2005; 185(6):1573–1574

Case 28

Rocky C. Saenz

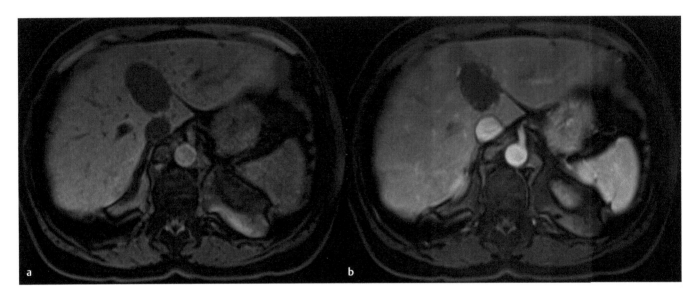

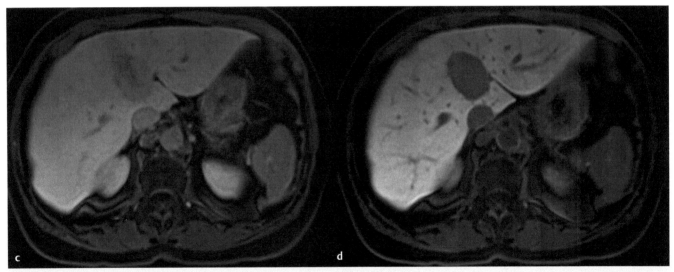

Fig. 28.1 MRI dynamic study utilizing intracellular hepatocyte imaging, precontrast T1 fat saturation image **(a)** demonstrates a T1 low signal mass bordering segments IVa and I. The mass demonstrates progressive, peripheral, nodular enhancement on arterial phase imaging **(b)** and equilibrium phase imaging **(c)**. On hepatocyte delayed imaging at 20 minutes **(d)**, the lesion is hypointense to liver parenchyma and is similar signal to the inferior vena cava (IVC).

■ Clinical History

A 43-year-old female with non-specific abdominal pain (▶Fig. 28.1).

■ Key Finding

Liver mass hypointense to liver parenchyma on hepatocyte imaging.

■ Top 3 Differential Diagnoses

- **Hemangioma:** Hemangiomas are the most common benign hepatic lesion. Hemangiomas do not have hepatocytes but are endothelial lined vascular channels with fibrous septa. On MRI, hemangiomas are hypointense on T1 imaging and hyperintense on T2 (light bulb sign differentiating it from focal nodular hyperplasia (FNH) and hepatic adenoma). On dynamic imaging, the arterial phase usually shows, peripheral, nodular enhancement. During the portal venous phase, the lesions have progressive, peripheral enhancement which fills the lesion. On the 20 minute delay hepatocyte/intracellular phase, the lesion is hypointense to liver parenchyma and is similar signal to the inferior vena cava (IVC) (blood pool).
- **Hepatocellular carcinoma (HCC):** HCC is the most common primary hepatic malignancy. Patients may present with a single lesion, multiple lesions, or diffuse involvement. On MRI, T1 imaging it is low signal and high signal on T2. On dynamic imaging, the arterial phase imaging classically demonstrates hyperintense enhancement. The portal venous phase shows the lesions washing out with a hypointense appearance. On the 20 minute delay hepatocyte/intracellular phase, the lesions typically do not enhance unless the HCC is well circumscribed. Since these well circumscribed HCCs may have remaining functioning hepatocytes which can enhance on the intracellular images but are usually heterogeneous.
- **Metastases:** Metastasis is the most common tumor and malignancy of the liver. Metastasis is more than 10 times more common than primary liver malignancies. Imaging findings is most dependent on the primary tumor type, but lesions are often poorly circumscribed, multiple, and have variable enhancement on dynamic studies. Metastatic disease has variable signal on T1 and T2 but is usually heterogeneous or high signal. Since metastasis have primarily an arterial blood supply, the majority enhance on the arterial phase with washout on delayed phase. On the 20 minute delay hepatocyte/intracellular phase, metastasis does not enhance and are hypointense.

■ Additional Diagnostic Considerations

Hepatic adenoma: Hepatic adenomas are benign lesions predominantly seen in women of reproductive age. These lesions are composed of hepatocytes arranged in cords separated by dilated sinusoids but do not contain bile ducts unlike FNH. On MRI, T1 imaging it is hypointense and on T2 it is hyperintense signal compared to the liver. The minority of hepatic adenoma on T1 images show hyperintensity due to macroscopic fat. On dynamic imaging hepatic adenoma enhancement pattern is variable, but typically on arterial phase imaging hyperintense enhancement is seen. The portal venous phase the lesions is hyperintense to isointense. On the 20 minute delay hepatocyte/intracellular phase, hepatic adenomas are hypointense.

■ Diagnosis

Hemangioma.

✓ Pearls

- Hemangiomas demonstrate progressive, peripheral, nodular, enhancement on dynamic imaging.
- Hemangiomas are homogeneous "light bulb" bright on T2.
- Lesions without hepatocytes are hypointense on hepatocyte/intracellular phase imaging.

Suggested Readings

Federle MP, Jeffrey RB, Woodward PJ, Borhani A. Diagnostic Imaging: Abdomen. 2nd ed. Philadelphia, PA: Lippincott Williams & Wilkins; 2009

Kamel IR, Lawler LP, Fishman EK. Comprehensive analysis of hypervascular liver lesions using 16-MDCT and advanced image processing. AJR Am J Roentgenol. 2004; 183(2):443–452

Saenz RC. MRI of benign liver lesions and metastatic disease characterization with gadoxetate disodium. J Am Osteopath Coll Radiol. 2012; 1(4):2–9

Case 29

Rocky C. Saenz

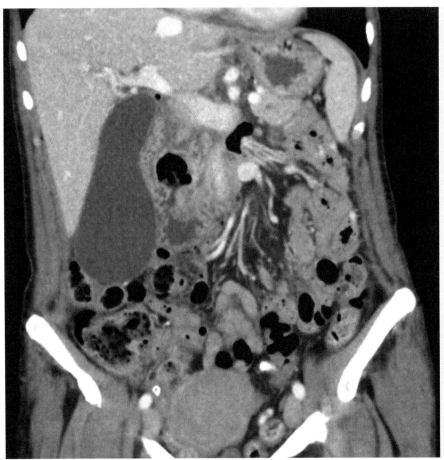

Fig. 29.1 CT coronal image with intravenous contrast demonstrates a markedly dilated gallbladder.

■ Clinical History

A 41-year-old female with right upper quadrant pain (▶Fig. 29.1).

■ Key Finding

Dilated gallbladder.

■ Top 3 Differential Diagnoses

- **Hydropic gallbladder:** Hydropic refers to a gallbladder that is dilated. It is typically larger than 10 cm in longitudinal dimension and 4 cm in transverse dimension. Most commonly this is a chronic obstructive process. The gallbladder usually is filled with nonpigmented mucin.
- **Acute cholecystitis:** Most frequent inflammatory condition of the gallbladder which is most commonly caused by gallbladder neck obstruction. Cholecystitis is suspected on CT when a thick-walled gallbladder and fat stranding are seen. Classically the gallbladder is dilated greater than 4 cm. CT is not as accurate as ultrasound for the diagnosis. The presence of cholelithiasis and a positive sonographic Murphy sign has high specificity for acute cholecystitis.
- **Chronic cholecystitis:** It is almost always caused by gallbladder stones that create transient obstruction which leads to prolonged inflammation and fibrosis. This fibrosis may lead to a contracted gallbladder, and is almost always seen with cholelithiasis. Imaging findings include gallstones in thick-walled gallbladder with no pericholecystic fluid and lack of wall hyperemia.

■ Additional Diagnostic Considerations

Gallbladder carcinoma: More than 90% are adenocarcinomas with a 5-year survival rate of less than 5%. This entity can appear as a mass replacing the gallbladder, an intraluminal polypoid mass, or wall thickening that is focal or diffuse. Gallbladder wall thickening greater than 10 mm is suspicious for malignancy. The majority of cases have gallstones.

■ Diagnosis

Hydropic gallbladder secondary to choledocholithiasis.

✓ Pearls

- When the gallbladder is dilated beyond 10 cm it is abnormal.
- Gallbladder hydrops is commonly due to chronic obstruction.
- The most common gallbladder carcinoma is adenocarcinoma.

Suggested Readings

Federle MP, Jeffrey RB, Woodward PJ, Borhani A. Diagnostic Imaging: Abdomen. 2nd ed. Philadelphia, PA: Lippincott Williams & Wilkins; 2009

Runner GJ, Corwin MT, Siewert B, Eisenberg RL. Gallbladder wall thickening. AJR Am J Roentgenol. 2014; 202(1):W1–W12

Queiroz AB, de Miranda JS. Images in clinical medicine. Hydropic gallbladder. N Engl J Med. 2011; 364(20):e43

Case 30

Rocky C. Saenz

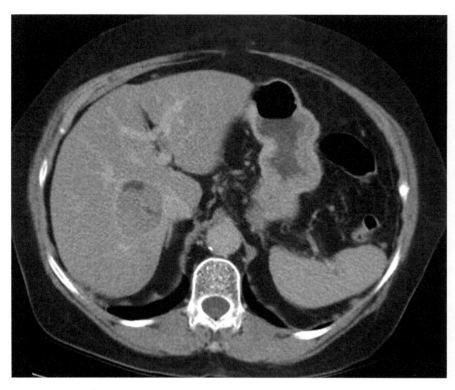

Fig. 30.1 CT with intravenous contrast from a dynamic study, delayed phase demonstrates an encapsulated, heterogeneous lesion in the right lobe of the liver.

■ Clinical History

A 41-year-old female without complaints (▶ Fig. 30.1).

■ Key Finding

Liver lesion with a capsule.

■ Top 3 Differential Diagnoses

- **Hepatocellular carcinoma (HCC):** HCC is the most common primary hepatic malignancy. The key imaging features include its characteristic enhancement pattern (early arterial phase enhancement with washout on delayed imaging) and a tumor capsule. The capsule is best seen on the portal venous and delayed images. A pseudocapsule, which mimics a true capsule, is usually only seen on the arterial phase and not on the later phases of a dynamic study. MRI has a high accuracy of identifying an HCC capsule. The capsule appearance is due to fibrous tissue and prominent sinusoids which derives its blood supply primarily from the portal venous system.
- **Metastases:** Metastasis is the most common lesion of the liver. Although the lesions do not have a true capsule, occasionally they can have a peripheral enhancement. Hepatic metastases on dynamic cross-sectional imaging commonly show enhancement on the early arterial phase. Imaging findings depend on the primary tumor type, but lesions are often poorly circumscribed with variable enhancement and typically multiple.
- **Hepatic adenoma:** Hepatic adenomas are benign lesions predominantly seen in women (90%). These lesions are usually seen in women on birth control, athletes on anabolic steroids, and patients with metabolic diseases. Hepatic adenomas have an increased risk of rupture when larger than 5 cm. At least four subtypes have been identified with the inflammatory subtype being most common and typically arise in steatotic livers. Intravoxel fat has been seen in 11 to 20% of the inflammatory subtype. Lesions usually are well-circumscribed with variable enhancement but can be heterogeneous due to prior internal hemorrhage.

■ Additional Diagnostic Considerations

Hepatic abscesses: Hepatic abscesses are uncommon and can be categorized into pyogenic (80%), amebic (10%), and fungal (10%). Pyogenic hepatic abscesses the most common are found in the setting of diverticulitis and sepsis. Amebic abscesses are prone to rupture. Imaging findings include thick-walled, hypoatten-uating liver masses with internal septations, peripheral lesion enhancement, and gas in up to 20% of cases. Pyogenic abscesses are commonly multilocular. Untreated, liver abscesses have a high mortality rate.

■ Diagnosis

Hepatic adenoma.

✓ Pearls

- A hepatic lesion with a capsule in a patient at risk for HCC should be considered HCC.
- Remember pseudocapsule enhancement is only seen during the arterial phase.
- Consider hepatic adenoma with an encapsulated hepatic lesion in a young female on contraceptive pills.

Suggested Readings

Coast, et al. Fat-containing liver lesions on imaging: detection and differential diagnosis. Am J Roentgen. 2018; 210:1–10

Saenz RC. MRI of benign liver lesions and metastatic disease characterization with gadoxetate disodium. J Am Osteopath Coll Radiol. 2012; 1(4):2–9

Tang A, Bashir MR, Corwin MT, et al. LI-RADS Evidence Working Group. Evidence supporting LI-RADS major features for CT- and MR imaging-based diagnosis of hepatocellular carcinoma: a systematic review. Radiology. 2018; 286(1):29–48

Case 31

Rocky C. Saenz

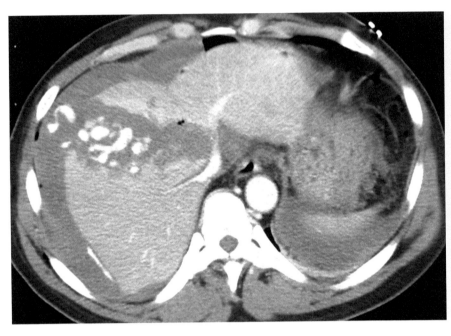

Fig. 31.1 CT with intravenous contrast of the abdomen shows the liver with a low attenuation band which has multiple foci of increased attenuation traversing it. Along the right lobe is free fluid with foci increased linear density representing hemoperitoneum. Punctate foci of free air are also seen.

■ Clinical History

A 36-year-old male with pain after motor vehicle accident (▶ Fig. 31.1).

■ Key Finding

Linear band of low attenuation.

■ Top 3 Differential Diagnoses

- **Laceration:** On CT, a laceration is usually a linear low attenuation on postcontrast images. Advanced lacerations can be large and may appear geographic in shape and are associated with hemoperitoneum. Imaging needs to be done in dual phase manner with delayed imaging in order to exclude vascular extravasation. On delayed images, extravasation is seen as foci of high density. Grading of injuries is done utilizing (American Association for Surgical Trauma) scale. The AAST grades are from I to VI with VI being the most severe. Treatment for patients with vascular extravasation who are unstable needs surgical intervention.
- **Metastases:** Metastasis is the most common lesion of the liver. The most common appearance of hepatic metastases on CT is a low-density lesion with respect to the liver parenchyma.

Metastasis is known to be unpredictable with regards to their appearance and can mimic a laceration. Metastasis is typically multiple and are much more common than primary liver malignancies.
- **Hepatic infarction:** Hepatic infarcts are not common due to the dual blood supply of the liver. Etiologies include post-surgical ligation, vasculitis, blunt trauma, hypercoagulable states and rarely infection. Hepatic artery occlusion is more common than portal vein thrombosis. The most reliable findings are wedge-shaped nonenhancement on all phases of a dynamic study. Angiography may be necessary to confirm hepatic artery occlusion. Treatment includes revascularization and transplantation.

■ Diagnosis

Liver laceration, grade V with extravasation.

✓ Pearls

- The key to diagnosis is linear, band like attenuation with a history of trauma.

- Low-grade liver injuries are usually treated conservatively.
- Always do delayed imaging with trauma.

Suggested Readings

Coast, et al. Fat-Containing Liver Lesions on Imaging: Detection and Differential Diagnosis. Am J Roentgen. 2018; 210:1–10

Federle MP, Jeffrey RB, Woodward PJ, Borhani A. Diagnostic Imaging: Abdomen. 2nd ed. Philadelphia, PA: Lippincott Williams & Wilkins; 2009

Saenz RC. MRI of benign liver lesions and metastatic disease characterization with gadoxetate disodium. J Am Osteopath Coll Radiol. 2012; 1(4):2–9

Case 32

Rocky C. Saenz

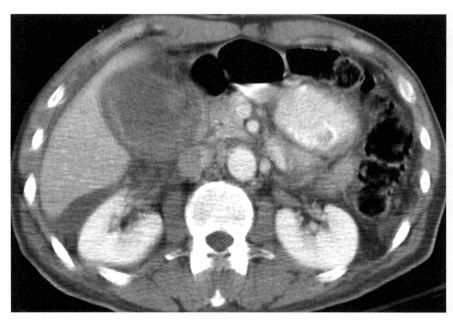

Fig. 32.1 CT image of the abdomen with IV and oral contrast demonstrates gallbladder wall thickening with areas which are ill-defined and nonenhancing.

■ Clinical History

A 44-year-old female with generalized abdominal pain (▶Fig. 32.1).

■ Key Finding

Gallbladder wall thickening with areas of nonenhancement.

■ Top 3 Differential Diagnoses

- **Gangrenous cholecystitis:** The most common complication of acute cholecystitis affecting a minority of patients. It is thought to occur secondary to increased distention with subsequent ischemia and necrosis of the gallbladder wall. These patients are typically more ill than patients with uncomplicated acute cholecystitis. CT signs include gallbladder wall or lumen gas, focal irregularity or defect in the gallbladder wall, intraluminal membranes, absence of wall enhancement, and pericholecystic abscess. Of these findings, the most accurate is noting irregularities in the wall of non-enhancement and or air.
- **Emphysematous cholecystitis:** Emphysematous cholecystitis is a rare form of acute cholecystitis complicated by secondary infection from a gas-forming organism. The most common organisms include *E. coli* and *Clostridium* species. On CT this is manifested by intramural air or intraluminal air. If both intramural and intraluminal air are present, it usually represents advanced disease. Emphysematous cholecystitis is considered a surgical emergency. If perforation occurs, then pneumoperitoneum may be seen. Septic shock and peritonitis are seen with perforation. Emphysematous cholecystitis most commonly occurs in elderly men or diabetic patients.
- **Gallbladder adenocarcinoma:** Adenocarcinoma is the most common gallbladder primary malignancy. This entity can appear as a diffuse mass replacing the gallbladder or as a focal lesion replacing or invading the gallbladder wall. The majority of cases have gallstones. Direct invasion can also be seen with the liver, duodenum, stomach, bile ducts, pancreas, and right kidney. Stage V disease is liver involvement or distant metastasis.

■ Additional Diagnostic Considerations

Cholecystitis: Cholecystitis is the most frequent inflammatory condition of the gallbladder. Acute cholecystitis is suspected on CT when a thick-walled gallbladder and fat stranding are noted but should be confirmed on ultrasound. Chronic cholecystitis is caused by gallbladder stones that create transient obstruction which leads to prolonged inflammation and biliary dyskinesia. Uncomplicated acute and chronic cholelithiasis should demonstrate good delineation of the gallbladder wall.

■ Diagnosis

Gangrenous cholecystitis.

✓ Pearls

- Gangrenous cholecystitis will have loss of wall enhancement.
- CT is the best modality for identifying intramural or intraluminal gas.
- In acute and chronic cholelithiasis, the gallbladder wall should be well delineated.

Suggested Readings

Federle MP, Jeffrey RB, Woodward PJ, Borhani A. Diagnostic Imaging: Abdomen. 2nd ed. Philadelphia, PA: Lippincott Williams & Wilkins; 2009

Grayson DE, Abbott RM, Levy AD, Sherman PM. Emphysematous infections of the abdomen and pelvis: a pictorial review. Radiographics. 2002; 22(3):543–561

Smith EA, Dillman JR, Elsayes KM, Menias CO, Bude RO. Cross-sectional imaging of acute and chronic gallbladder inflammatory disease. AJR Am J Roentgenol. 2009; 192(1):188–196

Case 33

Rocky C. Saenz

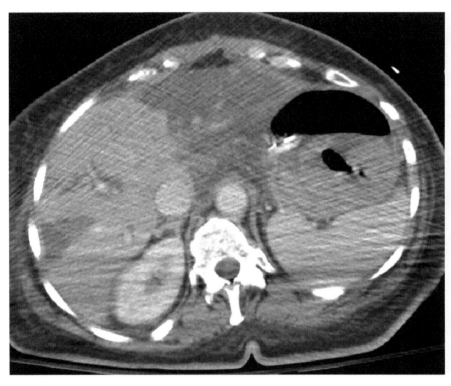

Fig. 33.1 CT axial image with intravenous contrast through the liver parenchyma shows a wedge-shaped area of low attenuation in the right lobe and low attenuation involving the left lobe.

■ Clinical History

A 49-year-old female with sharp upper quadrant pain after cholecystectomy last night (▶ Fig. 33.1).

■ **Key Finding**

Wedge shaped liver lesion.

■ **Top 3 Differential Diagnoses**

• **Laceration:** The most common cause of hepatic injury is blunt trauma. Most commonly the right lobe is injured. On CT, a laceration is usually a linear and of low attenuation on postcontrast images. Commonly complex ascites is noted indicative of hemoperitoneum. Imaging needs to be done in dual phase manner with delayed imaging in order to exclude vascular extravasation. Grading of injuries is done utilizing AAST (American Association for Surgical Trauma) scale. Treatment for patients with vascular extravasation includes angiointerventional embolization.

• **Steatosis:** Hepatic steatosis also known as fatty liver is due to the accumulation of triglycerides in the hepatocytes. Steatosis has many appearances including: diffuse, diffuse with sparring, focal, multifocal, and geographic. The diffuse form is the most common. A key imaging feature is noting normal vessels coursing through the lesion. On ultrasound, the involved liver will have a hyperechoic appearance compared to the remaining liver.

• **Infarction:** Hepatic infarcts are not common due to the dual blood supply of the liver. Etiologies include postsurgical ligation, vasculitis, blunt trauma, hypercoagulable states, and rarely infection. Hepatic artery occlusion is more common than portal vein thrombosis. The most reliable findings are wedge-shaped nonenhancement on all phases of a dynamic study. Angiography may be necessary to confirm hepatic artery occlusion. Treatment includes revascularization and transplantation.

■ **Additional Diagnostic Considerations**

• **Hepatic lymphoma:** Hepatic lymphoma may be primary or secondary. Secondary hepatic lymphoma is seen in greater than 50% of all lymphoma patients. Most often they are lobulated and are multiple. Non-Hodgkin's lymphoma (NHL) is more common to have hepatic involvement than Hodgkin.

• **Metastases:** Metastasis is the most common liver malignancy. The most common primary tumors include lung, breast, colon, melanoma and pancreas. These lesions are most easily detected on arterial phase imaging because malignancies primary blood supply is arterial. Utilizing gadoxetate disodium hepatocyte phase, metastatic lesions will not enhance because they do not have hepatocytes.

■ **Diagnosis**

Liver infarction, postsurgical ligation.

✓ **Pearls**

• Wedge-shaped nonenhancement should be considered infarction.
• Typically AAST grades I to III liver injuries are treated conservatively.

• Metastasis is always a consideration when there is a primary cancer but should enhance.

Suggested Readings

Federle MP, Jeffrey RB, Woodward PJ, Borhani A. Diagnostic Imaging: Abdomen. 2nd ed. Philadelphia, PA: Lippincott Williams & Wilkins; 2009

Saenz RC. MRI of benign liver lesions and metastatic disease characterization with gadoxetate disodium. J Am Osteopath Coll Radiol. 2012; 1(4):2–9

Yoon W, Jeong YY, Kim JK, et al. CT in blunt liver trauma. Radiographics. 2005; 25(1):87–104

Case 34

Timothy McKnight

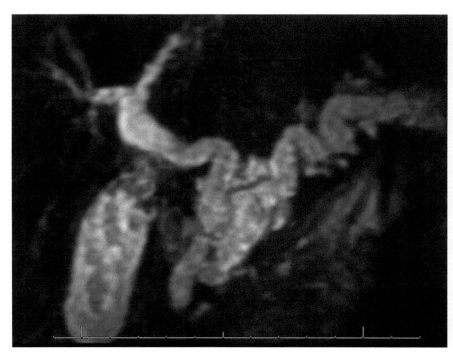

Fig. 34.1 T2-weighted coronal maximum intensity projection through the extrahepatic ducts. Significant dilation is seen of the common hepatic and common bile duct. In addition, the main pancreatic duct and its side branches are also markedly dilated. (Image courtesy of Rocky C. Saenz.)

■ Clinical History

A 70-year-old female with recurrent abdominal pain (▶ Fig. 34.1).

■ Key Finding

Dilated common bile and pancreatic ducts, the "double duct" sign.

■ Top 3 Differential Diagnoses

- **Ductal adenocarcinoma:** An obstructing pancreatic head mass may occlude the extrahepatic ductal system with dilation of both the common bile duct and pancreatic duct (double duct sign). Most of these tumors are mucinous adenocarcinomas. Primary tumor location is most common in the head (60%), followed by the body (second most common, 15%) and then the tail (least common, 5%). Diffuse tumor involvement is seen in 20%.
- **Acute pancreatitis:** Interstitial edematous pancreatitis represents majority of pancreatitis. The most common causes include alcoholism and gallstones. Typical imaging features are pancreatic focal or diffuse enlargement and peripancreatic fat stranding. Acute peripancreatic nonencapsulated fluid collections (APFC) are common and may develop into pseudo-

cysts. If areas of parenchymal nonenhancement are seen, then necrosis is present (acutely termed acute necrotic collections; chronically termed walled of necrosis).
- **Choledocholithiasis:** Obstructing biliary stones may present with a double duct sign when the stone is at or near the ampulla. Approximately 10% of cholelithiasis patients have choledocholithiasis. Endoscopic retrograde cholangiopancreatography (ERCP) is the gold standard for duct imaging, but it is usually reserved for therapy as it is invasive. Therefore, magnetic resonance cholangiopancreatography (MRCP) is utilized when choledocholithiasis is not seen on ultrasound. On ultrasound, the stones will appear hyperechoic with posterior acoustic shadowing.

■ Additional Diagnostic Considerations

- **Chronic pancreatitis:** Multiple bouts of pancreatitis over time can lead to chronic extrahepatic ductal dilation. Other classic findings of chronic pancreatitis include parenchymal and intraductal calcifications (54%) and parenchymal atrophy (50%). Patients usually have a history of chronic alcoholism (70% of cases), obstructing biliary stones, chronic smoking, or cystic fibrosis.

- **Metastasis:** Metastatic disease involving the pancreas is uncommon and typically seen in cases of disseminated metastases. Most common primaries include renal cell, lung, breast, colon, and melanoma. The most common presentation is a solitary lesion (70% of cases).

■ Diagnosis

Choledocholithiasis.

✓ Pearls

- Careful assessment for a pancreatic head mass for adenocarcinoma should be done with any ductal abnormality.
- Areas of absent pancreatic parenchymal enhancement indicate necrosis.

- Acute pancreatitis often has associated fluid collections and history of alcoholism or obstructing stone.

Suggested Readings

Borghei P, Sokhandon F, Shirkhoda A, Morgan DE. Anomalies, anatomic variants, and sources of diagnostic pitfalls in pancreatic imaging. Radiology. 2013; 266(1):28–36

Tirkes T, Sandrasegaran K, Sanyal R, et al. Secretin-enhanced MR cholangiopancreatography: spectrum of findings. Radiographics. 2013; 33(7):1889–1906

Zhao K, Adam SZ, Keswani RN, Horowitz JM, Miller FH. Acute pancreatitis: revised Atlanta classification and the role of cross-sectional imaging. AJR Am J Roentgenol. 2015; 205(1):W32–41

Case 35

Rocky C. Saenz

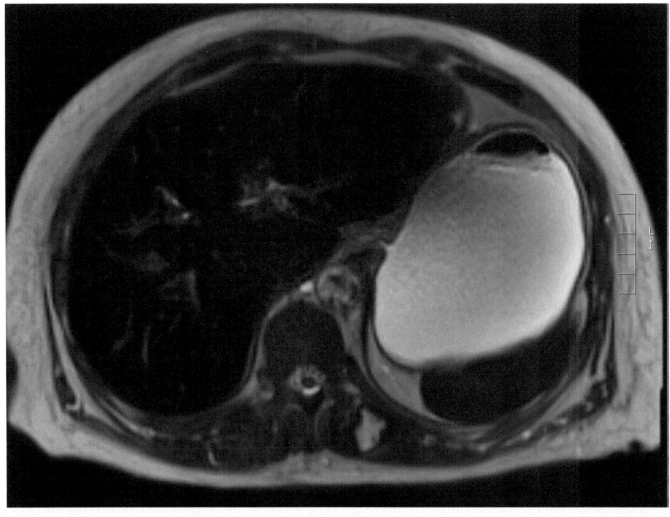

Fig. 35.1 MRI T2 axial image of the liver demonstrates diffuse low signal of the liver and spleen. In addition, a 1.5 cm left paraspinal hematoma is seen.

■ Clinical History

A 65-year-old man with sickle cell anemia (▶ Fig. 35.1).

■ Key Finding

Diffuse low T2 signal of liver.

■ Diagnosis

Hemochromatosis: Hemochromatosis may be either primary or secondary. Primary is less common than secondary and is autosomal recessive. Primary hemochromatosis results from increased iron absorption by small bowel with resulting deposition within the parenchymal cells of the liver, pancreas, and heart. Primary iron overload is most often associated with hereditary hemochromatosis. Classic MRI features in primary hemochromatosis are diffuse parenchymal low T2 signal intensity of the liver, pancreas, and cardiac myocardial. T2 gradient recalled echo images are more sensitive to magnetic susceptibility effects of the iron deposition. The iron deposition in the liver parenchyma causes a paramagnetic effect resulting in hypointense appearance on T2-weighted images.

Secondary hemochromatosis initially involves iron deposition of the reticuloendothelial system (liver and spleen) and later may affect pancreas, myocardium, endocrine glands, and kidneys. Etiologies include: increased iron oral intake, multiple blood transfusions (typically associated with dialysis or chronic anemia), alcoholic cirrhosis, portacaval shunts, or ineffective erythropoiesis (thalassemia, sideroblastic anemia). Secondary iron overload is most commonly associated with multiple red blood cell transfusions. The classic MRI features include dark/low hepatic parenchymal signal intensity on T2-weighted imaging sequences due to the superparamagnetic effect of iron. In addition, decreased T2 signal intensity in the spleen is characteristic of secondary hemochromatosis (as in this case). Noninvasive quantification of iron overload with MR imaging is considered the standard of care in diagnosis and monitoring.

✓ Pearls

- Hemochromatosis has an increased risk of hepatocellular carcinoma (HCC) so monitor for it.
- Primary hemochromatosis affects pancreas, while secondary hemochromatosis affects spleen.
- Secondary hemochromatosis is more common.

Suggested Readings

Labranche R, Gilbert G, Cerny M, et al. Liver iron quantification with MR imaging: a primer for radiologists. Radiographics. 2018; 38(2):392–412

Lim RP, Tuvia K, Hajdu CH, et al. Quantification of hepatic iron deposition in patients with liver disease: comparison of chemical shift imaging with single-echo T2*-weighted imaging. AJR Am J Roentgenol. 2010; 194(5):1288–1295

Tani I, Kurihara Y, Kawaguchi A, et al. MR imaging of diffuse liver disease. AJR Am J Roentgenol. 2000; 174(4):965–971

Case 36

Rocky C. Saenz

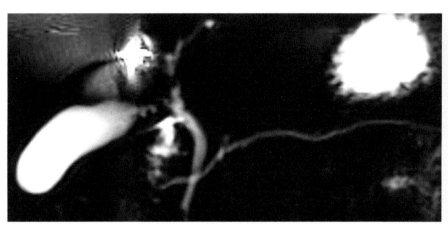

Fig. 36.1 MRCP T2-weighted maximum intensity projection image shows an abnormal course of the pancreatic duct crossing over the common bile duct. The pancreatic duct also has a couple of dilated side branches along the pancreatic body.

■ **Clinical History**

A 24-year-old male with occasional right upper quadrant pain (▶Fig. 36.1).

■ Key Finding

Pancreatic duct crossing over the common bile duct.

■ Top 3 Differential Diagnoses

• **Pancreatic divisum:** Pancreatic divisum is an anatomical variant which is seen in 4 to 10% of the population. It occurs when the ventral and dorsal duct moieties do not fuse. The dorsal duct (duct of Santorini) will be seen draining into the minor papilla and does not communicate to the ventral duct (duct of Wirsung). Magnetic resonance cholangiopancreatography (MRCP) has high accuracy to diagnosis pancreatic divisum. The key to the diagnosis is noting the ducts (pancreatic dorsal and common bile duct) crossing each other which is known as the "duct crossing or crossover" sign. Pancreatic divisum can also have associated ductal dilation. The majority of these patients are asymptomatic, but they can have intermittent pain secondary to idiopathic recurrent pancreatitis. Also, the dorsal duct near them minor papilla can become dilated which is termed "santorinicele." Treatment is usually conservative but surgical minor papillectomy and stenting may also be needed.

• **Annular pancreas:** Congenital rare anomaly with pancreatic parenchyma wrapping around the duodenum. Main pancreatic duct extends around to right side of duodenum. There are two distinct types of annular pancreas. The extramural type having dorsal and ventral ducts joining on right side of duodenum before common drainage pathway into duodenum, presents as bowel obstruction from the encircling pancreas narrowing the duodenum. The intramural type has the pancreatic tissue intermingled in duodenal muscle fibers with multiple distal small ducts from the dorsal and ventral systems draining directly into the duodenum, and usually presents with symptoms of duodenal ulceration. Treatment for both types of annular pancreas is surgical.

• **Ansa pancreatica:** This is a rare ductal variant with absence of the distal portion of the dorsal duct (the main duct of Santorini) with the proximal dorsal duct (the minor duct of Santorini) connecting to the ventral duct. This communication is via a "loop-shaped" collateral to small inferior side branch of ventral duct. This variant can also be associated with idiopathic pancreatitis.

■ Diagnosis

Pancreatic divisum.

✓ Pearls

• Duct "crossover" sign is pathognomic for pancreatic divisum.
• Pancreatic divisum can result in recurrent pancreatitis.
• Pancreas and duct encircle the duodenum is pathognomic of annular pancreas.

Suggested Readings

Borghei P, Sokhandon F, Shirkhoda A, Morgan DE. Anomalies, anatomic variants, and sources of diagnostic pitfalls in pancreatic imaging. Radiology. 2013; 266(1):28–36

Leyendecker JR, Elsayes KM, Gratz BI, Brown JJ. MR cholangiopancreatography: spectrum of pancreatic duct abnormalities. AJR Am J Roentgenol. 2002; 179(6):1465–1471

Soto JA, Lucey BC, Stuhlfaut JW. Pancreas divisum: depiction with multi-detector row CT. Radiology. 2005; 235(2):503–508

Case 37

Rocky C. Saenz

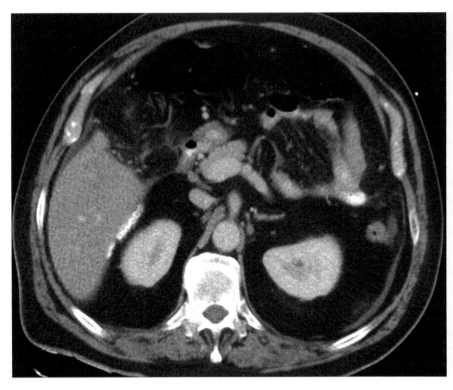

Fig. 37.1 CT axial image with intravenous and oral contrast of the abdomen shows multiple subcentimeter calcified foci in Morrison's pouch.

■ Clinical History

A 53-year-old male with generalized abdominal pain, postchole-cystectomy (▶ Fig. 37.1).

■ Key Finding

Calcified densities free in the abdomen in a postcholecystectomy patient.

■ Diagnosis

Dropped gallstones: Dropped gallstones occur in 7% of laparoscopic cholecystectomies. The majority of patients are asymptomatic. The highest risk of dropped gallstones is seen in elderly patients, obese patients, difficult surgeries, patients undergoing emergent procedure, and patients with multiple adhesions. These gallstones can act as an inflammatory nidus. In most patients, asymptomatic soft tissue granulomas are created. If an abscess, sinus track or fistula develops, then the patient becomes symptomatic.

When dropped gallstones become infected, abscess formation can be seen. When infection occurs, the diagnosis of dropped gallstones can then become challenging. These dropped stones with abscess can then mimic carcinomas. Dropped gallstones can become symptomatic many years after surgery, the median interval is 5 months. When infected, surgical treatment is indicated.

✓ Pearls

• The diagnosis of dropped gallstones can only be made in postcholecystectomy patients.

• Dropped gallstones with surrounding fluid attenuation and fat stranding are likely infected.

Suggested Reading

Ramamurthy NK, Rudralingam V, Martin DF, Galloway SW, Sukumar SA. Out of sight but kept in mind: complications and imitations of dropped gallstones. AJR Am J Roentgenol. 2013; 200(6):1244–1253

Case 38

Zophia Martinez

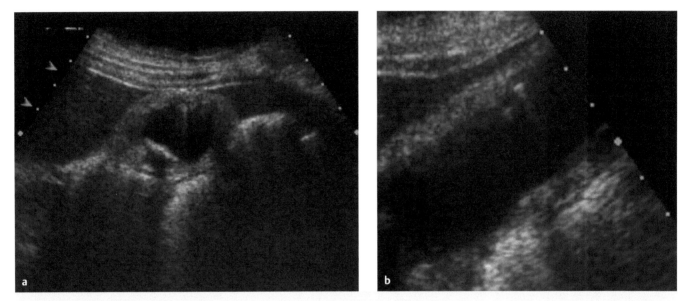

Fig. 38.1 Abdominal ultrasound of the right upper quadrant reveals gallbladder wall thickening with internal echogenic areas producing comet-tail reverberation artifact (a). The second image is a close up of the gallbladder showing reverb artifact from the nondependent wall (b).

■ Clinical History

A 74-year-old male with weight loss (▶Fig. 38.1).

■ Key Finding

Gallbladder wall "comet tail" artifact.

■ Top 3 Differential Diagnoses

- **Adenomyomatosis:** This is a relatively common condition found in at least 5% of gallbladder specimens and is usually an incidental finding requiring no further treatment or follow up. A key feature is the formation of intramural diverticula referred to as Rokitansky–Aschoff sinuses. Crystal precipitates forms are responsible for the intramural echogenic foci and V-shaped comet-tail artifact is seen on ultrasound. Gallbladder wall thickening is typically present and can be diffuse, fundal, or segmental in distribution.
- **Cholesterol polyps:** Similar to adenomyomatosis, cholesterolosis is a benign hyperplastic process that is virtually always incidental and of no clinical significance. It is characterized by numerous small cholesterol polyps and/or superficial cholesterol deposits. Ultrasound findings include multiple small (< 10 mm) nonshadowing, nonmobile iso- to hyperechoic polyps with posterior comet-tail artifact. The gallbladder wall is usually normal in thickness.
- **Emphysematous cholecystitis:** This is a rare form of acute cholecystitis. It is important to identify as it holds a high risk of gangrene, perforation, and sepsis. It is caused by ischemia with secondary infection by gas-forming organisms usually leading to the development of intramural and intraluminal gas within the gallbladder. Sonographic findings include nondependent echogenic reflectors with dirty shadowing and ring-down artifact which can appear similar to comet-tail artifact.

■ Additional Diagnostic Considerations

Gallbladder carcinoma: Focal, mass-like gallbladder wall thickening or large polyps in the absence of comet-tail artifact should be considered suspicious for carcinoma. The presence of comet-tail artifact effectively rules out malignancy and recognition of this finding can prevent unnecessary workup.

■ Diagnosis

Adenomyomatosis of the gallbladder.

✓ Pearls

- Unlike malignancy, there is no color Doppler vascularity within areas of wall thickening in adenomyomatosis.
- Ring-down artifact is typically longer than comet-tail artifact and lacks the characteristic "V" shape.
- If emphysematous cholecystitis is of concern, the intramural/ intraluminal air can be confirmed easily on noncontrast CT.

Suggested Readings

Boscak AR, Al-Hawary M, Ramsburgh SR. Best cases from the AFIP: Adenomyomatosis of the gallbladder. Radiographics. 2006; 26(3):941–946

Hammad AY, Miura JT, Turaga KK, Johnston FM, Hohenwalter MD, Gamblin TC. A literature review of radiological findings to guide the diagnosis of gallbladder adenomyomatosis. HPB (Oxford). 2016; 18(2):129–135

Hertzberg BS, Middleton WD. Ultrasound: The Requisites. 3rd ed. Philadelphia, PA: Elsevier; 2016

Case 39

Shaun Loh

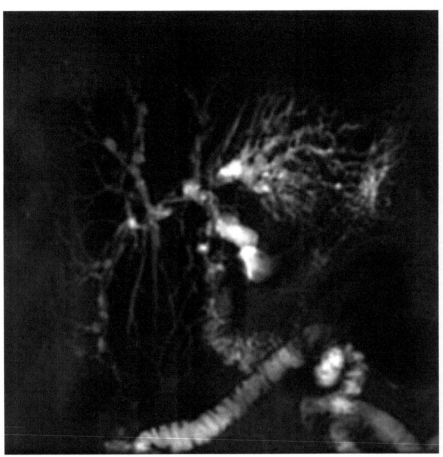

Fig. 39.1 Maximum intensity projection image from an MRCP study demonstrate a "string-of-beads" appearance with an alternating pattern of dilated and strictured intrahepatic bile ducts.

■ **Clinical History**

A 45-year-old woman with jaundice (▶ Fig. 39.1).

■ Key Finding

Intrahepatic biliary ductal strictures.

■ Top 3 Differential Diagnoses

- **Primary sclerosing cholangitis:** Primary sclerosing cholangitis is a chronic idiopathic inflammatory disease involving the bile ducts, which may progress to biliary ductal destruction, cholestasis, biliary cirrhosis, and cholangiocarcinoma. It is highly associated with ulcerative colitis. Classic findings include a "string-of-beads" appearance with an alternating pattern of dilation and stenosis of the intrahepatic and extrahepatic bile ducts. Diverticular outpouchings of the biliary tree on cholangiography are pathognomonic. Hypertrophy of the caudate lobe occurs in more advanced cases of primary sclerosing cholangitis. Periportal fibrosis may occur and appears on MR as areas of decreased periportal signal on T1 with increased signal on T2-weighted imaging.
- **Ascending cholangitis:** Ascending cholangitis is a bacterial infection of an obstructed biliary system. Patients may present with Charcot's triad: pain, fever, and jaundice. Choledocholithiasis and strictures from prior surgery may result in biliary obstruction with biliary stasis and infection. The intrahepatic and extrahepatic bile ducts are frequently dilated with high-density purulent bile and thickened walls. Left untreated, complications such as liver abscesses, sepsis, and even death may occur.
- **AIDS cholangiopathy:** This cholangiopathy results from strictures caused by AIDS related opportunistic infections, usually Cytomegalovirus (CMV) or Cryptosporidium. It is characterized by multiple intrahepatic biliary strictures, distal ampullary stenosis, or cholecystitis. The common bile duct is often involved with irregular areas of thickening and/or ulcerations. MRI reveals asymmetric intrahepatic and extrahepatic bile ducts ductal dilatation with pericholecystic inflammatory changes. On magnetic resonance cholangiopancreatography (MRCP) an alternating pattern of high signal biliary ductal dilatation and intrahepatic and extrahepatic biliary strictures may be present. Prognosis is poor as the cholangiopathy presents in late stage AIDS.

■ Additional Diagnostic Considerations

- **Neoplasm:** Neoplasms, such as cholangiocarcinoma and metastases, are another cause of intrahepatic biliary strictures. In cholangiocarcinoma, long strictures and prestenotic ductal dilatation with wall thickening may be the only findings. Malignant strictures may also result from pancreatic or ampullary carcinomas, as well as metastatic disease from colorectal, lung, breast cancer, and lymphoma.
- **Posttransplant arterial ischemia:** Intrahepatic biliary strictures may occur after liver transplantation and are thought to be secondary to hepatic artery occlusion and ischemia. The intrahepatic bile ducts are dilated with additional narrowed segments. Doppler ultrasound may show signs of hepatic artery occlusion or stenosis (such as a tardus/parvus waveform).

■ Diagnosis

Primary sclerosing cholangitis.

✓ Pearls

- Primary sclerosing cholangitis is characterized by a "string-of-beads" appearance of the intrahepatic bile ducts.
- Biliary strictures may be seen as either a cause or complication of ascending cholangitis.
- Care must be taken to assess for cholangiocarcinoma or metastases in the setting of a focal biliary stricture.
- Hepatic artery occlusion complicating liver transplantation leads to biliary necrosis with strictures.

Suggested Readings

Bilgin M, Balci NC, Erdogan A, Momtahen AJ, Alkaade S, Rau WS. Hepatobiliary and pancreatic MRI and MRCP findings in patients with HIV infection. AJR Am J Roentgenol. 2008; 191(1):228–232

Vitellas KM, Keogan MT, Freed KS, et al. Radiologic manifestations of sclerosing cholangitis with emphasis on MR cholangiopancreatography. Radiographics. 2000; 20(4):959–975, quiz 1108–1109, 1112

Case 40

Elias Antypas

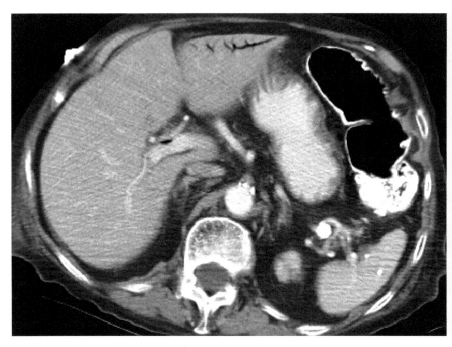

Fig. 40.1 CT axial image with intravenous and oral contrast shows air in the portal vein and air in the periphery of the left lobe of the liver (in intrahepatic portal veins). (Image courtesy of Rocky C. Saenz.)

■ **Clinical History**

A 79-year-old female with abdominal pain (▶Fig. 40.1).

■ Key Finding

Air within the portal venous system.

■ Diagnosis

Bowel ischemia: Portomesenteric gas most commonly develops because of bowel ischemia. Other etiologies of portomesenteric gas include iatrogenic, traumatic, inflammatory, infectious, neoplastic, obstructive, and idiopathic etiology. Portal venous gas on CT has been associated with a mortality rate in three-fourth of patients. Pneumatosis is associated with transmural bowel infarction in three-fourth of patients. When both portomesenteric gas and pneumatosis are present on CT bowel infarct is present in greater than 90% of patients.

On CT, portal venous gas may appear in the liver or as pneumatosis with a linear or curvilinear distribution of gas within the bowel wall. Other worrisome features for pneumatosis include mesenteric or portal venous gas or pneumoperitoneum. Note that portal venous gas flows toward the periphery of the liver. CT evaluation with wide windows is best to detect pneumatosis and portal venous gas. On radiographs, pneumatosis may demonstrate fine linear lucency representing air within bowel wall.

Be cautious of pseudopneumatosis, which occurs when gas is trapped against the mucosal surface of the bowel wall by semisolid feces. This is most commonly seen in cecum and ascending colon. Gas bubbles will not be seen beyond an air fluid level due to their intraluminal location. The air bubbles will be punctate and separated by mucosal folds rather than a linear or curvilinear pattern. The most reliable portion of the bowel to diagnose pneumatosis is identifying it along the dependent bowel wall. The treatment of pneumatosis depends on the etiology. If it is a nonischemic cause, then treatment is conservative. However, if bowel necrosis is suspected, then urgent surgical resection of necrotic bowel is necessary.

✓ Pearls

- Portal venous gas is suspicious for bowel ischemia.
- Portal venous gas collects in the liver periphery.
- Utilize the dependent bowel wall to diagnose pneumatosis.
- Pneumobilia gas is seen centrally near porta hepatis.

Suggested Readings

Faberman RS, Mayo-Smith WW. Outcome of 17 patients with portal venous gas detected by CT. AJR Am J Roentgenol. 1997; 169(6):1535–1538

Milone M, et al. CT findings of pneumatosis and portomesenteric venous gas in acute bowel ischemia. World J Gastroenterol. 2013; 19(39):6579–6584

Moisidou R, Gounos D, Tepetes K. Typical CT findings of pneumatosis intestinalis and portal venous air in intestinal necrosis. Dig Surg. 2004; 21(3):184

Pickhardt PJ, Kim DH, Taylor AJ. Asymptomatic pneumatosis at CT colonography: a benign self-limited imaging finding distinct from perforation. AJR Am J Roentgenol. 2008; 190(2):W112–7

Case 41

Rocky C. Saenz

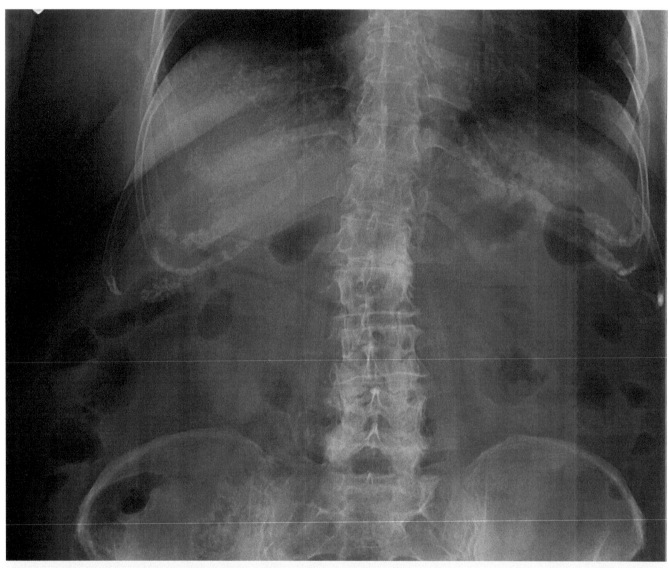

Fig. 41.1 Frontal radiograph of the abdomen demonstrates multiple, grouped, round, dense calcifications in the right upper quadrant. These are along the inferior margin of the liver.

■ **Clinical History**

A 47-year-old female with occasional postprandial pain (▶ Fig. 41.1).

■ Key Finding

Right upper quadrant multiple, grouped calcifications.

■ Diagnosis

Cholelithiasis: Gallstones are the diagnosis when multiple, grouped right upper quadrant calcifications are seen. The minority of gallstones, approximately 20%, are visible on X-ray. Gallstones are gravity dependent in the gallbladder and can be seen changing orientation on different abdominal X-ray views. Cholelithiasis is associated with cholecystitis, but cholecystitis is not an X-ray diagnosis. The majority of gallstones are not calcified as 80% are cholesterol stones. Therefore, CT and X-ray are not reliable to exclude gallstones. So, ultrasound is the gold standard for gallstone evaluation. On ultrasound, gallstones are hyperechoic with posterior acoustic shadowing. ultrasound signs of an obstructing gallstone include: hydropic dilatation of the gallbladder, pericholecystic fluid, and positive sonographic Murphy sign (most reliable).

The "Mercedes-Benz" sign is a CT finding of cholelithiasis caused by nitrogen gas within a degenerating gallstones. A porcelain gallbladder refers to calcification of the gallbladder wall. So it appears as a single oval usually greater than 3 cm calcified density. Acute cholecystitis and chronic cholecystitis are not X-ray diagnoses. Both acute and chronic cholecystitis can be easily differentiated with a nuclear hepatobiliary scan.

✓ Pearls

- X-ray cannot exclude cholelithiasis as the majority of gallstones are noncalcified.
- X-ray cannot diagnosis cholecystitis.

- If acute cholecystitis is suspected it should be confirmed on ultrasound.

Suggested Readings

Bortoff GA, Chen MYM, Ott DJ, Wolfman NT, Routh WD. Gallbladder stones: imaging and intervention. Radiographics. 2000; 20(3):751–766

Dyer RB, Chen MY, Zagoria RJ. Abnormal calcifications in the urinary tract. Radiographics. 1998; 18(6):1405–1424

Stoupis C, Taylor HM, Paley MR, et al. The Rocky liver: radiologic-pathologic correlation of calcified hepatic masses. Radiographics. 1998; 18(3):675–685, quiz 726

Case 42

Robert A. Jesinger

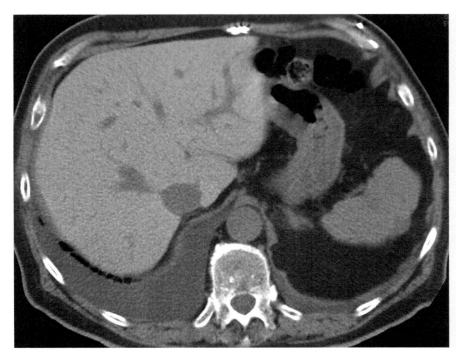

Fig. 42.1 Unenhanced CT image of the liver demonstrates diffuse increased attenuation (> 80 HU). Small layering bilateral pleural effusions are noted, as is metallic artifact along the anterior chest wall.

■ Clinical History

A 65-year-old man with recurrent congestive heart failure (▶Fig. 42.1).

■ Key Finding

Hyperdense liver.

■ Top 3 Differential Diagnoses

• **Iron deposition:** Iron deposition in the liver, commonly in the reticuloendothelial system, can be seen as a consequence of increased oral intake, multiple blood transfusions (usually in the setting of dialysis or chronic anemia), ineffective erythropoiesis (thalassemia, sideroblastic anemia), or from the more rare disorder of primary hemochromatosis. Hepatic enlargement, increased parenchymal attenuation (HU > 80), and cirrhotic liver morphology can be key visual markers, as can laboratory markers of impaired hepatic function. Careful detection of liver masses is important due to increased risk of hepatocellular carcinoma (HCC). Classic MRI features of iron deposition include decreased hepatic parenchymal signal intensity on T2-weighted imaging sequences due to the superparamagnetic effect of iron. Decreased myocardial and pancreatic parenchymal T2 signal intensity is a classic MRI feature in primary hemochromatosis, while decreased T2 signal intensity in the spleen is characteristic of secondary hemochromatosis.

• **Amiodarone therapy:** Amiodarone is an antiarrhythmic medication that is 40% iodine by weight. It has primary hepatic and biliary metabolism and is slowly excreted into bile by the liver. Hence, chronic amiodarone therapy increases hepatic parenchymal attenuation; normalization occurs over weeks to months after the medication is discontinued. In addition to a hyperdense liver, amiodarone therapy is associated with lower lobe pulmonary interstitial lung disease, as well as focal pulmonary infiltrates with characteristic increased attenuation.

• **Glycogen storage disease:** There are multiple subtypes of glycogen storage disease, many of which can result in decreased liver density similar to hepatic steatosis. Types I (von Gierke) and IV, however, are subtypes that are associated with increased hepatic attenuation. Type IV in particular may result in cirrhosis with an increased incidence of HCC. Unlike hemochromatosis, the classic MRI feature is increased hepatic parenchymal signal on T1-weighted imaging sequences.

■ Additional Diagnostic Considerations

• **Gold therapy:** Intramuscular gold therapy was commonly used to treat patients with rheumatoid arthritis until approximately the 1990s. Agents with less toxicity are now routinely used as disease modifying agents for rheumatoid arthritis in place of gold therapy. Chronic accumulation of gold salts results in a hyperdense liver.

• **Thoratrast:** Thoratrast is a radioactive material (alpha emitter) that was used as a contrast agent for several decades (1920–1950s). The agent is taken up by the reticuloendothelial system, resulting in dense opacities within the liver, spleen, and lymph nodes. There is an increased risk of malignancy, especially angiosarcoma.

■ Diagnosis

Amiodarone therapy.

✓ Pearls

• Primary hemochromatosis affects pancreas, while secondary hemochromatosis affects spleen.
• Amiodarone may cause a hyperdense liver, high attenuation pulmonary infiltrates and interstitial lung disease.

• Hepatoma and angiosarcoma may arise in the setting of a hyperdense liver.

Suggested Readings

Guyader D, Gandon Y, Deugnier Y, et al. Evaluation of computed tomography in the assessment of liver iron overload. A study of 46 cases of idiopathic hemochromatosis. Gastroenterology. 1989; 97(3):737–743

Lim RP, Tuvia K, Hajdu CH, et al. Quantification of hepatic iron deposition in patients with liver disease: comparison of chemical shift imaging with single-echo T2*-weighted imaging. AJR Am J Roentgenol. 2010; 194(5):1288–1295

Tani I, Kurihara Y, Kawaguchi A, et al. MR imaging of diffuse liver disease. AJR Am J Roentgenol. 2000; 174(4):965–971

Case 43

Sharon Kreuer

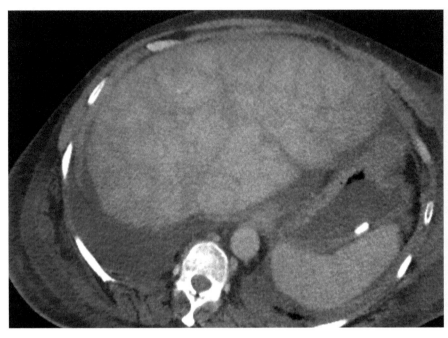

Fig. 43.1 CT of the upper abdomen with intravenous contrast shows the liver to have heterogeneous, "nutmeg" enhancement pattern. In addition, there are partially seen small bilateral pleural effusions, a small amount of free fluid around the liver, and anasarca. (Image courtesy of Rocky C. Saenz.)

■ Clinical History

A 67-year-old male with abdominal fullness (▶Fig. 43.1).

■ Key Finding

Liver parenchymal heterogeneous, "nutmeg" enhancement pattern.

■ Top 3 Differential Diagnoses

- **Congestive Heart Failure:** Passive hepatic congestion is also known as nutmeg liver. Decreased cardiac output results in venous stasis in the inferior vena cava (IVC), hepatic veins, and sinusoids with perisinusoidal edema and thrombosis of the sinusoidal vessels. Enlarged IVC and hepatic veins can be seen on CT or MRI showing nonspecific reflux of contrast on early phase imaging. The congested liver has a very heterogeneous enhancement pattern related to delayed enhancement adjacent to the hepatic veins. Chronic congestion can progress to cirrhosis. Treatment is targeted toward improvement of cardiac function.
- **Budd–Chiari syndrome:** Occurs with vascular occlusion of the hepatic veins, IVC, or both resulting in obstructed venous flow from the liver to the heart. Causes are numerous and are generally classified as primary versus secondary. Vascular imaging findings are that of venous occlusion in both the acute or chronic setting and collateral vessels and portal hypertension in more long standing disease. Enhanced CT shows decreased peripheral enhancement with increased central enhancement of the caudate lobe. Treatment is specific to the cause of occlusion and includes anticoagulation, shunt placement and liver transplantation.
- **Cirrhosis:** A process of fibrotic and nodular regeneration of the liver secondary to hepatocellular insult. The most common causes are alcohol abuse, viral hepatitis, and steatosis. Imaging findings include altered morphology with nodular contour and a pattern of lateral segment/caudate lobe hypertrophy and medial segment/anterior right hepatic lobe atrophy. The unenhanced and enhanced appearance of the cirrhotic liver can be heterogeneous, mimicking passive hepatic congestion. Close inspection should be made for hepatocellular carcinoma (HCC), portal vein thrombosis and associated findings of portal hypertension.

■ Additional Diagnostic Considerations

- **Pseudocirrhosis:** Pseudocirrhosis gives the appearance of cirrhosis without fibrosis or regenerative nodules. It classically is associated with treated breast cancer, although has been described with other treated cancers. In the setting of metastasis, multiple liver tumors give a nodular appearance to the liver. Nodularity can also be seen with pseudomyxoma peritonei and sarcoid.
- **Viral hepatitis:** Acute infection results in hepatocyte injury. On CT and ultrasound, hepatic edema seen as decreased attenuation and echogenicity respectively. Hepatomegaly is also seen. Chronic viral hepatitis B and C can progress to cirrhosis.

■ Diagnosis

Passive hepatic congestion.

✓ Pearls

- Hepatic congestion of cardiac origin is secondary to venous stasis and can progress to cirrhosis. Look for secondary imaging findings of congestive heart failure to diagnosis and distinguish from other etiologies of cirrhosis.
- Typical imaging appearance of Budd–Chiari is of decreased peripheral and increased central enhancement.
- Imaging in cirrhosis is used for assessing portal hypertension, portal vein thrombosis, and HCC.

Suggested Readings

Brancatelli G, Vilgrain V, Federle MP, et al. Budd-Chiari syndrome: spectrum of imaging findings. AJR Am J Roentgenol. 2007; 188(2):W168:W76

Dalrymple NC, Leyendecker JR, Oliphant M. Problem Solving in Abdominal Imaging. 1st ed. Philadelphia, PA: Mosby Elsevier; 2009

Wells ML, Fenstad ER, Poterucha JT, et al. Imaging findings of congestive hepatopathy. Radiographics. 2016; 36(4):1024–1037

Case 44

Grant E. Lattin, Jr.

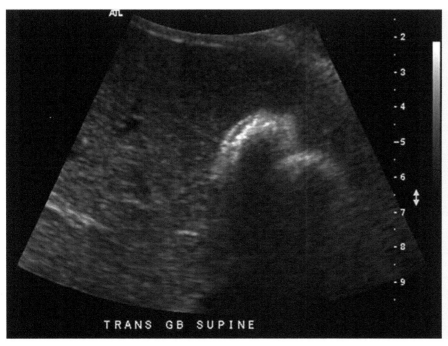

Fig. 44.1 Sonographic image of the gallbladder demonstrates the gallbladder wall (linear hyperechoic focus) with a second thin curvilinear hyperechoic focus just deep to this and posterior acoustic shadowing. This appearance of two curvilinear echogenic lines with an intervening area of decreased echotexture is commonly described as the "WES" sign.

■ Clinical History

A 47-year-old woman with right upper quadrant pain (▶Fig. 44.1).

■ Key Finding

Wall-echo-shadow (WES) sign.

■ Diagnosis

Cholelithiasis

■ Discussion

The WES sign is characterized by two curvilinear echogenic lines created by the gallbladder wall and a gallbladder lumen filled with stones. These hyperechoic foci are separated by an intervening sonolucent region of bile within the gallbladder lumen. The gallstones cause posterior acoustic shadowing.

Gallstones commonly present in women in their 40s with right upper quadrant discomfort following a fatty meal. The evaluation of gallstones is best performed by ultrasound. Decubitus imaging should be performed to look for mobility, as impacted stones may result in concurrent cholecystitis. Likewise, the common bile duct should be imaged as well to exclude choledocholithiasis. Ultrasound findings which may indicate associated cholecystitis include pericholecystic fluid, a gallbladder wall measuring greater than 3 mm in diameter, and a sonographic Murphy sign.

CT is less sensitive than ultrasound in the evaluation of gallstones. T2-weighted image on MRI will show the stones as areas of signal void surrounded by hyperintense bile. Hepatobiliary scintigraphy may be of benefit if concern exists for an obstructing stone and ultrasound findings are equivocal for cholecystitis.

Although the WES sign is classic for cholelithiasis, care should be taken to exclude potential mimickers, such as emphysematous cholecystitis or porcelain gallbladder. Emphysematous cholecystitis presents with gas within the gallbladder wall and associated "dirty" posterior shadowing, as opposed to the "clean" shadowing seen with calcifications. Porcelain gallbladder is characterized by calcification within the gallbladder wall with posterior shadowing. Since the calcification is within the wall and not the gallbladder lumen, there is absence of the second hyperechoic focus which makes up the WES sign. If uncertain, CT will help evaluate for gas or calcifications within the gallbladder wall.

Treatment of cholelithiasis may be conservative if asymptomatic. If symptomatic, surgical removal of the gallbladder is usually performed.

✓ Pearls

- The WES sign is caused by a gallbladder lumen full of gallstones.
- Ultrasound is more sensitive than CT in the evaluation of cholecystitis.

- WES sign mimickers, such as emphysematous cholecystitis and porcelain gallbladder, can be easily excluded with noncontrast CT.

Suggested Readings

Bortoff GA, Chen MY, Ott DJ, Wolfman NT, Routh WD. Gallbladder stones: imaging and intervention. Radiographics. 2000; 20(3):751–766

Duncan CB, Riall TS. Evidence-based current surgical practice: calculous gallbladder disease. J Gastrointest Surg. 2012; 16(11):2011–2025

Rosenthal SJ, Cox GG, Wetzel LH, Batnitzky S. Pitfalls and differential diagnosis in biliary sonography. Radiographics. 1990; 10(2):285–311

Part 2

Pancreas and Spleen

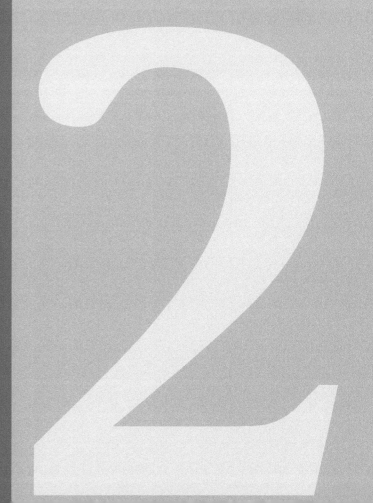

Case 45

Rocky C. Saenz

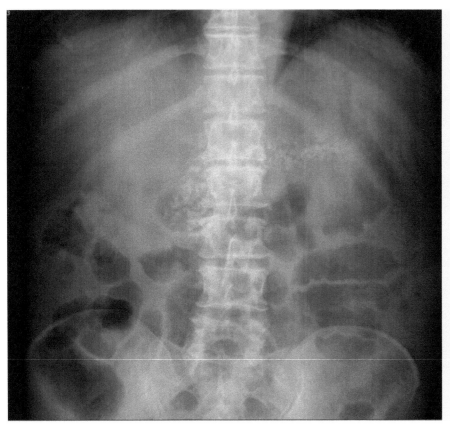

Fig. 45.1 Abdominal X-ray has multiple subcentimeter central calcifications in the midabdomen.

■ Clinical History

A 45-year-old male with history of alcohol abuse (▶ Fig. 45.1).

■ Key Finding

Central abdominal grouped calcifications.

■ Diagnosis

• **Chronic pancreatitis:** Chronic pancreatitis is the most common cause of pancreatic parenchymal calcifications. It is most commonly related to alcoholic pancreatitis. These calcifications typically are subcentimeter in size and spherical to oval in morphology. Chronic pancreatitis is caused by repeated episodes of pancreatic inflammation, which can cause proteinaceous material and calcium carbonate to obstruct small ducts resulting in ductal ectasia and progressive periductal fibrosis. These parenchymal calcifications are easily seen on X-rays.

On cross-sectional imaging, other findings of chronic pancreatitis may be seen including pancreatic ductal dilation and pancreatic atrophy. The most common finding in chronic pancreatitis is ductal dilation. The ducal dilation can often involve dilated side branches (which are typically seen in the body of the pancreas and are perpendicular to the long axis of the main duct). The key finding on an X-ray is noting calcifications in the anatomical location of the pancreas. Therefore, other diagnoses are highly unlikely such as calcified lymph nodes (spherical with an egg-shell appearance) and arteriosclerosis (linear following arterial distributions).

✓ Pearls

• Pancreatic parenchymal calcifications are a classic X-ray finding of chronic pancreatitis.
• Chronic pancreatitis is typically related to alcoholism.

• Arterial calcifications are linear and should not be confused for chronic pancreatitis.

Suggested Readings

Federle MP, Jeffrey RB, Woodward PJ, Borhani A. Diagnostic Imaging: Abdomen. 2nd ed. Philadelphia, PA: Lippincott Williams & Wilkins; 2009

Javadi S, Menias CO, Korivi BR, et al. Pancreatic calcifications and calcified pancreatic masses: pattern recognition approach on CT. AJR Am J Roentgenol. 2017; 209(1):77–87

Case 46

Michael Legacy

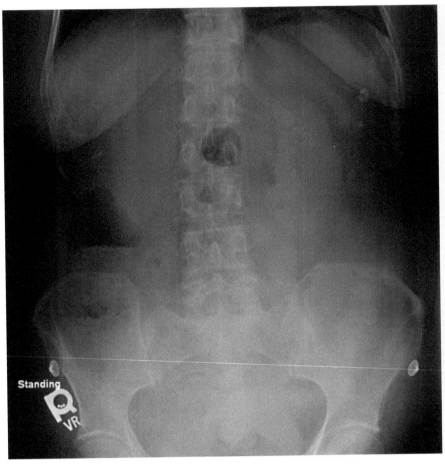

Fig. 46.1 Abdominal X-ray demonstrates two calcific densities in the left upper quadrant. (Image courtesy of Rocky C. Saenz.)

■ **Clinical History**

A 48-year-old female with general abdominal pain (▶ Fig. 46.1).

■ Key Finding

Left upper quadrant calcifications.

■ Top 3 Differential Diagnoses

- **Pancreatic calcifications:** Chronic pancreatitis is the most common cause of pancreatic parenchymal calcifications and most commonly related to alcoholic pancreatitis. Look for small irregular calcific densities in the anatomical location of the pancreas. Less commonly, pancreatic calcifications can be due to cystic fibrosis, neuroendocrine tumors (e.g., insulinomas), and pancreatic cancer.
- **Nephrolithiasis:** Most renal stones are calcium based with the most common being calcium oxalate. Calcium stones are seen on X-rays and typically are oval in shape and overlying the kidney silhouette. Less commonly, the morphology may be staghorn when composed of magnesium ammonium phosphate (struvite stone). The majority of patients will present with hematuria and flank pain.
- **Splenic calcifications:** Most commonly healed granulomatous infections from histoplasmosis, tuberculosis, brucellosis, toxoplasmosis, candidiasis, and fungal infections. Histoplasmosis is the most common in the United States and typically presents with multiple small round calcifications. Calcific densities overlying the splenic silhouette are seen on an X-ray.

■ Additional Diagnostic Considerations

- **Atherosclerosis:** Atherosclerotic disease (ASD) appears as curvilinear parallel lines of calcification in the expected location of vascularity. Considering left upper quadrant calcifications, splenic artery involvement is a consideration but is usually tortuous.
- **Ingested pills/foreign bodies:** The key to diagnosis is the angular margins and irregular nonanatomical morphologies. Swallowed pills/objects will most likely move location on repeat studies. Metallic objects will be more radiopaque compared to bones and calcic densities.

■ Diagnosis

Splenic granulomas.

✓ Pearls

- Nephrolithiasis on an X-ray should be further evaluated on ultrasound/CT to exclude obstructive uropathy.
- Pancreatic calcifications are one of the three findings of chronic pancreatitis.
- Splenic granulomas are benign and require no follow-ups.

Suggested Readings

Dyer RB, Chen MY, Zagoria RJ. Classic signs in uroradiology. Radiographics. 2004; 24(Suppl 1):S247–S280

Federle MP, Jeffrey RB, Woodward PJ, Borhani A. Diagnostic Imaging: Abdomen. 2nd ed. Philadelphia, PA: Lippincott Williams & Wilkins; 2009

Guelfguat M, Kaplinskiy V, Reddy SH, DiPoce J. Clinical guidelines for imaging and reporting ingested foreign bodies. AJR Am J Roentgenol. 2014; 203(1):37–53

Javadi S, Menias CO, Korivi BR, et al. Pancreatic calcifications and calcified pancreatic masses: pattern recognition approach on CT. AJR Am J Roentgenol. 2017; 209(1):77–87

Thipphavong S, Duigenan S, Schindera ST, Gee MS, Philips S. Nonneoplastic, benign, and malignant splenic diseases: cross-sectional imaging findings and rare disease entities. AJR Am J Roentgenol. 2014; 203(2):315–322

Case 47

Rocky C. Saenz

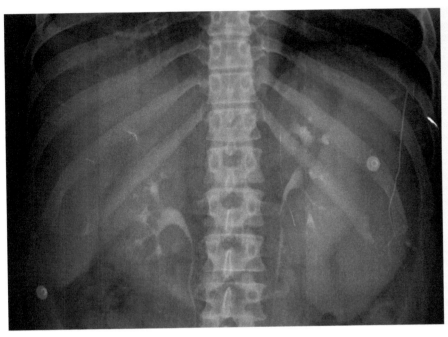

Fig. 47.1 Abdominal X-ray demonstrates the splenic shadow extending below the left renal shadow. Contrast is noted within both collecting systems.

■ Clinical History

A 38-year-old male with abdominal fullness (▶Fig. 47.1).

■ Key Finding

Spleen inferior margin extends below the left renal shadow.

■ Diagnosis

Splenomegaly: Splenomegaly is defined as a spleen larger than 14 cm. It can be diagnosed on X-ray when the inferior splenic margin extends below the left renal shadow. Common causes for splenomegaly include portal hypertension, anemia, infection, and tumor. Portal hypertension is the most common cause of splenomegaly that is classically due to hepatic cirrhosis. Any cause of extramedullary hematopoiesis can result in hepatosplenomegaly. Hemolytic anemias such as thalassemia enlarge the spleen due to sequestration of red blood cells. A common infectious cause of splenomegaly is mononucleosis from Epstein–Barr virus. Any tumor can result in spleen enlargement. Lymphoma is the most common malignancy in the spleen. Primary splenic lymphoma is much less common than secondary lymphoma (commonly seen in HIV/AIDS [human immunodeficiency virus/acquired immunodeficiency syndrome] patients). Hemangiomas are the most common benign splenic neoplasms and when large can result in splenomegaly. When splenomegaly is suspected on X-ray, it should be further investigated with cross-sectional imaging.

✓ Pearls

- Spleen greater than 14 cm is splenomegaly.
- The most common cause of splenomegaly is portal hypertension.

- Splenomegaly on X-ray should be further investigated with cross-sectional imaging.

Suggested Readings

Cheson BD, Fisher RI, Barrington SF, et al. Alliance, Australasian Leukaemia and Lymphoma Group, Eastern Cooperative Oncology Group, European Mantle Cell Lymphoma Consortium, Italian Lymphoma Foundation, European Organisation for Research, Treatment of Cancer/Dutch Hemato-Oncology Group, Grupo Español de Médula Ósea, German High-Grade Lymphoma Study Group, German Hodgkin's Study Group, Japanese Lymphorra Study Group, Lymphoma Study Association, NCIC Clinical Trials Group, Nordic Lymphoma Study Group, Southwest Oncology Group, United Kingdom National Cancer Research Institute. Recommendations for initial evaluation, staging, and response assessment of Hodgkin and non-Hodgkin lymphoma: the Lugano classification. J Clin Oncol. 2014; 32(27):3059–3068

Federle MP, Jeffrey RB, Woodward PJ, Borhani A. Diagnostic Imaging: Abdomen. 2nd ed. Philadelphia, PA: Lippincott Williams & Wilkins; 2009

Thipphavong S, Duigenan S, Schindera ST, Gee MS, Philips S. Nonneoplastic, benign, and malignant splenic diseases: cross-sectional imaging findings and rare disease entities. AJR Am J Roentgenol. 2014; 203(2):315–322

Case 48

Rocky C. Saenz

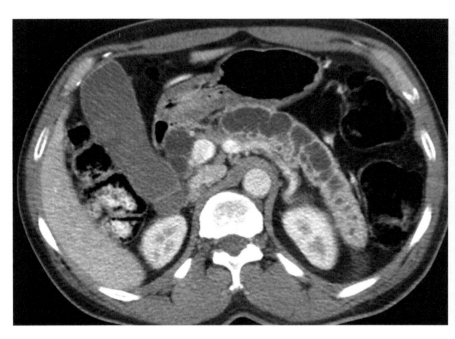

Fig. 48.1 CT axial image, with intravenous and oral contrast, demonstrates significant pancreatic duct dilation with pancreatic atrophy. The gallbladder is elongated and the common bile duct is also dilated.

■ **Clinical History**

A 44-year-old male with occasional epigastric pain (▶ Fig. 48.1).

■ Key Finding

Pancreatic duct dilatation.

■ Top 3 Differential Diagnoses

• **Acute pancreatitis:** Interstitial edematous pancreatitis represents majority of pancreatitis. The focal or diffuse pancreatic edema can result in portions of the narrowing and poststenotic dilation. When pancreatitis is focal (e.g., groove pancreatitis), it can mimic a mass. Cross-sectional imaging is only used to evaluate the severity of disease. Pancreatitis is a clinical and laboratory diagnosis. Patients usually present with epigastric pain radiating to the back. Acute pancreatitis is usually treated with bowel rest (nothing by mouth, NPO) and supportive therapy. Surgical intervention may be needed in advanced cases.

• **Chronic pancreatitis:** Multiple bouts of pancreatitis over time can lead to chronic extrahepatic ductal dilation. The classic triad of findings of chronic pancreatitis is parenchymal calcifications, parenchymal atrophy, and ductal dilation (> 4 mm). Another chronic pancreatitis finding is side branch ductal dilation. The most common etiology is chronic alcoholism.

• **Neoplasm:** Tumors such as cholangiocarcinoma, pancreatic adenocarcinoma, gallbladder malignancies, and metastasis may invade the biliary system. Malignant tumors involving the common bile duct create an abrupt caliber change with shouldering and asymmetry. There is usually a transition point between the dilated obstructed duct and the smaller caliber decompressed duct. Extrinsic compression from malignant masses, lymphadenopathy, or dilated collateral vasculature may also produce poststenotic ductal dilation.

■ Additional Diagnostic Considerations

Papillary stenosis: Defined as obstruction of bile flow at the sphincter of Oddi without the presence of a mass or inflammation at the ampulla, papillary stenosis appears as common bile duct dilation on magnetic resonance cholangiopancreatography (MRCP). The most common cause is dysfunction of the sphincter of Oddi and patients typically present clinically with jaundice and pancreatitis. Papillary size less than 12 mm suggests an underlying benign cause. Endoscopic retrograde cholangiopancreatography (ERCP) is useful in determining the cause.

■ Diagnosis

Chronic pancreatitis.

✓ Pearls

• Acute pancreatitis cannot be diagnosed on imaging without peripancreatic fat stranding.
• Chronic pancreatitis is the diagnosis when the triad of parenchymal calcifications, atrophy, and ductal dilation is seen.

• Neoplasm must be excluded when pancreatic ductal dilation is seen.

Suggested Readings

Leyendecker JR, Elsayes KM, Gratz BI, Brown JJ. MR cholangiopancreatography: spectrum of pancreatic duct abnormalities. AJR Am J Roentgenol. 2002; 179(6):1465–1471

Nikolaidis P, Hammond NA, Day K, et al. Imaging features of benign and malignant ampullary and periampullary lesions. Radiographics. 2014; 34(3):624–641

O'Connor OJ, O'Neill S, Maher MM. Imaging of biliary tract disease. AJR Am J Roentgenol. 2011; 197(4):W551–8

Case 49

Sarika N. Joshi

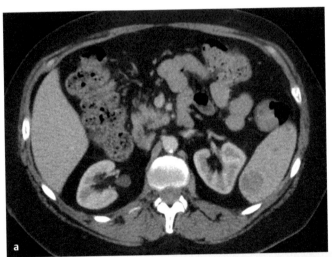 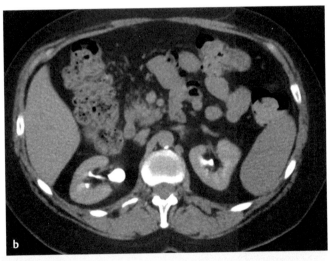

Fig. 49.1 Top image, CT axial, with intravenous contrast in the portal venous phase, shows a round low-density lesion in the posterior spleen. Bottom image, is a CT axial delayed image that demonstrates the lesion to be isodense to the spleen. (Image courtesy of Rocky C. Saenz.)

■ Clinical History

A 54-year-old male with occasional left upper quadrant pain
(▶Fig. 49.1).

■ Key Finding

Solitary solid splenic lesion.

■ Top 3 Differential Diagnoses

• **Infarct:** An infarction can mimic a solid mass; however, there will be no internal enhancement. Capsular enhancement may be observed. The classical appearance is similar to that of other organs as a peripherally based wedge-shaped hypodensity. Atypical presentations such as an irregular or linear shape are common. Extension to the capsular is a more reliable indicator but not always seen. Many infarcts are occult by imaging. The cause may be idiopathic or from a predisposing factor such as sickle-cell disease or embolic phenomenon.

• **Hemangioma:** This benign mass is the most common primary splenic neoplasm. The characteristic liver findings of peripheral nodular discontinuous enhancement pattern and high T2 signal on MR are less commonly seen in the spleen. The CT appearance is often homogeneously hypodense lesion with soft-tissue attenuation. On delayed imaging, the lesion can become isodense to the spleen. Central punctate or peripheral curvilinear calcifications can also present. The imaging appearance is indistinguishable from hamartoma (which is rare). This usually has no clinical significance; however, in large lesions thrombocytopenia from Kasabach–Merritt syndrome (consumptive coagulopathy) can rarely occur.

• **Lymphoma:** This is the most common malignancy to affect the spleen. A solitary hypodense mass is one of four major appearances in the spleen. The others include diffuse infiltration, multiple focal lesions, and miliary involvement. Primary splenic lymphoma is often associated with AIDS. Concurrent adenopathy is helpful in narrowing the differential diagnosis.

■ Additional Diagnostic Considerations

• **Solitary Metastasis:** Hematogenous metastasis occurs due to the rich arterial supply, although they are infrequent compared to liver metastasis. The imaging appearance can range from solid to cystic, single lesions or multiple, with variable enhancement. Most commonly these are from melanoma, breast, lung, gastrointestinal, or ovarian malignancies.

• **Angiosarcoma:** Rare, however the most common primary malignancy of the spleen after lymphoma. Splenomegaly should also be present. There is high metastatic potential to multiple organs and a poor prognosis.

■ Diagnosis

Hemangioma.

✓ Pearls

• Splenic hemangiomas are frequently atypical but may retain contrast on delayed images.
• Extrasplenic manifestations are helpful in detecting lymphoma or metastases.

• Consider infarction if there is no appreciable enhancement.

Suggested Readings

Luna A, Ribes R, Caro P, Luna L, Aumente E, Ros PR. MRI of focal splenic lesions without and with dynamic gadolinium enhancement. AJR Am J Roentgenol. 2006; 186(6):1533–1547

Ricci ZJ, Mazzariol FS, Flusberg M, et al. Improving diagnosis of atraumatic splenic lesions, part II: benign neoplasms/nonneoplastic mass-like lesions. Clin Imaging. 2016; 40(4):691–704

Thipphavong S, Duigenan S, Schindera ST, Gee MS, Philips S. Nonneoplastic, benign, and malignant splenic diseases: cross-sectional imaging findings and rare disease entities. AJR Am J Roentgenol. 2014; 203(2):315–322

Case 50

Timothy McKnight

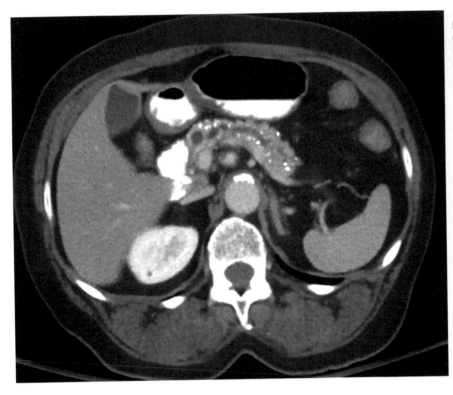

Fig. 50.1 Intravenous contrast enhanced axial CT image through the pancreas demonstrates innumerable diffuse pancreatic parenchymal calcifications and irregular dilation of the main pancreatic duct and common bile duct dilation.

■ Clinical History

A 67-year-old male with recurrent abdominal pain (▶ Fig. 50.1).

■ Key Finding

Pancreatic calcifications.

■ Top 3 Differential Diagnoses

- **Chronic pancreatitis:** Repeated episodes of inflammation cause proteinaceous material and calcium carbonate to obstruct small ducts, resulting in ductal ectasia and progressive periductal fibrosis. This results in the classic appearance of irregular ductal dilation (68%) often including side branches, parenchymal and intraductal calcifications (54%), and parenchymal atrophy (50%). Patients usually have a history of chronic alcoholism (70% of cases), obstructing biliary stones, chronic smoking, or cystic fibrosis.
- **Vascular:** Calcified atheromatous plaque along the course of the splenic artery, gastroduodenal, superior mesenteric, and pancreaticoduodenal branches may mimic and are more common than parenchymal calcifications. These calcifications have tram track configuration. Focal aneurysms, most commonly splenic, have usual peripheral or eggshell calcifications. Chronic venous thrombosis, usually superior mesenteric vein (SMV) or splenic, may have intraluminal calcification and mural thickening.
- **Choledocholithiasis:** Coexisting biliary dilatation, cholelithiasis (95%), and clinical obstructive jaundice. The gold standard is endoscopic retrograde cholangiopancreatography (ERCP) but magnetic resonance cholangiopancreatography (MRCP) sensitivity and specificity are both 80 to 100%. CT "bull's-eye" sign with rim of low-density bile around calcified stone is 60 to 80% sensitive. Choledocolithiasis is usually solitary, but when multiple, they are clustered typically within the distal common bile duct.

■ Additional Diagnostic Considerations

- **Serous cystadenoma (SCA):** Complex microcystic, multilocular cystic lesion with a "honeycomb" appearance, typically more than six locules each less than 2 cm, usually less than 1 cm, and may be so small as to give appearance of solid lesion. A central scar is present in 20 to 30% with calcifications. It presents in the sixth to seventh decade in women. Vascular encasement and ductal dilation are rare.
- **Islet cell/neuroendocrine tumor:** These appear as hypervascular tumors with intense arterial phase enhancement. Calcifications are seen in 20% usually either with insulinomas or larger nonfunctional tumors (usually coarse irregular central calcification). Lesions less than 3 cm are more likely to be functional or syndromic. Insulinoma is the most common representing 50% of these tumors.
- **Other tumors:** Pancreatic adenocarcinoma very rarely has calcifications. Mucinous tumors such as intraductal papillary mucinous neoplasm (IPMN) and mucinous cystic neoplasm (MCN) have calcifications in 16 to 20% peripheral or septal. Solid pseudopapillary neoplasms have calcifications in 50% but this tumor is rare, always in women less than 35 years of age.

■ Diagnosis

Chronic pancreatitis.

✓ Pearls

- Pancreatic calcifications, atrophy, and ductal dilatation are characteristic of chronic pancreatitis.
- Vascular calcifications are most common overall with a typical tram track configuration and intravenous contrast will typically define the vessel of origin.
- Choledocholithiasis on ultrasound can be confirmed with either MRCP or ERCP.

Suggested Readings

Anderson SW, Lucey BC, Varghese JC, Soto JA. Accuracy of MDCT in the diagnosis of choledocholithiasis. AJR Am J Roentgenol. 2006; 187(1):174–180

Lesniak RJ, Hohenwalter MD, Taylor AJ. Spectrum of causes of pancreatic calcifications. AJR Am J Roentgenol. 2002; 178(1):79–86

Miller FH, Keppke AL, Wadhwa A, Ly JN, Dalal K, Kamler VA. MRI of pancreatitis and its complications: part 2, chronic pancreatitis. AJR Am J Roentgenol. 2004; 183(6):1645–1652

Case 51

Sarika N. Joshi

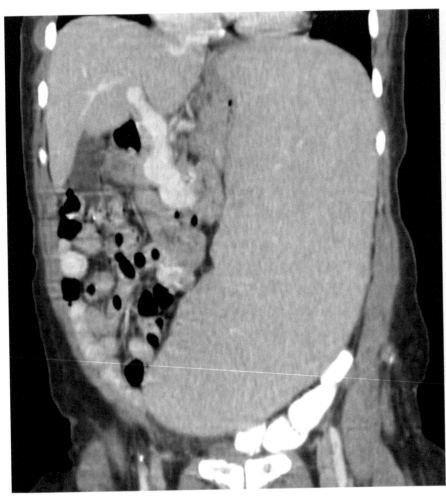

Fig. 51.1 CT coronal image with intravenous and oral contrast demonstrates marked enlargement of the spleen. (Image courtesy of Rocky C. Saenz.)

■ Clinical History

A 43-year-old female with abdominal fullness (▶Fig. 51.1).

■ Key Finding

Global enlargement of the spleen.

■ Top 3 Differential Diagnoses

- **Portal hypertension:** Portal hypertension is the most common cause of splenomegaly. This is classically due to hepatic cirrhosis; however, other causes of portal hypertension include right-sided heart failure, portal vein thrombosis, Budd–Chiari syndrome, and hepatic fibrosis. MRI may demonstrate characteristic Gamma–Gandy bodies, seen as multiple foci of low T1 and T2 signal. Clinch the diagnosis with associated findings of cirrhosis such as a shrunken liver with nodular surface contour, ascites, and varices.
- **Lymphoma:** Lymphoma is most common malignancy in the spleen. The imaging appearance includes diffuse splenic enlargement, solitary mass, or multiple masses. Other patterns of splenic involvement include solitary mass, multiple masses, or miliary appearance. Enlarged extrasplenic lymph nodes are typically seen. Primary splenic lymphoma is much less common than secondary lymphoma, and should prompt consideration for HIV/AIDS (human immunodeficiency virus/acquired immunodeficiency syndrome). Leukemia is typically a diffuse infiltrative process that can result in massive splenomegaly.
- **Infection:** Infectious splenomegaly often has concurrent hepatomegaly. Consider mononucleosis from Epstein–Barr virus in a young and otherwise healthy patient. In this context, the spleen is particularly susceptible to rupture. Splenomegaly in parasitic involvement can be due to sequestration of the parasitic agent or the immunoglobulin M response from splenic infiltration. Bacterial and fungal etiologies typically result in focal lesions rather than splenomegaly.

■ Additional Diagnostic Considerations

- **Hematologic disorders:** Any cause of extramedullary hematopoiesis can result in hepatosplenomegaly. Hemolytic anemias such as thalassemia are also a cause due to increased sequestration of defective red blood cells. Early in life sickle-cell disease causes splenic enlargement; however, eventually autosplenectomy occurs from repeated infarction.
- **Sarcoidosis:** Hepatosplenomegaly is a frequent manifestation. Numerous hypodense lesions, calcifications, and adenopathy may also be present.

■ Diagnosis

Splenomegaly secondary to leukemia.

✓ Pearls

- Differential for splenomegaly is vast, look for associated imaging findings such as hepatomegaly and adenopathy to narrow the etiologies.
- Splenomegaly often results in convexity of the medial surface (normally concave).
- Complications include splenic rupture and hyperfunctioning spleen resulting in pancytopenia (hypersplenism).

Suggested Readings

Cheson BD, Fisher RI, Barrington SF, et al. Alliance, Australasian Leukaemia and Lymphoma Group. Eastern Cooperative Oncology Group. European Mantle Cell Lymphoma Consortium. Italian Lymphoma Foundation. European Organisation for Research, Treatment of Cancer/Dutch Hemato-Oncology Group, Grupo Español de Médula Ósea, German High-Grade Lymphoma Study Group, German Hodgkin's Study Group, Japanese Lymphorra Study Group, Lymphoma Study Association, NCIC Clinical Trials Group, Nordic Lymphoma Study Group, Southwest Oncology Group, United Kingdom National Cancer Research Institute. Recommendations for initial evaluation, staging, and response assessment of Hodgkin and non-Hodgkin lymphoma: the Lugano classification. J Clin Oncol. 2014; 32(27):3059–3068

Federle MP, Jeffrey RB, Woodward PJ, Borhani A. Diagnostic Imaging: Abdomen. 2nd ed. Philadelphia, PA: Lippincott Williams & Wilkins; 2009

Thipphavong S, Duigenan S, Schindera ST, Gee MS, Philips S. Nonneoplastic, benign, and malignant splenic diseases: cross-sectional imaging findings and rare disease entities. AJR Am J Roentgenol. 2014; 203(2):315–322

Case 52

Timothy McKnight

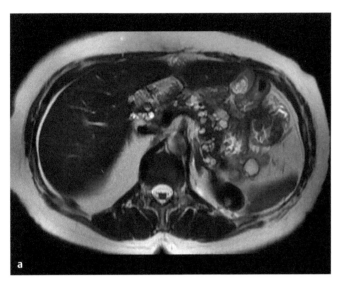

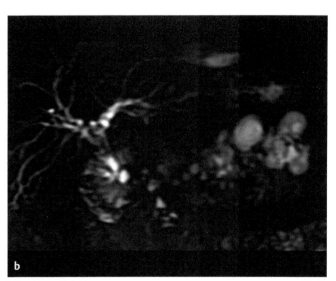

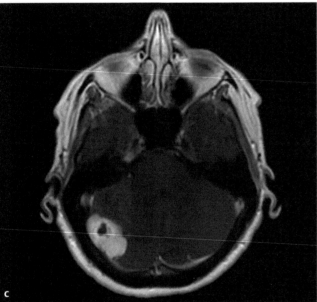

Fig. 52.1 Axial T2 MR image **(a)** and coronal T2 maximum intensity projection MRCP (magnetic resonance cholangiopancreatography) **(b)** images through the pancreas. Innumerable simple cystic lesions throughout the pancreas, no ductal dilation or communication. Axial T1 postgadolinium MR **(c)** patient revealed a cystic enhancing extraaxial neoplasm in the right posterior fossa, subsequently proven to be a hemangioblastoma.

■ Clinical History

A 42-year-old male with abdominal pain (▶ Fig. 52.1).

■ Key Finding

Multiple pancreatic cysts.

■ Top 3 Differential Diagnoses

- **Pseudocysts:** The most common pancreatic cystic lesion and most commonly are multiple. These are the sequelae of pancreatitis beginning as acute peripancreatic fluid collections that persist after 4 weeks organizing with an enhancing pseudocapsule and no internal complex septations or any soft-tissue nodules. Ductal communication is often visible. Pseudocysts may appear complex if complicated by infection or hemorrhage. Present in 20 to 40% of cases of chronic pancreatitis. Most are asymptomatic and nearly 40% will regress spontaneously with no intervention. Complications, symptoms, and failure to regress are more common with size greater than 4 cm.
- **Intraductal papillary mucinous neoplasm (IPMN):** Side branch ductal type IPMN have a unilocular or multilocular cluster of grapes appearance, typically smaller than 3 cm, may communicate with main duct, calcifications in 20%, and typically low grade. There may be multiple small separate clusters suggestive of this diagnosis. Main duct type presents as irregular diffuse ductal dilation usually not as a focal lesion. Both types are present in older patients (sixth to seventh decade). Features of malignant conversion include large size greater than 3 cm, mural nodularity, main duct dilatation greater than 1 cm, mural nodularity, peripheral wall thickening or enhancement, and developing focal distal pancreatic atrophy.
- **Congenital cysts:** Rare, less than 1% of pancreatic cystic lesions, with simple unilocular cysts either solitary or multiple throughout the pancreas. No ductal communication, nodules, calcifications, or septations. These are associated with congenital disorders such as autosomal dominant polycystic kidney disease (ADPCKD), von Hippel–Lindau disease, and cystic fibrosis. Other characteristic imaging features of these disorders offer a clue to diagnosis, such as numerous renal/hepatic cysts for ADPCKD, central nervous system hemangioblastomas, pheochromocytomas, or renal cell carcinoma (RCC) for von Hippel–Lindau, or diffuse fatty replacement of pancreas with cystic fibrosis. There is no neoplastic potential and rarely are symptomatic.

■ Diagnosis

Congenital cysts secondary to von Hippel–Lindau.

✓ Pearls

- Pseudocysts are the most common pancreatic cysts.
- IPMN side branch type will have discrete separate clusters of cysts with ductal communication.
- Congenital cysts are rare, simple, unilocular and have other imaging findings characteristic of the underlying congenital disorder.
- Consider a solitary cluster of cysts as a single complex mass and distinct from this differential. More likely to be neoplastic, either microcystic or macrocystic, in morphology.

Suggested Readings

Demos TC, Posniak HV, Harmath C, Olson MC, Aranha G. Cystic lesions of the pancreas. AJR Am J Roentgenol. 2002; 179(6):1375–1388

Kalb B, Sarmiento JM, Kooby DA, Adsay NV, Martin DR. MR imaging of cystic lesions of the pancreas. Radiographics. 2009; 29(6):1749–1765

Sahani DV, Kambadakone A, Macari M, Takahashi N, Chari S, Fernandez-del Castillo C. Diagnosis and management of cystic pancreatic lesions. AJR Am J Roentgenol. 2013; 200(2):343–354

Case 53

Timothy McKnight

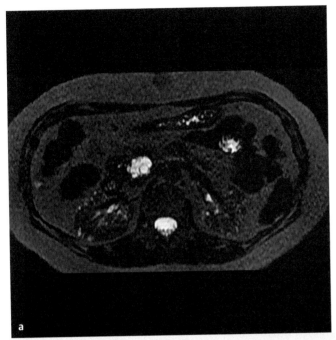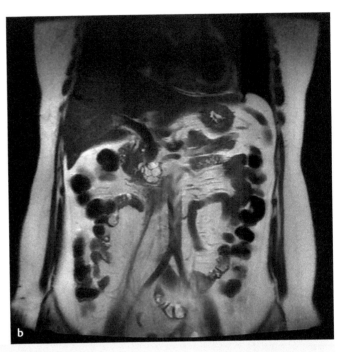

Fig. 53.1 MRI axial (**a**) heavy T2-weighted and (**b**) coronal T2 HASTE (Half-Fourier Acquisition Single-shot Turbo spin Echo) from through the pancreas demonstrates a complex multilocular cystic mass in the pancreatic uncinate process.

■ Clinical History

A 68-year-old female with abdominal pain (▶ Fig. 53.1).

■ Key Finding

Multilocular cystic pancreatic head/uncinate lesion.

■ Top 3 Differential Diagnoses

- **Intraductal papillary mucinous neoplasm (IPMN):** Side branch ductal type IPMN have a unilocular or multilocular cluster of grapes appearance, typically smaller than 3 cm, may communicate with main duct, calcifications in 20%, and typically low grade. Main duct type presents as irregular diffuse ductal dilation usually not as a focal mass/cysts. Both types are present in older patients (sixth to seventh decade). Worrisome features for conversion to invasive malignancy requiring resection include large size greater than 3 cm, mural nodularity, main duct dilatation greater than 1 cm, mural nodularity, peripheral wall thickening or enhancement, and developing focal distal pancreatic atrophy.
- **Serous cystadenoma (SCA):** Complex microcystic, multilocular cystic lesion with a "honeycomb" appearance, typically more than six locules each less than 2 cm, usually less than 1 cm, and may be so small, as to give one the appearance of solid lesion. A central scar is present in 20 to 30% with calcifications.

SCA presents sixth to seventh decade in women, 3:1 over men, and 70% found in body/tail and 30% in pancreatic head. The cyst content is high glycogen, low mucin, and low CEA (< 5 ng/mL). SCA has a low malignant potential and is usually followed with serial imaging. It is resected when it is larger than 4 cm or becomes symptomatic.
- **Mucinous cystic neoplasm (MCN):** Unilocular or multilocular cystic mass with septations, which may be thick or calcify, no main duct communication and is considered premalignant. Any mural nodularity suggests conversion to invasive malignancy. Typically, MCN is oligocystic with less than six locules that are macrocystic, less than 2 cm each. Most are in the pancreatic body and tail. It is most commonly seen in women (fourth to sixth decade). Cystic contents include elevate mucin, absent glycogen, and elevated CEA (> 192 ng/mL). Resection is usually performed due to the malignant potential.

■ Additional Diagnostic Considerations

- **Pseudocyst:** Most common pancreatic cystic lesion. Usually unilocular with simple fluid density, but may appear complex if complicated by infection or hemorrhage. Present in 20 to 40% of cases of chronic pancreatitis. A sequelae of pancreatitis beginning as acute peripancreatic fluid collection that persists after 4 weeks organizing with an enhancing pseudocapsule and no internal complex septations nor any soft-tissue nodules. Ductal communication is often visible.
- **Cystic neuroendocrine tumor:** Larger lesions more than 5 cm more likely to be heterogeneous, cystic, necrotic, with

calcifications and less likely to be clinically functional. Hypervascular solid mass areas will still likely be visible. Insulinoma is the most common (50%), followed by gastrinoma (25%). Gastrinomas are more likely to demonstrate malignant behavior, approximately 60%, than insulinomas, only 10%. Associated syndromes include multiple endocrine neoplasia type 1, von Hippel–Lindau disease, neurofibromatosis type 1, and tuberous sclerosis.

■ Diagnosis

IPMN, side branch type.

✓ Pearls

- Side branch IPMN likely with cluster of grapes morphology, older patient, and ductal communication.

- SCA has many locules each less than 2 cm, a central scar, older women, and high glycogen.
- MCN presents in middle age women.

Suggested Readings

Brounts LR, Lehmann RK, Causey MW, Sebesta JA, Brown TA. Natural course and outcome of cystic lesions in the pancreas. Am J Surg. 2009; 197(5):619–622, discussion 622–623

Kalb B, Sarmiento JM, Kooby DA, Adsay NV, Martin DR. MR imaging of cystic lesions of the pancreas. Radiographics. 2009; 29(6):1749–1765

Sahani DV, Kambadakone A, Macari M, Takahashi N, Chari S, Fernandez-del Castillo C. Diagnosis and management of cystic pancreatic lesions. AJR Am J Roentgenol. 2013; 200(2):343–354

Case 54

Rocky C. Saenz

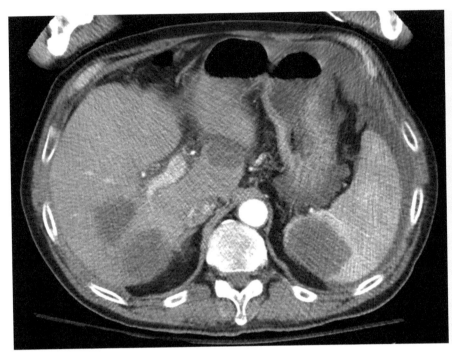

Fig. 54.1 Contrast enhanced axial CT image through the liver and spleen demonstrate a single hypodense splenic lesion and multiple hypodense liver lesions. Free fluid is seen in the left upper quadrant.

■ Clinical History

A 55-year-old male with weight loss (▶ Fig. 54.1).

■ Key Finding

Splenic low-density lesion.

■ Top 3 Differential Diagnoses

- **Metastases:** Any primary malignancy can metastasize to the spleen, but the more common primary malignancies involved include malignant melanoma, lung, and breast carcinomas. Metastatic disease to the spleen is often asymptomatic and is usually found in later stage cancers. Imaging findings depend on the primary tumor type, but lesions are often hypoattenuating and multiple. An exceedingly rare complication of splenic metastases is spontaneous splenic rupture, with metastatic choriocarcinoma, melanoma, and lung cancer accounting for the majority of the cases.
- **Cyst:** Splenic cyst includes true, epithelial cell lined and false or pseudocysts. These lesions on MRI follow fluid signal on T1- and T2-weighted imaging. Most importantly, on CT and MRI no contrast enhancement is seen. Pseudocysts on CT may show peripheral calcifications, which are typically not seen with epithelial cysts. False cysts are usually related to a history of trauma.
- **Abscess:** Splenic abscesses are relatively rare, except in the setting of trauma with superimposed infection or in immunosuppressed patients. In the immunosuppressed patient population, candidiasis is a leading cause of splenic abscess formation. Characteristic imaging findings are ring-enhancing, less than a centimeter in diameter lesions, usually round in shape. Ultrasound reveals multiple target lesions. Antimicrobial therapy is first-line treatment; percutaneous drainage is employed for larger organized collections.

■ Additional Diagnostic Considerations

- **Lymphoma/leukemia:** Lymphomatous/leukemic involvement of the spleen is relatively common. Although splenomegaly is the most common manifestation, the presence of multiple hypoattenuating splenic masses is not unusual. Extrasplenic nodal enlargement supports the diagnosis of lymphoma.
- **Multiple splenic infarcts:** Splenic infarcts typically present as irregularly shaped, peripherally based hypoattenuating lesions. Hematologic disorders (e.g., sickle cell anemia) and embolization of arterial clots (e.g., left heart thrombi in the setting of myocardial infarction) are frequent etiologies. Splenic infarcts are clinically occult in approximately 30% of cases. Prognosis depends on the underlying cause, but most cases result in no significant long-term sequelae.

■ Diagnosis

Metastasis.

✓ Pearls

- Splenic metastasis usually occurs after the liver is involved.
- Candidiasis is the favored diagnosis in the immunosuppressed patients.
- Splenic cysts should be considered with nonenhancing lesions.

Suggested Readings

Elsayes KM, Narra VR, Mukundan G, Lewis JS, Jr, Menias CO, Heiken JP. MR imaging of the spleen: spectrum of abnormalities. Radiographics. 2005; 25(4):967–982
Federle MP, Jeffrey RB, Woodward PJ, Borhani A. Diagnostic Imaging: Abdomen. 2nd ed. Philadelphia, PA: Lippincott Williams & Wilkins; 2009
Rabushka LS, Kawashima A, Fishman EK. Imaging of the spleen: CT with supplemental MR examination. Radiographics. 1994; 14(2):307–332

Case 55

Timothy McKnight

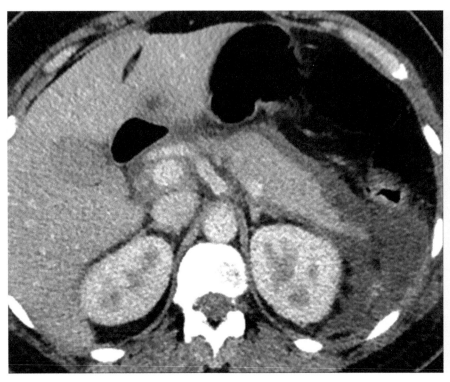

Fig. 55.1 Contrast enhanced axial CT image through the pancreas demonstrates pancreatic diffuse enlargement with extensive peripancreatic inflammatory fat stranding and peripancreatic nonencapsulated fluid collection extending across anterior pararenal space to lateral conal fascia.

■ Clinical History

A 30-year-old with acute epigastric pain (▶ Fig. 55.1).

■ Key Finding

Pancreatic peripheral fat stranding.

■ Top 3 Differential Diagnoses

- **Acute pancreatitis:** Interstitial edematous pancreatitis represents majority of pancreatitis (80%) using the Revised Atlanta Criteria Nomenclature. The most common causes include alcoholism and common duct obstruction from gallstones. Typical features on CT and MR are pancreatic focal or diffuse enlargement with interstitial and peripancreatic fat stranding/edema. Acute peripancreatic nonencapsulated fluid collections are common and when persistent they may develop into pseudocysts. Combined intra- and peripancreatic collections (70%) or areas of absent parenchymal enhancement indicate necrosis, acutely termed acute necrotic collections or chronically termed walled of necrosis. Other complications include infected necrosis, venous thrombosis, and pseudoaneurysm.
- **Autoimmune pancreatitis:** Pancreatic manifestation of immunoglobulin G4 sclerosing disease. It may be associated with other autoimmune disorders including inflammatory bowel disease, Sjogren, retroperitoneal fibrosis, primary biliary cirrhosis, primary sclerosing cholangitis, and systemic lupus erythematosus. It is also seen with 2 to 11% of recurrent pancreatitis. The male to female ratio is 15:2. A diffuse pattern is the most common with a swollen *sausage-like* pancreas (in the absence of atrophy, peripancreatic fluid, and duct dilation). When it is focal, it appears as hypodense "mass" with delayed enhancement and areas of ductal stenosis (can mimic carcinoma).
- **Pancreatic adenocarcinoma:** Glandular histology embedded in desmoplastic stroma accounts for the typical hypodense appearance on CT. Primary tumor location: 60% head, 15% body, 5% tail, and 20% diffuse involvement. Diffuse involvement may mimic pancreatitis. Secondary signs of carcinoma include focal pancreatic enlargement, upstream pancreas atrophy, and dilated or abrupt cutoff of main pancreatic and common bile ducts.

■ Additional Diagnostic Considerations

- **Duodenal ulcer:** Duodenal bulb most common location (95%). Inflammatory fat stranding, edema, and extravasated fluid around the bulb, which can extend across anterior pararenal space to secondarily, involve the pancreatic region. Most common etiologies include *Helicobacter pylori* and nonsteroidal anti-inflammatory drugs (NSAIDs).
- **Lymphoma:** Primary pancreatic lymphoma is rare, less than 1% of pancreatic tumors, more commonly seen with secondary involvement from diffuse abdominal lymphoma. Two forms include solitary mildly hypodense mass with minimal enhancement and diffuse pancreatic involvement with enlargement. It can mimic pancreatitis. Lymphoma classically encases surrounding vessels but rarely narrows or occludes. Ductal dilation and parenchymal atrophy are rarely seen.

■ Diagnosis

Acute pancreatitis (interstitial edematous pancreatitis).

✓ Pearls

- Acute pancreatitis often has associated fluid collections and history of alcoholism or obstructing stone.
- Autoimmune pancreatitis has *sausage*-shaped enlarged pancreas and elevated immunoglobulin G4.
- Infiltrating neoplasms have secondary signs such as ductal dilation, atrophy, metastases, or adenopathy.

Suggested Readings

Al-Hawary MM, Francis IR, Chari ST, et al. Pancreatic ductal adenocarcinoma radiology reporting template: consensus statement of the Society of Abdominal Radiology and the American Pancreatic Association. Radiology. 2014; 270(1):248–260

Jayaraman MV, Mayo-Smith WW, Movson JS, Dupuy DE, Wallach MT. CT of the duodenum: an overlooked segment gets its due. Radiographics. 2001; 21(Spec No):S147–S160

Zhao K, Adam SZ, Keswani RN, Horowitz JM, Miller FH. Acute pancreatitis: Revised Atlanta Classification and the role of cross-sectional imaging. AJR Am J Roentgenol. 2015; 205(1):W32–41

Case 56

Timothy McKnight

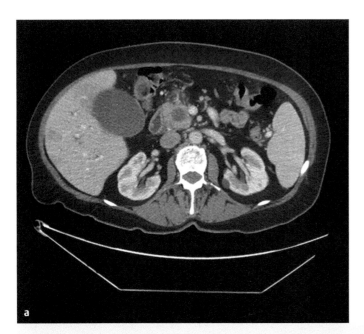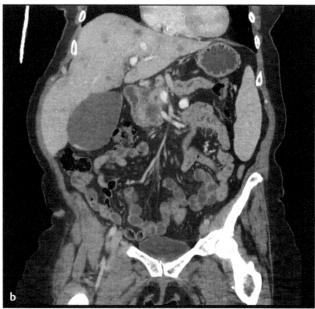

Fig. 56.1 (a) Intravenous contrast enhanced axial CT through the pancreatic head demonstrates a solitary hypodense lesion. The fat planes around the superior mesenteric artery (SMA) and superior mesenteric vein (SMV) are preserved. A vague hypodense lesion in the right hepatic lobe is present. **(b)** Intravenous contrast-enhanced abdominal coronal CT reformats again demonstrates the solitary hypodense pancreas lesion. Also noted is associated mild pancreatic ductal dilation, multiple hypodense liver lesions (metastases), and cholelithiasis.

▪ Clinical History

A 60-year-old with abdominal pain and weight loss (▶Fig. 56.1).

■ Key Finding

Solitary solid pancreas mass.

■ Top 3 Differential Diagnoses

- **Pancreatic adenocarcinoma:** Glandular histology embedded in desmoplastic stroma accounts for the typical hypodense appearance on CT. Contrast-enhanced multiphase CT sensitivity and specificity 85 and 95%, respectively. Primary tumor location: 60% head, 15% body, 5% tail, and 20% diffuse involvement. Secondary signs include focal pancreatic enlargement, upstream pancreas atrophy, and dilated or abrupt cutoff of main pancreatic and common bile ducts ("double duct" sign), present in up to 50% of cases. CA19–9 serum marker may be elevated. Known risk factors include smoking, chronic pancreatitis, gastric surgery, diabetes, radiation, industrial chemical exposure, and syndromes such as hereditary non-polyposis colorectal cancer (HNPCC) or Peutz–Jeghers.
- **Islet cell/neuroendocrine tumor:** These are hypervascular tumors with intense arterial phase enhancement. Metastatic lesions usually involve the liver and lymph nodes, which are also hypervascular. Lesions less than 3 cm more likely to be functional/syndromic. Insulinoma is the most common (50%) and the second most common is gastrinoma (25%). Associated hereditary syndromes include multiple endocrine neoplasia type 1 and von Hippel–Lindau disease.
- **Metastasis:** Metastatic disease involving the pancreas is uncommon and typically seen in cases of disseminated metastases. Most common primaries include renal cell, lung, breast, colon, and melanoma. Metastasis are usually solitary approximately 70% of cases with multiple lesions seen less commonly. Secondary signs of ductal dilation and vessel encasement are uncommon with metastasis. CT enhancement characteristics are variable but similar to the primary carcinoma.

■ Additional Diagnostic Considerations

Lymphoma: Primary pancreatic lymphoma is rare, less than 1% of pancreatic tumors, more commonly seen with secondary involvement from diffuse abdominal lymphoma. Non-Hodgkin's B-cell type with increased incidence in immunocompromised patients and elderly patients. Two forms include solitary mildly hypodense mass with minimal enhancement and diffuse pancreatic involvement with enlargement. May mimic pancreatitis. May encase surrounding vessels but rarely narrow or occlude. Ductal dilation and parenchymal atrophy are rarely seen.

■ Diagnosis

Pancreatic ductal adenocarcinoma.

✓ Pearls

- Pancreatic adenocarcinoma is typically a solitary hypodense mass with ductal dilation.
- Neuroendocrine tumors are classically hypervascular.
- Metastases and lymphoma most commonly seen with disseminated disease.

Suggested Readings

Al-Hawary MM, Francis IR, Chari ST, et al. Pancreatic ductal adenocarcinoma radiology reporting template: consensus statement of the Society of Abdominal Radiology and the American Pancreatic Association. Radiology. 2014; 270(1):248–260

Tamm EP, Balachandran A, Bhosale PR, et al. Imaging of pancreatic adenocarcinoma: update on staging/resectability. Radiol Clin North Am. 2012; 50(3):407–428

Tamm EP, Silverman PM, Charnsangavej C, Evans DB. Diagnosis, staging, and surveillance of pancreatic cancer. AJR Am J Roentgenol. 2003; 180(5):1311–1323

Case 57

Rocky C. Saenz

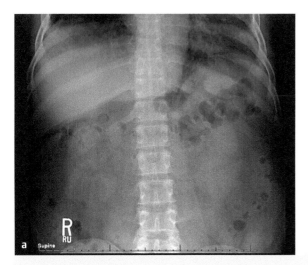 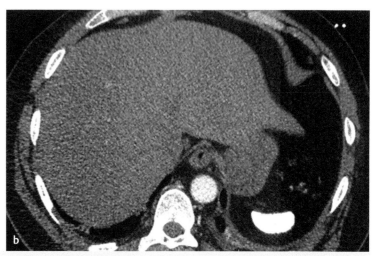

Fig. 57.1 **(a)** Abdominal X-ray demonstrates an oval shaped calcific density in the left upper quadrant. **(b)** CT axial image with intravenous contrast shows a shrunken, calcified spleen.

■ Clinical History

A 48-year-old female with general abdominal pain (▶ Fig. 57.1).

■ Key Finding

Shrunken calcified spleen.

■ Diagnosis

- **Autosplenectomy:** Autosplenectomy refers to infarction of the spleen leading to a calcified shrunken appearance. This classically occurs with homozygous sickle cell patients. The distorted red blood cells have a sickle shape that leads to accumulation, sickling. Sickling then leads to microvascular obstruction leading to infarction. This may occur in multiple organs. Sickle cell disease is autosomal recessive. Other complications include seen on imaging are cholelithiasis, papillary necrosis, salmonella osteomyelitis, and acute chest syndrome.

  On X-ray and CT, the spleen will be high density secondary to calcifications. On MRI, it is of low signal on T1- and T2-weighted images. Low T2 signal on MRI involving the splenic parenchyma can also be seen with secondary hemochromatosis. No enhancement is seen within the parenchyma.

✓ Pearls

- Autosplenectomy most commonly is secondary to homozygous sickle cell disease.
- Secondary signs of sickle cell disease such as "H-shaped" vertebral bodies maybe helpful.
- Low T2 signal within the spleen can also be seen with secondary hemochromatosis.

Suggested Readings

Adler DD, Glazer GM, Aisen AM. MRI of the spleen: normal appearance and findings in sickle-cell anemia. AJR Am J Roentgenol. 1986; 147(4):843–845

Magid D, Fishman EK, Siegelman SS. Computed tomography of the spleen and liver in sickle cell disease. AJR Am J Roentgenol. 1984; 143(2):245–249

Thipphavong S, Duigenan S, Schindera ST, Gee MS, Philips S. Nonneoplastic, benign, and malignant splenic diseases: cross-sectional imaging findings and rare disease entities. AJR Am J Roentgenol. 2014; 203(2):315–322

Case 58

Rocky C. Saenz

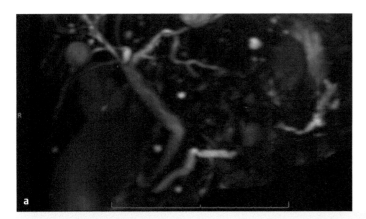
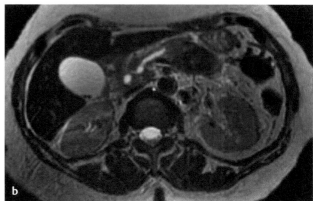

Fig. 58.1 Top, MRI T2-weighted maximum intensity projection through the extrahepatic ducts shows a portion of the pancreatic duct not visible with dilation in the tail with side-branch dilation. Bottom, T2-weighted axial image shows a low signal lesion in the pancreatic duct and its side branches are also markedly dilated. Also seen are choleliths.

■ **Clinical History**

A 80-year-old female with epigastric pain (▶ Fig. 58.1).

■ Key Finding

A portion of the pancreatic ducts is not visible, the "duct cutoff" sign.

■ Top 3 Differential Diagnoses

- **Pancreatic carcinoma:** It represents the most common malignant exocrine pancreatic tumor (>75%). A pancreatic mass can obstruct the pancreatic duct and may result in non-visualization of a portion of the duct (the duct cutoff sign). The overwhelming majority of these tumors are ductal adenocarcinomas. These are considered nonresectable when there is vascular encasement or distant metastasis. Risk factors include smoking, recurrent pancreatitis, fatty diet, and diabetes. Poor prognosis despite surgical intervention (20% in 5 years). Tumors are treated with a Whipple's resection (pancreaticoduodenectomy).
- **Acute pancreatitis:** Interstitial edematous pancreatitis represents majority of pancreatitis. The focal or diffuse pancreatic edema can result in portions of the narrowing and post-stenotic dilation. When pancreatitis is focal (e.g., groove pancreatitis), it can mimic a mass. Cross-sectional imaging is only used to evaluate the severity of the disease. Pancreatitis is a clinical and laboratory diagnosis. Patients usually present with epigastric pain radiating to the back. Acute pancreatitis is usually treated with bowel rest (NPO) and supportive therapy. Surgical intervention may be needed in advanced cases.
- **Islet cell/neuroendocrine neoplasm (NEN):** NENs are endocrine tumors divided into hyperfunctioning and nonhyperfunctioning (the former being most common). The most common hyperfunctioning tumor is insulinoma followed by gastrinoma, glucagonoma, and vasoactive intestinal peptideoma. Insulinomas uncommonly have metastasis while the majority of all other hyperfunctioning NEN have metastasis. Insulinomas are usually less than 2 cm in size. All NEN are hypervascular on dynamic liver studies. Nonhyperfunctioning NENs tend to be larger in size with the absence of vascular encasement.

■ Additional Diagnostic Considerations

- **Lymphoma:** Primary pancreatic lymphoma is rare, representing less than 1% of pancreatic tumors. It is more commonly seen with secondary involvement from diffuse abdominal lymphoma. Non-Hodgkin's B-cell type with increased incidence in immunocompromised patients and very elderly patients. Two forms include solitary mildly hypodense mass with minimal enhancement and diffuse pancreatic involvement with enlargement. It can mimic pancreatitis and can also encase surrounding vessels. Ductal dilation and parenchymal atrophy are rarely seen.
- **Metastasis:** Metastatic disease involving the pancreas is uncommon and typically seen in cases of advanced metastatic disease. Most common primaries include renal cell, lung, breast, colon, and melanoma. The most common presentation is a solitary lesion (70% of cases).

■ Diagnosis

Pancreatic adenocarcinoma.

✓ Pearls

- Pancreatic "duct cutoff" sign is seen, a mass must be excluded.
- Only consider a metastatic pancreatic lesion with advanced metastasis.
- NENs represent 5% of all pancreatic tumors.

Suggested Readings

Federle MP, Jeffrey RB, Woodward PJ, Borhani A. Diagnostic Imaging: Abdomen. 2nd ed. Philadelphia, PA: Lippincott Williams & Wilkins; 2009

Tamm EP, Balachandran A, Bhosale PR, et al. Imaging of pancreatic adenocarcinoma: update on staging/resectability. Radiol Clin North Am. 2012; 50(3):407–428

Theoni R. Pancreatic neoplasms. J Am Osteopath Coll Radiol. 2012; 1(4):10–21

Case 59

Timothy McKnight

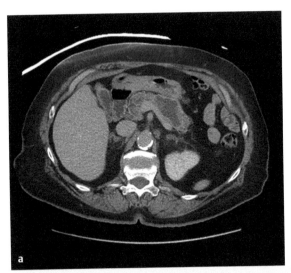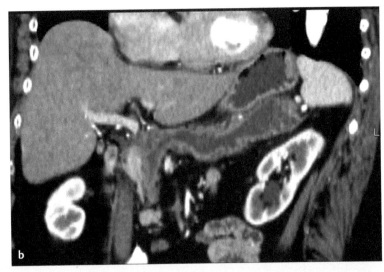

Fig. 59.1 Intravenous contrast-enhanced axial **(a)** and coronal curve planar reformat **(b)**. CT images through the pancreas demonstrate diffuse irregular marked ductal dilation with intraductal mural nodules.

■ Clinical History

An 85-year-old female with abdominal pain (▶ Fig. 59.1).

■ Key Finding

Pancreatic ductal dilation.

■ Top 3 Differential Diagnoses

- **Ductal adenocarcinoma:** Glandular histology embedded in desmoplastic stroma accounts for the typical hypodense appearance on CT. Ductal adenocarcinoma usually has no intraductal nodularity, and its degree of dilation not as severe as intraductal papillary mucinous neoplasm (IPMN). Secondary signs include focal pancreatic enlargement, upstream pancreas atrophy, and dilated or abrupt cutoff of main pancreatic and common bile ducts ("double duct" sign), present in up to 50% of cases. CA19–9 serum marker may be elevated. Known risk factors include smoking, chronic pancreatitis, gastric surgery, diabetes, radiation, industrial chemical exposure, and syndromes such as hereditary non-polyposis colorectal cancer (HNPCC) or Peutz–Jeghers.
- **Chronic pancreatitis:** Repeated episodes of inflammation cause proteinaceous material and calcium carbonate to obstruct the ducts resulting in ductal ectasia and progressive periductal fibrosis. This results in classic appearance with irregular ductal dilation (68%) often including side branches, parenchymal and intraductal calcifications (54%), and parenchymal atrophy (50%). Patients usually have a history of chronic alcoholism (70% of cases), obstructing biliary stones, chronic smoking, or cystic fibrosis.
- **Intraductal papillary mucinous tumor (IPMT):** Cystic neoplasm with three types: main duct, side branch, and mixed type. Age is typically over 65 years and more common in men 2:1. Main duct type causes diffuse main duct dilation. Small IPMTs are usually benign. Increased risk of malignancy is associated with ductal dilation 1cm or greater, intraductal nodules, or intraductal calcifications seen in only 20%. Frank mucin pouring out of the ampulla is evident on endoscopy.

■ Additional Diagnostic Considerations

- **Choledocholithiasis:** Typically seen is biliary dilatation, cholelithiasis (95%) and clinical obstructive jaundice. Detection gold standard is endoscopic retrograde cholangiopancreatography (ERCP), but magnetic resonance cholangiopancreatography (MRCP) sensitivity and specificity are both 80 to 100%. CT "bull's-eye" sign with rim of low-density bile around calcified stone is 60 to 80% sensitive.
- **Ampullary carcinoma:** Imaging features overlap with pancreatic ductal adenocarcinoma. CT findings of low-density mass at the ampulla of Vater and common bile duct dilation are seen in most cases, whereas pancreatic duct obstruction in only 50%. Pancreatic atrophy is uncommon. There is increased risk of hereditary polyposis syndromes. The survival rate is usually better than pancreatic carcinoma due to earlier ductal obstruction and earlier detection.

■ Diagnosis

Intraductal papillary mucinous tumor, main duct type.

✓ Pearls

- Ductal dilation over 1cm with intraductal nodules favors IPMT main duct type.
- Solid low-density mass on CT with ductal dilation is most likely ductal adenocarcinoma.
- Pancreatic ductal dilation, atrophy, and calcifications favors chronic pancreatitis.

Suggested Readings

Edge MD, Hoteit M, Patel AP, Wang X, Baumgarten DA, Cai Q. Clinical significance of main pancreatic duct dilation on computed tomography: single and double duct dilation. World J Gastroenterol. 2007; 13(11):1701–1705

Javadi S, Menias CO, Korivi BR, et al. Pancreatic Calcifications and Calcified Pancreatic Masses: Pattern Recognition Approach on CT. AJR Am J Roentgenol. 2017; 209(1):77–87

Kim JH, Hong SS, Kim YJ, Kim JK, Eun HW. Intraductal papillary mucinous neoplasm of the pancreas: differentiate from chronic pancreatitis by MR imaging. Eur J Radiol. 2012; 81(4):671–676

Case 60

Sarika N. Joshi

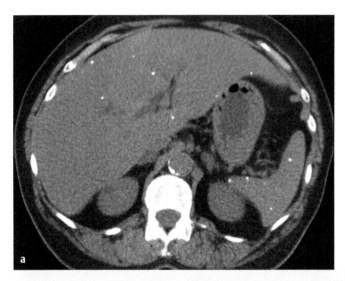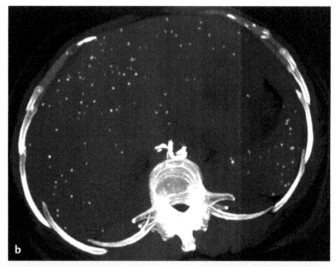

Fig. 60.1 Top image, CT axial image without contrast demonstrates scattered punctate calcifications involving the spleen and liver. Bottom image, CT maximum intensity projection shows more extensive involvement with parenchymal calcifications in the liver and spleen. (Images courtesy of Rocky C. Saenz.)

■ **Clinical History**

A 67-year-old female with abdominal pain (▶ Fig. 60.1).

■ Key Finding

Multiple splenic parenchymal calcifications.

■ Top 3 Differential Diagnoses

- **Sequelae of microabscesses:** This represents the significant majority of causes of calcified granulomas. Histoplasmosis is the most common and the favored diagnosis if more than five calcifications are present. Immunocompromised patients may have mycobacterial infection or less commonly seen pneumocystic infection.
- **Sarcoidosis:** Splenic calcifications may be seen as a chronic manifestation of sarcoidosis. Multiple small hypodense nodules can eventually calcify leading to this appearance.

- **Treated lymphoma:** One of the many manifestations of splenic lymphoma is multiple parenchymal lesions. After successful treatment of the splenic lesions, some may calcify. In addition, lymphoma will typically have abdominal lymph nodes that when treated may also have calcifications.

■ Additional Diagnostic Considerations

Brucellosis: Brucellosis is a rare bacterial infection typically acquired from infected animals. It can cause splenic calcifications that are large chunky calcifications.

■ Diagnosis

Calcified granulomas from histoplasmosis.

✓ Pearls

- Calcified splenic foci are most commonly secondary to old healed histoplasmosis.
- Lymphoma will typically have calcified abdominal lymph nodes.

- Splenic granulomas are typically benign.

Suggested Readings

Johnson C. Mayo Clinic Gastrointestinal Imaging Review. Rochester, MN: Mayo Clinic Scientific Press; 2005

Ricci ZJ, Oh SK, Chernyak V, et al. Improving diagnosis of atraumatic splenic lesions, part I: nonneoplastic lesions. Clin Imaging. 2016; 40(4):769–779

Case 61

Timothy McKnight

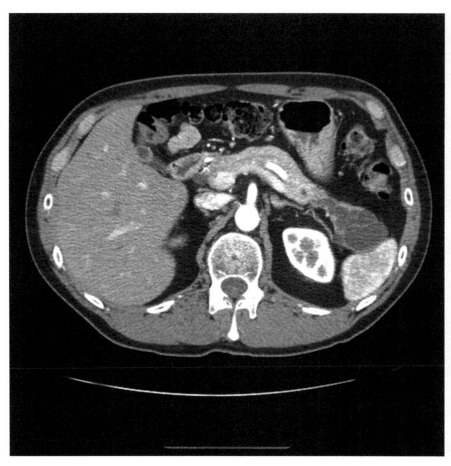

Fig. 61.1 Intravenous contrast-enhanced axial CT image through the pancreas demonstrates a complex multilocular cystic lesion in the tail. Multiple large locules and no focal duct communication. No mural nodules or calcifications are seen.

■ Clinical History

A 52-year-old female with nausea (▶Fig. 61.1).

■ Key Finding

Multilocular cystic pancreatic tail lesion.

■ Top 3 Differential Diagnoses

- **Mucinous cystic neoplasm (MCN):** Unilocular or multilocular cystic mass with septations, which may be thick or calcify, no main duct communication, and is considered premalignant. Any mural nodularity suggests conversion to invasive malignancy. Typically, MCN is oligocystic with less than six locules, which are macrocystic (> 2 cm each). Most are in the pancreatic body and tail. It is most commonly seen in middle-aged women (fourth to sixth decade). Cystic contents include elevate mucin, absent glycogen, and elevated CEA (> 192 ng/mL). Resection is usually performed due to the malignant potential.
- **Intraductal papillary mucinous neoplasm (IPMN):** Side branch ductal type IPMN have a unilocular or multilocular cluster of grapes appearance, typically smaller than 3 cm, may communicate with main duct, calcifications in 20%, and typically low grade. Main duct type presents as irregular diffuse ductal dilation usually not as a focal mass/cysts. Both types present in older patients (sixth to seventh decade). Worrisome features for conversion to invasive malignancy requiring resection include large size more than 3 cm, mural nodularity, main duct dilatation more than 1 cm, mural nodularity, peripheral wall thickening or enhancement, and developing focal distal pancreatic atrophy.
- **Serous cystadenoma (SCA):** Complex microcystic, multilocular cystic lesion with a "honeycomb" appearance, typically more than six locules each less than 2 cm, usually less than 1 cm, and may be so small as to give appearance of solid lesion. A central scar is present in 20 to 30% with calcifications. It presents in older women (sixth to seventh decade) and occurs three times more often than for men. Approximately 70% are found in body/tail and 30% in pancreatic head. The cyst content is high glycogen, low mucin, and low CEA (< 5 ng/mL). SCA has a low malignant potential and is usually followed with serial imaging. It is resected when it is larger than 4 cm or becomes symptomatic.

■ Additional Diagnostic Considerations

- **Pseudocyst:** Most common pancreatic cystic lesion. Usually unilocular with simple fluid density but may be complex appearing if complicated by infection or hemorrhage. Present in 20 to 40% of cases of chronic pancreatitis. A sequelae of pancreatitis beginning as acute peripancreatic fluid collection that persists after 4 weeks organizing with an enhancing pseudocapsule and no internal complex septations nor any soft tissue nodules. Ductal communication is often visible.
- **Cystic neuroendocrine tumor:** Larger lesions greater than 5 cm more likely to be heterogeneous, cystic, necrotic, have calcifications, and less likely to be clinically functional. Hypervascular solid mass areas will still likely be visible. Insulinoma is most common (50%) followed by gastrinoma (25%). Gastrinomas are more likely to demonstrate malignant behavior, approximately 60%, than insulinomas, only 10%. Associated syndromes include multiple endocrine neoplasia type 1, von Hippel–Lindau disease, neurofibromatosis type 1, and tuberous sclerosis.

■ Diagnosis

MCN.

✓ Pearls

- MCN has few locules each greater than 2 cm, variable mural nodularity, high mucin and CEA.
- MCN was previously termed macrocystic adenoma.
- MCN presents in middle age women while IPMN and SCA are more common in elderly patients.

Suggested Readings

Brounts LR, Lehmann RK, Causey MW, Sebesta JA, Brown TA. Natural course and outcome of cystic lesions in the pancreas. Am J Surg. 2009; 197(5):619–622, discussion 622–623

Kalb B, Sarmiento JM, Kooby DA, Adsay NV, Martin DR. MR imaging of cystic lesions of the pancreas. Radiographics. 2009; 29(6):1749–1765

Sahani DV, Kambadakone A, Macari M, Takahashi N, Chari S, Fernandez-del Castillo C. Diagnosis and management of cystic pancreatic lesions. AJR Am J Roentgenol. 2013; 200(2):343–354

Case 62

Timothy McKnight

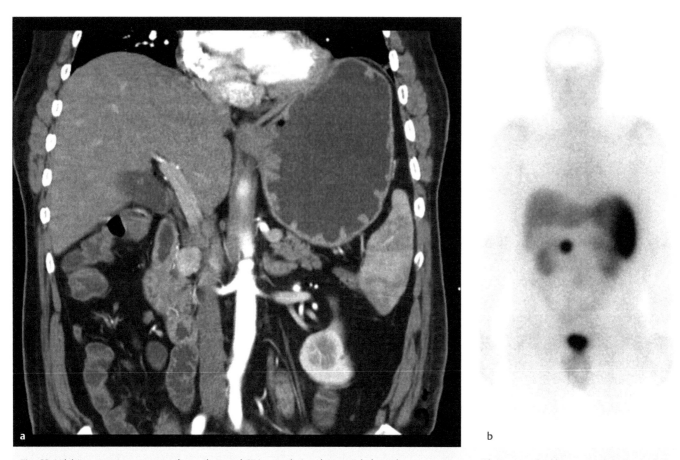

Fig. 62.1 **(a)** Intravenous contrast-enhanced coronal CT image during the arterial phase demonstrates an ovoid circumscribed hypervascular mass in the pancreatic head. **(b)** In-111 OctreoScan planar coronal image through the abdomen demonstrates focal intense uptake in the pancreatic head region corresponding to the mass seen on CT.

■ Clinical History

A 52-year-old male with vague abdominal pain (▶ Fig. 62.1).

■ Key Finding

Solid hypervascular pancreatic mass.

■ Top 3 Differential Diagnoses

- **Islet cell/neuroendocrine tumor:** These appear as hypervascular tumors with intense arterial phase enhancement on CT and MR. Metastases usually involve the liver and lymph nodes and are hypervascular. Lesions greater than 3 cm are more likely to be functional or syndromic. Larger lesions (> 5 cm) are more likely to be heterogeneous, cystic, necrotic, and have calcifications. Insulinoma is the most common (50%), followed by gastrinoma (25%). Gastrinomas are more likely to demonstrate malignant behavior, approximately 60%, than insulinomas, only 10%. Associated syndromes include multiple endocrine neoplasia type 1, von Hippel–Lindau disease, neurofibromatosis type 1, and tuberous sclerosis.
- **Metastasis:** Metastatic disease involving the pancreas is uncommon and typically seen in cases of disseminated metastases. CT enhancement characteristics are variable usually similar to that of a known primary lesion. Renal cell carcinoma (RCC) with hypervascular appearance is the most common and may be indistinguishable from islet cell tumor in absence of visible renal mass. Others including lung, breast, and colon are more commonly hypoattenuating. Metastasis are usually solitary approximately 70% of cases with multiple lesions seen less commonly. Secondary signs of ductal dilation and vessel encasement are uncommon with metastasis. Ductal dilation and vascular encasement are less commonly seen than with primary adenocarcinoma.
- **Pancreatic adenocarcinoma:** Glandular histology embedded in desmoplastic stroma accounts for the typical hypodense appearance on CT. On contrast enhanced multiphase CT, 5 to 11% of lesions may be isoattenuating. Primary tumor location: 60% head, 15% body, 5% tail, and 20% diffuse involvement. Secondary signs include focal pancreatic enlargement, upstream pancreas atrophy, and dilated or abrupt cutoff of main pancreatic and common bile ducts ("double duct" sign), present in up to 50% of cases. CA19–9 serum marker may be elevated. Known risk factors include smoking, chronic pancreatitis, gastric surgery, diabetes, radiation, industrial chemical exposure, and syndromes such as hereditary non-polyposis colorectal cancer (HNPCC) or Peutz–Jeghers.

■ Additional Diagnostic Considerations

- **Serous cystadenoma (SCA):** Coalescence of innumerable small, honeycomb, cystic components and calcified central scar may mimic a solid appearance. The numerous internal enhancing septa may mimic a hypervascular appearance. SCA are benign slow growing and typically asymptomatic. Located in the body and tail (70%), and only 30% in the head. Calcifications is common (40% vs. 16%) in mucinous neoplasm. Most common in elderly females, over 60 years old. Vascular encasement and ductal dilation are rare.
- **Pseudoaneurysm:** In the pancreatic region, it represents a contained arterial rupture most commonly of gastroduodenal or splenic arteries. Etiologies include most commonly acute or chronic pancreatitis, followed by trauma, or iatrogenic. Variable amounts of peripheral mural thrombus present. Hypervascular enhancement equivalent to adjacent arterial contrast and may see direct communication. Significant overall increased mortality of 11%. Treatment with endovascular embolization or surgery.

■ Diagnosis

Gastrinoma.

✓ Pearls

- Neuroendocrine metastases are also hypervascular.
- Metastatic renal cell may be indistinguishable from an islet cell tumor.
- Ductal adenocarcinoma more likely to be hypodense or isoattenuating.

Suggested Readings

Heller MT, Shah AB. Imaging of neuroendocrine tumors. Radiol Clin North Am. 2011; 49(3):529–548, vii

Lewis RB, Lattin GE, Jr, Paal E. Pancreatic endocrine tumors: radiologic-clinicopathologic correlation. Radiographics. 2010; 30(6):1445–1464

Raman SP, Hruban RH, Cameron JL, Wolfgang CL, Fishman EK. Pancreatic imaging mimics: part 2, pancreatic neuroendocrine tumors and their mimics. AJR Am J Roentgenol. 2012; 199(2):309–318

Case 63

Sarika N. Joshi

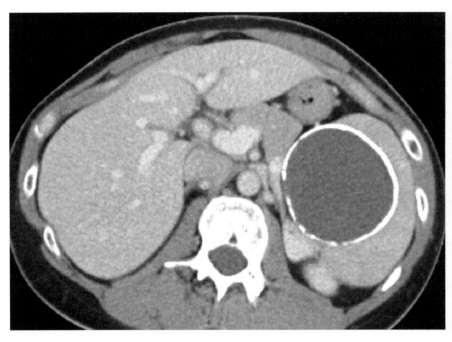

Fig. 63.1 CT axial image with intravenous contrast shows a mostly cystic lesion in the spleen with peripheral calcifications. (Images courtesy of Rocky C. Saenz.)

■ Clinical History

A 31-year-old male with a remote abdominal injury (▶Fig. 63.1).

■ Key Finding

Cystic splenic lesion.

■ Top 3 Differential Diagnoses

• **Splenic cyst:** Posttraumatic cysts represent approximately 75% of all cystic lesions in the spleen. These are considered "false" or pseudocysts because there is no epithelial lining. A "true" epithelial cyst, also called epidermoid cyst, is thought to be congenital. They have a benign appearance with a well-defined margin, thin wall, internal fluid contents, and no enhancement. Posttraumatic cysts may have this manifestation or a more complex appearance with internal debris, a thicker wall, or peripheral calcification. Most are discovered incidentally and of no clinical consequence. Rarely larger cysts may rupture or become superinfected requiring treatment.

• **Pyogenic abscess:** Splenic macroabscess is most commonly bacterial from hematogenous seeding of infection. The imaging appearance is that of a single or multiple hypodense fluid collections that do not internally enhance. Cross-sectional findings include peripheral enhancement, adjacent inflammatory changes or infrequently internal gas. A rare complication is rupture, which can manifest as adjacent complex free fluid or subcapsular fluid.

• **Splenic infarction:** Infarcts are peripherally based lesions with no internal enhancement. Capsular enhancement may be observed due to a separate blood supply. Subacute or chronic infarcts will often have fluid attenuation. Infarcts are classically wedge-shaped but in the spleen are often irregular or linear. Most are idiopathic and clinically occult. A predisposing factor may be present such as sickle-cell disease or embolic phenomenon.

■ Additional Diagnostic Considerations

• **Lymphoma:** Larger lesions can appear cystic or rarely undergo internal necrosis. Clinical features can mimic that of splenic abscess.

• **Splenic laceration:** Appears on CT as an irregular area of hypoattenuation in the splenic parenchyma that is linear or branching. High attenuation on precontrast images suggests hematoma. There is no enhancement on postcontrast images. Look for active extravasation as a change in morphology from arterial to delayed phase images, which is a critical imaging finding.

■ Diagnosis

Posttraumatic cyst.

✓ Pearls

• Posttraumatic cyst is the most common splenic cystic lesion.
• Consider abscess in cystic lesions with peripheral fat stranding or internal gas.
• Straight margins favor an infarction rather than mass or cystic lesion.

Suggested Readings

Boland G. Gastrointestinal Imaging: The Requisites. 4th ed. Philadelphia, PA: Elsevier/Saunders 2014

Hamilton JD, Kumaravel M, Censullo ML, Cohen AM, Kievlan DS, West OC. Multidetector CT evaluation of active extravasation in blunt abdominal and pelvic trauma patients. Radiographics. 2008; 28(6):1603–1616

Ricci ZJ, Mazzariol FS, Flusberg M, et al. Improving diagnosis of atraumatic splenic lesions, part II: benign neoplasms/nonneoplastic mass-like lesions. Clin Imaging. 2016; 40(4):691–704

Case 64

Timothy McKnight

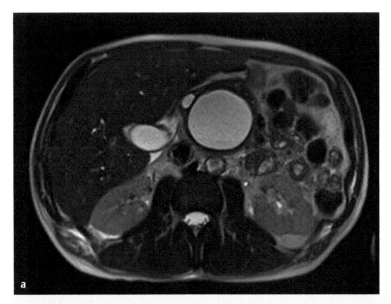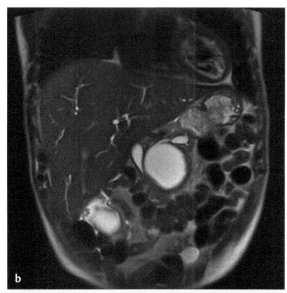

Fig. 64.1 **(a)** Axial T2 HASTE (Half-Fourier Acquisition Single-shot Turbo spin Echo) and **(b)** coronal T2 HASTE MRI images through the pancreas both show a large solitary simple cyst. There is associated ductal dilatation of the common bile duct and main pancreatic duct from regional mass effect. Potential ductal communication visible on the coronal image.

■ **Clinical History**

A 48-year-old male with recurrent abdominal pain (▶Fig. 64.1).

■ Key Finding

Solitary pancreatic unilocular cyst.

■ Top 3 Differential Diagnoses

- **Pseudocyst:** The most common pancreatic cystic lesion and most commonly are multiple. These are the sequelae of pancreatitis beginning as acute peripancreatic fluid collections that persist after 4 weeks organizing with an enhancing pseudocapsule and no internal complex septations or any soft-tissue nodules (ductal communication often visible). Pseudocysts may appear complex if complicated by infection or hemorrhage. Present in 20 to 40% of cases of chronic pancreatitis. Most are asymptomatic and nearly 40% will regress spontaneously with no intervention. Complications, symptoms, and failure to regress are more common with size greater than 4 cm.
- **Mucinous cystic neoplasm (MCN):** Unilocular or multilocular cystic mass with septations, which may be thick or calcify, no main duct communication, and is considered premalignant. Any mural nodularity suggests conversion to invasive malignancy. Typically, MCN is oligocystic with less than six locules; which are macrocystic (> 2 cm each). Most are in the pancreatic body and tail. It is most commonly seen in women (fourth to sixth decade).
- **Intraductal papillary mucinous neoplasm (IPMN):** Side branch ductal type IPMN have a unilocular or multilocular cluster of grapes appearance, typically smaller than 3 cm, may communicate with main duct, calcifications in 20%, and typically low grade. Main duct type presents as irregular diffuse ductal dilation usually not as a focal mass/cysts. Both types present in older patients (sixth to seventh decade). Worrisome features for conversion to invasive malignancy requiring resection include large size greater than 3 cm, mural nodularity, main duct dilatation greater than 1 cm, mural nodularity, peripheral wall thickening or enhancement, and developing focal distal pancreatic atrophy.

■ Additional Diagnostic Considerations

- **Necrotizing Pancreatitis:** Complex fluid collections also resulting from pancreatitis are likely the result of necrosis and include acute necrotic collection if less than 4 weeks old and walled off necrosis if persisting beyond 4 weeks. The may involve parenchyma, peripancreatic fat, or most commonly both (> 75%). Complex fluid may contain nests of partially necrosed fat or blood products. Most are sterile but may become infected, with air bubbles as most specific sign but only present in 15%.
- **Cystic neuroendocrine neoplasm (NEN):** Larger lesions greater than 5 cm more likely to be heterogeneous, cystic, necrotic, have calcifications, and less likely to be clinically functional. Hypervascular solid mass areas will still likely be visible. Insulinoma is most common (50%), followed by gastrinoma (25%). Gastrinomas are more likely to demonstrate malignant behavior, approximately 60%, than insulinomas, only 10%. Associated syndromes include multiple endocrine neoplasia type 1, von Hippel–Lindau disease, neurofibromatosis type 1, and tuberous sclerosis.

■ Diagnosis

Pseudocyst.

✓ Pearls

- Solitary unilocular cyst with a history of pancreatitis is almost always a pseudocyst.
- Solitary large multilocular mass with septations or nodules is suspicious for MCN.
- Complex fluid collections with pancreatitis should raise concern for either necrosis or infection.

Suggested Readings

Kalb B, Sarmiento JM, Kooby DA, Adsay NV, Martin DR. MR imaging of cystic lesions of the pancreas. Radiographics. 2009; 29(6):1749–1765

Sahani DV, Kambadakone A, Macari M, Takahashi N, Chari S, Fernandez-del Castillo C. Diagnosis and management of cystic pancreatic lesions. AJR Am J Roentgenol. 2013; 200(2):343–354

Zhao K, Adam SZ, Keswani RN, Horowitz JM, Miller FH. Acute pancreatitis: Revised Atlanta Classification and the role of cross-sectional imaging. AJR Am J Roentgenol. 2015; 205(1):W32–41

Case 65

Rocky C. Saenz

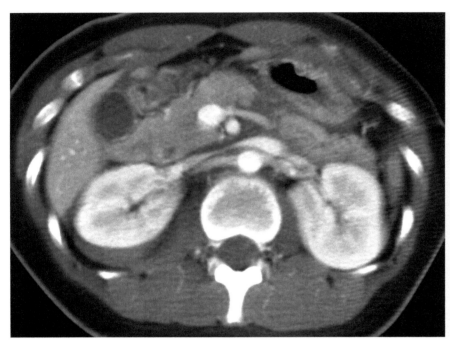

Fig. 65.1 Intravenous contrast-enhanced axial CT through the pancreas demonstrates a pancreatic body focal linear defect which extends thru the pancreatic duct. The fat planes around the SMA and SMV are attenuated. Also noted is a subcapsular hematoma involving the right kidney.

■ **Clinical History**

A 22-year-old male with abdominal pain post trauma (▶Fig. 65.1).

■ Key Finding

Pancreatic parenchymal linear defect.

■ Diagnosis

Pancreatic laceration: Pancreatic injury is not common and only represents 5% of abdominal injuries. Due to its central location in the abdomen, the pancreas is well protected from blunt trauma. It becomes vulnerable in thin and young patients that lack intra-abdominal fat. These injuries occur from direct blunt trauma. Pancreatic injuries are thought to be secondary to compression by the blunt force vector and the spine. Typically, pancreatic injuries occur with other visceral injuries. The pancreatic body is the most common part injured. CT has a sensitivity and specificity of greater than 90% for diagnosing pancreatic injuries.

On CT, hematomas and contusions are hypodense collections involving the pancreatic parenchyma. Lacerations appear as linear defects traversing the pancreas. Commonly peripancreatic fat stranding is seen. When there is loss of attenuation between the pancreas and vessels (SMV [superior mesenteric vein], SMA [superior mesenteric artery], and splenic vein) an injury is likely present. It is imperative to decipher if the laceration involves the pancreatic duct.

These injuries are graded utilizing the American Association for the Surgery of Trauma (AAST). AAST grades are I to V, with V being the most severe. Grades I and II are usually treated conservatively. Grades III to V are parenchymal injuries that include injury to the pancreatic duct. The more serve injuries, grades III to V require surgical intervention due to transection of the pancreatic duct. These injuries increase the morbidity and mortality especially without treatment.

■ Diagnosis

Pancreatic laceration.

✓ Pearls

- Pancreatic laceration extending from the anterior to the posterior margin signifies ductal transection.
- Low attenuation with loss of the fat planes between the pancreas and the vessels is highly suspicious for a pancreatic injury.
- Pancreatic laceration is usually associated with other visceral injuries.

Suggested Readings

Daly KP, Ho CP, Persson DL, Gay SB. Traumatic retroperitoneal injuries: review of multidetector CT findings. Radiographics. 2008; 28(6):1571–1590

Federle MP, Jeffrey RB, Woodward PJ, Borhani A. Diagnostic Imaging: Abdomen. 2nd ed. Philadelphia, PA: Lippincott Williams & Wilkins; 2009

Case 66

Sarika N. Joshi

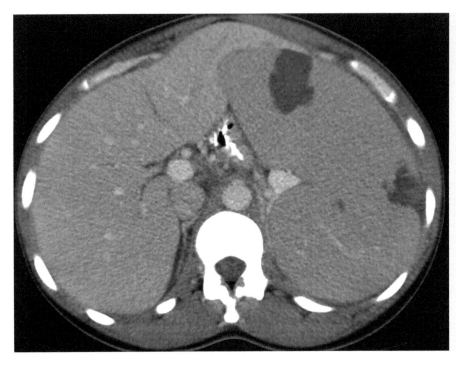

Fig. 66.1 CT axial image with intravenous and oral contrast shows two cystic lesions in the periphery of the spleen. Also, note the enlarged size of the spleen. (Images courtesy of Rocky C. Saenz.)

■ **Clinical History**

A 41-year-old male with left upper quadrant pain (▶ Fig. 66.1).

■ Key Finding

Multiple cystic lesions in the spleen.

■ Top 3 Differential Diagnoses

• **Microabscesses:** These are frequently fungal due to *Candida albicans*, and seen in immunocompromised patients. They are typically multiple, round, and small measuring 5 to 10 mm. Ultrasound demonstrates a characteristic target or bull's-eye lesion with a hyperechoic center and surrounding hypoechoic band. On CT they are usually hypodense but may demonstrate peripheral enhancement. MRI is more sensitive due to the increased T2 signal. Similar appearing lesions can occur in the liver or kidney.

• **Hydatid cysts:** Also called echinococcal cysts, these are due to infection from the tapeworm *Echinococcus granulosus*. Splenic involvement is uncommon, and concomitant liver lesions are usually present. The classic appearance is a sharply defined cystic lesion with or without internal daughter cysts. Collapsed internal membranes can form the "water lily" sign. Peripheral calcification is common. These have traditionally been treated surgically due to the risk of anaphylaxis from spillage of cyst contents. Current treatment options also include percutaneous management and/or drug therapy.

• **Cystic metastases:** The most common primary malignancies to metastasize to the spleen include melanoma, lung, and breast carcinoma. Of these, melanoma has a propensity to form cystic lesions although all can develop internal necrosis. Metastases can also have a target appearance.

■ Additional Diagnostic Considerations

• **Lymphoma:** Larger lesions can appear cystic or rarely undergo internal necrosis. Clinical features can mimic that of splenic abscess.

• **Splenic infarcts:** Splenic infarcts typically present as irregularly shaped, peripherally based hypoattenuating lesions. Subacute to chronic phases can have near fluid attenuation. Hematologic disorders and embolization of arterial clots are frequent etiologies.

■ Diagnosis

Splenic infarcts.

✓ Pearls

• Candidiasis is the favored diagnosis in immunosuppressed patients.

• A target appearance is associated with Candida microabscesses and metastatic lesions.

• Splenic infarcts typically are irregularly shaped and peripherally based.

Suggested Readings

Federle MP, Jeffrey RB, Woodward PJ, Borhani A. Diagnostic Imaging: Abdomen. 2nd ed. Philadelphia, PA: Lippincott Williams & Wilkins; 2009

Johnson C. Mayo Clinic Gastrointestinal Imaging Review. Rochester, MN: Mayo Clinic Scientific Press; 2005

Ricci ZJ, Oh SK, Chernyak V, et al. Improving diagnosis of atraumatic splenic lesions, part I: nonneoplastic lesions. Clin Imaging. 2016; 40(4):769–779

Case 67

Rocky C. Saenz

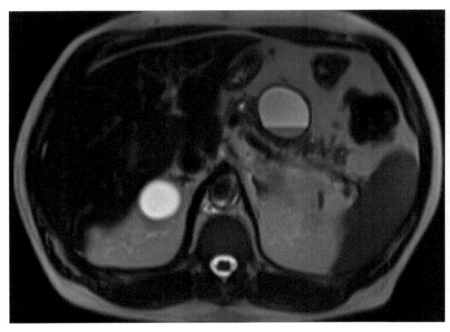

Fig. 67.1 Axial T2 MR images through the pancreas shows a large cyst with a fluid-fluid level. There is pancreatic parenchymal atrophy. Incidentally noted is a cyst projecting from the right kidney.

■ **Clinical History**

A 52-year-old male with recurrent abdominal pain (▶ Fig. 67.1).

■ Key Finding

Pancreatic cyst with a fluid–fluid level.

■ Diagnosis

Pseudocyst: Pseudocysts are the most common pancreatic cystic lesions and most commonly are multiple. These are the sequelae of pancreatitis beginning as acute peripancreatic fluid collections. The fluid persists after 4 weeks organizing with an enhancing pseudocapsule (no internal complex septations or soft-tissue nodules). Pseudocysts may appear complex if complicated by infection or hemorrhage. They are seen in 20 to 40% of chronic pancreatitis cases. Most are asymptomatic and nearly 40% will regress spontaneously with no intervention. Typically, these lesions follow fluid on all cross-sectional studies. When a fluid–fluid level is present the diagnosis is pathognomonic for a pseudocyst. Internal debris is seen layering dependently. Pseudocysts have ductal communication in many cases. When there are communicating lesions with the duct, they tend to reoccur. Complications, symptoms, and failure to regress are more common with size greater than 4 cm.

Interstitial edematous pancreatitis represents majority of pancreatitis using the Revised Atlanta Criteria Nomenclature. Repeated episodes of inflammation cause proteinaceous material and calcium carbonate to obstruct small ducts, resulting in ductal ectasia and progressive periductal fibrosis. This results in the classic triad of findings for chronic pancreatitis: ductal dilation (often including side branches), parenchymal calcifications, and pancreatic atrophy. Patients usually have a history of chronic alcoholism, obstructing biliary stones, chronic smoking, or cystic fibrosis. Pseudocysts that have air are concerning for infection. When pseudocysts become infected or enlarge resulting in mass effect drainage may be indicated.

✓ Pearls

- Fluid–fluid levels in a cyst almost always represent a pseudocyst.
- Pancreatic calcifications, atrophy, and ductal dilatation are characteristic of chronic pancreatitis.

- Air in a pseudocyst should raise concern for an infection.

Suggested Readings

Kalb B, Sarmiento JM, Kooby DA, Adsay NV, Martin DR. MR imaging of cystic lesions of the pancreas. Radiographics. 2009; 29(6):1749–1765

Sahani DV, Kambadakone A, Macari M, Takahashi N, Chari S, Fernandez-del Castillo C. Diagnosis and management of cystic pancreatic lesions. AJR Am J Roentgenol. 2013; 200(2):343–354

Zhao K, Adam SZ, Keswani RN, Horowitz JM, Miller FH. Acute pancreatitis: Revised Atlanta Classification and the role of cross-sectional imaging. AJR Am J Roentgenol. 2015; 205(1):W32:W41

Case 68

Sarika N. Joshi

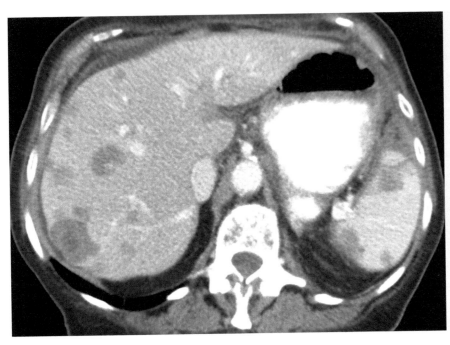

Fig. 68.1 CT axial image with intravenous and oral contrast demonstrates multiple lesions in the liver and spleen. Also seen is free fluid. (Images courtesy of Rocky C. Saenz.)

■ Clinical History

A 77-year-old female with abdominal fullness (▶Fig. 68.1).

■ Key Finding

Multiple splenic masses.

■ Top 3 Differential Diagnoses

• **Metastases:** Splenic metastases are usually found in widespread disseminated malignancy. Isolated splenic metastases are rare and usually asymptomatic. Hematogenous spread is most common due to the rich vascular supply. The most common etiologies of metastasis include melanoma, lung, and breast carcinoma. The imaging appearance varies with the primary neoplasm and can be solid or cystic. Lesions are typically multiple and hypodense on CT with variable enhancement. Percutaneous image-guided biopsy was historically viewed to have a high risk of hemorrhage, but it is now being increasingly performed for diagnosis with low rates of complications.

• **Lymphoma:** This is the most common malignant lesion to affect the spleen. Multifocal lesions are one of four major manifestations in the spleen. The others include diffuse infiltration, solitary lesion, and miliary involvement. Calcification in lesions is rarely seen but can occur after treatment. CT and MRI have low sensitivity for focal involvement as many lesions are infiltrative or subcentimeter. PET/CT has high sensitivity and specificity for splenic involvement and is useful for staging. Concurrent adenopathy is helpful in narrowing the differential diagnosis.

• **Sarcoidosis:** Hepatosplenic involvement of sarcoidosis is present in more than half of autopsy specimens but is usually asymptomatic and occult on imaging. When visible, hepatosplenic nodules are usually numerous, hypodense on CT, and hypointense on all MRI sequences. The nodules hypoenhance relative to splenic parenchyma and tend to be best seen on early phase postcontrast images, becoming less conspicuous on delayed phases. Otherwise imaging findings are nonspecific, including hepatosplenomegaly and lymphadenopathy.

■ Additional Diagnostic Considerations

Multiple splenic infarcts: The classical appearance is a peripherally based wedge-shaped hypodensity. In the spleen atypical presentations such as an irregular or linear shape are common. An infarction can mimic a solid mass; however, there will be no internal enhancement. Capsular enhancement may be observed due to separate blood supply. Arterial thrombosis is commonly due to embolic phenomenon. Venous thrombosis is usually from splenomegaly and diffuse infiltrative disease.

■ Diagnosis

Metastases from ovarian carcinoma.

✓ Pearls

• Splenic metastases occur in advanced cancers with other organs involved.
• PET/CT has significantly higher sensitivity in detecting splenic lymphoma than CT or MRI.

• Percutaneous splenic biopsy and other interventions are being increasingly performed with low rates of complications.

Suggested Readings

Boland G. (2014). Gastrointestinal Imaging: The Requisites. 4th ed. Philadelphia, PA: Elsevier/Saunders

Ricci ZJ, Kaul B, Stein MW, et al. Improving diagnosis of atraumatic splenic lesions, Part III: malignant lesions. Clin Imaging. 2016; 40(5):846–855

Singh AK, Shankar S, Gervais DA, Hahn PF, Mueller PR. Image-guided percutaneous splenic interventions. Radiographics. 2012; 32(2):523–534

Part 3

Gastrointestinal Tract

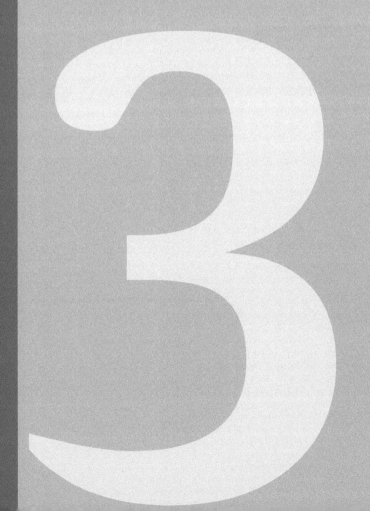

Case 70

Alex R. Martin

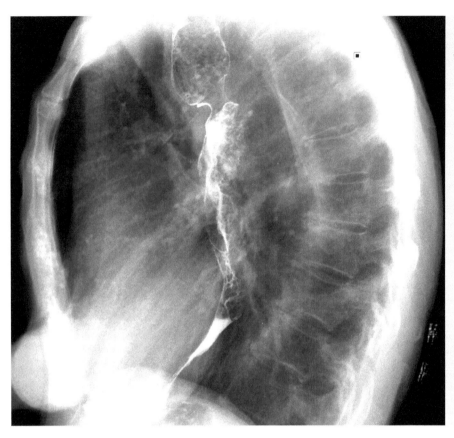

Fig. 70.1 Lateral X-ray obtained from a barium esophagram demonstrates abrupt narrowing with a long segment of stenosis and irregular mucosa. There is proximal esophagus dilation.

■ Clinical History

An 83-year-old male with dysphagia (▶Fig. 70.1).

■ Key Finding

Irregular distal esophageal mucosa with stricturing.

■ Top 3 Differential Diagnoses

- **Esophageal carcinoma:** Squamous cell carcinoma (SCC) is the most common carcinoma and typically occurs in the upper and midesophagus while adenocarcinoma typically occurs distally. For SCC, the most common risk factors are smoking and alcohol while adenocarcinoma arises from Barrett's esophagus due to chronic reflux. Most appear as an irregular mass causing stricture with ulceration and shouldered edges. Superficial carcinomas can also have a plaque-like, polypoid, or ulcerative appearance. A rare varicoid type can appear similar to esophageal varices, but does not change with peristalsis.
- **Metastasis:** The esophagus is most commonly involved by direct invasion, hematogenous metastases are rare. Lung and breast primaries typically involve the midesophagus through mediastinal lymph node metastases while gastric primaries directly invade the lower esophagus. The esophagus is the least common gastrointestinal location for lymphoma. Imaging features overlap with primary esophageal carcinoma.
- **Benign esophageal neoplasms:** Represent approximately one-fourth of esophageal neoplasms and are typically asymptomatic. Leiomyoma is the most common mesenchymal tumor while gastric gastrointestinal stromal tumors (GISTs) predominate in the rest of the gastrointestinal tract. Additional benign tumors include adenomas, polyps, and foregut duplication cysts. Imaging findings are typically a smooth intramural or intraluminal mass without ulceration or nodularity.

■ Additional Diagnostic Considerations

- **Foreign body:** History is often diagnostic except in children or the mentally impaired. Radiopaque foreign bodies are easily diagnosed with plain film. Large food boluses may appear as an irregular polypoid mass on barium examination. On resolution, the patient should be evaluated for underlying stricture or motility disorder.
- **Radiation esophagitis:** Barium examination demonstrates a long smooth narrow stricture with small shallow ulcers and granular mucosa that can mimic a circumferential mass. The location should correspond to a known radiation port. Strictures develop approximately 4 to 8 months following a radiation dose of at least 50 Gy.

■ Diagnosis

Esophageal carcinoma.

✓ Pearls

- Irregular esophageal stricturing is concerning for esophageal carcinoma.
- Metastatic involvement of the esophagus is almost always through direct extension.

- Benign tumors should have smooth margins.

Suggested Readings

Collazzo LA, Levine MS, Rubesin SE, Laufer I. Acute radiation esophagitis: radiographic findings. AJR Am J Roentgenol. 1997; 169(4):1067–1070

Gupta S, Levine MS, Rubesin SE, Katzka DA, Laufer I. Usefulness of barium studies for differentiating benign and malignant strictures of the esophagus. AJR Am J Roentgenol. 2003; 180(3):737–744

Lewis RB, Mehrotra AK, Rodriguez P, Levine MS. From the radiologic pathology archives: esophageal neoplasms: radiologic-pathologic correlation. Radiographics. 2013; 33(4):1083–1108

Case 71

Michael Legacy

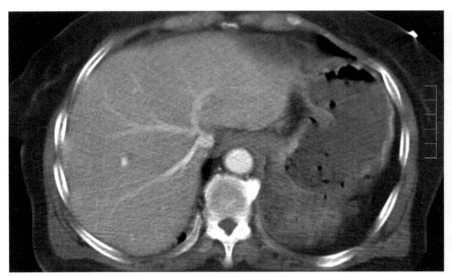

Fig. 71.1 CT of the upper abdomen with intravenous contrast shows left upper quadrant fat stranding. (Image courtesy of Rocky C. Saenz.)

■ **Clinical History**

A 35-year-old female with left upper quadrant pain (▶Fig. 71.1).

■ Key Finding

Left upper quadrant fat stranding.

■ Top 3 Differential Diagnoses

- **Acute pancreatitis:** Most commonly caused by alcohol abuse or gallstones. Patients present with epigastric pain radiating to the back. There are two main subtypes, interstitial edematous and necrotizing. Interstitial edematous pancreatitis represents the majority of cases and demonstrates loss of the normal fatty lobulated contour with peripancreatic fat stranding. Necrotizing pancreatitis demonstrates areas of parenchymal necrosis, which will be nonenhancing and poorly circumscribed, along with a greater degree of peripancreatic fat stranding.
- **Diverticulitis:** Diverticular disease most commonly affects the sigmoid colon. CT is used for evaluation of acute diverticulitis. Findings include segmental wall thickening and adjacent pericolonic inflammatory changes. Complications include perforation with pneumoperitoneum, abscess, and fistula formation. On CT, colonic wall thickening and pericolonic fat stranding are centered on the inflamed diverticulum.
- **Perforated gastric ulcer/gastritis:** Gastritis can be associated with ulcers; the majority (95%) is benign in etiology. Associations include epigastric pain, nonsteroidal anti-inflammatory drug (NSAID) use, and *H. pylori* infection. On CT, findings include epigastric fat stranding, gastric wall thickening, and free intraperitoneal air (when perforated).

■ Additional Diagnostic Considerations

- **Abscess:** On CT, findings include loculated, low-density fluid collection with peripheral rim enhancement, increased incidence in immunocompromised, diabetics, and postoperative patients. Prior to full abscess formation, phlegmon appears more like focal fat stranding without a discrete fluid collection.
- **Omental Infarct:** A portion of the omental fat is infarcted secondary to arterial insult. The most common location is in the right lower quadrant. Patients present with acute right lower quadrant pain, fever, and a palpable mass. On CT, findings include focal fat stranding. Treatment is conservative and centers on pain management.

■ Diagnosis

Gastritis secondary to peptic ulcer disease.

✓ Pearls

- Gastritis typically needs further evaluation with a barium fluoroscopy study.
- Pancreatitis is a clinical diagnosis and CT only serves to exclude its sequelae.
- When fat stranding is centered in the fat and not an organ consider omental infarct.

Suggested Readings

Federle MP, Jeffrey RB, Woodward PJ, Borhani A. Diagnostic Imaging: Abdomen. 2nd ed. Philadelphia, PA: Lippincott Williams & Wilkins; 2009

Pereira JM, Sirlin CB, Pinto PS, Jeffrey RB, Stella DL, Casola G. Disproportionate fat stranding: a helpful CT sign in patients with acute abdominal pain. Radiographics. 2004; 24(3):703–715

Thornton E, Mendiratta-Lala M, Siewert B, Eisenberg RL. Patterns of fat stranding. AJR Am J Roentgenol. 2011; 197(1):W1:W14

Case 72

Andrew Mizzi

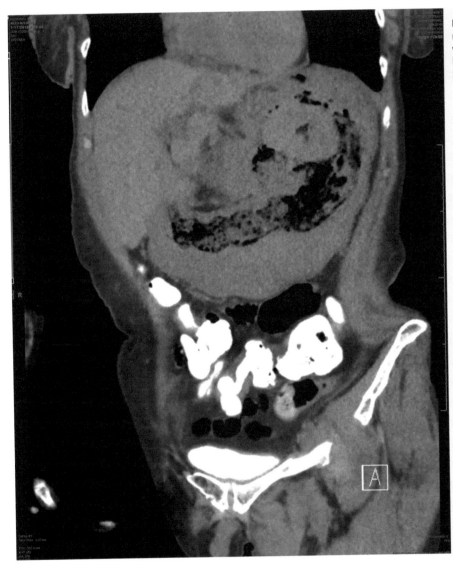

Fig. 72.1 CT abdomen with oral contrast, coronal reformat image demonstrates marked eccentric wall thickening along the greater curvature with luminal narrowing. (Image courtesy of Rocky C. Saenz.)

■ **Clinical History**

An 83-year-old male with early satiety (▶ Fig. 72.1).

■ Key Finding

Diffuse stomach wall thickening with luminal narrowing (linitis plastica).

■ Top 3 Differential Diagnoses

- **Gastric adenocarcinoma:** Gastric adenocarcinoma is the most common malignancy of the stomach (≈ 90%). When it infiltrates the muscular layer of the stomach it results in muscular dysfunction. This muscular infiltration prevents normal gastric distention and results in narrowing of the lumen. This nondistensibility has been described as a "leather bottle" appearance (linitis plastica). Scirrhous carcinoma (disseminated) accounts for 5 to 15% of cases and usually begins in the pylorus and extends superiorly. Gastric carcinoma risk factors include nitrites, salted, and smoked foods. On CT, there is diffuse thickening of the stomach with disappearance of the rugal folds and a small lumen. Linitis plastica is indicative of advanced disease.

- **Metastasis:** Metastatic disease to the stomach is relatively rare and only seen in 2% of cancer patients. It typically is a sign of stage IV disease with poor prognosis. The most common primary carcinoma that leads to gastric metastases is breast carcinoma. Breast metastasis can present as multiple small lesions or linitis plastica (leather bottle) appearance. Hematogenous spread of metastasis is the most common route for metastatic spread to the stomach. The most common carcinomas to spread hematogenously to the stomach are malignant melanoma, lung, and breast cancer.

- **Lymphoma:** Lymphoma is the second most common malignancy of the stomach. Gastrointestinal lymphoma is most commonly seen in the stomach. Most commonly it is non-Hodgkin's B-cell lymphoma (diffuse large B-cell lymphoma [DLBCL] and extranodal marginal zone C-cell previously MALT [mucosa associated lymphoid tissue]). Significant abdominal adenopathy may also be seen with lymphoma. Menetrier's disease can mimic lymphoma of the stomach due to rugal fold thickening.

■ Additional Diagnostic Considerations

Sarcoid: Involvement of the gastrointestinal tract is rare but when it occurs it most commonly involves the stomach. Signs of sarcoid involvement are nonspecific and include mucosal or wall thickening or gastric ulcers. Gastrointestinal manifestations of sarcoid are usually associated with pulmonary disease.

■ Diagnosis

Gastric adenocarcinoma.

✓ Pearls

- Gastric adenocarcinoma, lymphoma, and metastasis can all appear similar.
- Linitis plastic tends to cause loss of rugal folds whereas lymphoma, Menetrier's disease, and inflammatory processes of the stomach tend to accentuate them.

- Gastric mass or wall thickening with significant adenopathy is considered to be lymphoma.

Suggested Readings

Federle MP, Jeffrey RB, Woodward PJ, Borhani A. Diagnostic Imaging: Abdomen. 2nd ed. Philadelphia, PA: Lippincott Williams & Wilkins; 2009

Lewis RB, Mehrotra AK, Rodríguez P, Manning MA, Levine MS. From the radiologic pathology archives: gastrointestinal lymphoma: radiologic and pathologic findings. Radiographics. 2014; 34(7):1934–1953

Whitty LA, Crawford DL, Woodland JH, Patel JC, Nattier B, Thomas CR, Jr. Metastatic breast cancer presenting as linitis plastica of the stomach. Gastric Cancer. 2005; 8(3):193–197

Case 73

Vernon F. Williams, Jr.

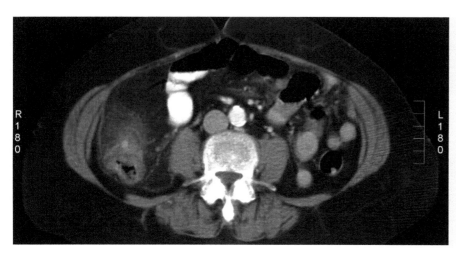

Fig. 73.1 CT axial image with intravenous and oral contrast through the mid abdomen demonstrating right lower quadrant stranding. (Image courtesy of Rocky C. Saenz.)

■ **Clinical History**

A 55-year-old female with right lower quadrant pain (▶ Fig. 73.1).

■ Key Finding

Right lower quadrant fat stranding.

■ Top 3 Differential Diagnoses

- **Inflammatory disease:** Crohn's disease is an idiopathic condition leading to transmural bowel wall inflammation. Crohn's disease may involve any portion of the gastrointestinal tract from the esophagus to the anus (most commonly involves the terminal ileum) and will demonstrate "skip lesions." In contrast, ulcerative colitis inflammation is limited to the mucosa and it has continuous involvement from the rectum. Imaging features of Crohn's disease include mucosal ulcerations (cobblestone appearance), fibrofatty proliferation (creeping fat), thickened/edematous folds, bowel wall enhancement, mesenteric fatty proliferation (comb sign), and submucosal thickening with fat/edema (fat halo sign/target sign).
- **Appendicitis:** Acute appendicitis is inflammation of the appendix and is one of the most common reasons for abdominal surgery in young patients. It occurs after obstruction of the appendiceal lumen (appendicoliths account for one-third of cases) leading to transmural inflammation and eventually infarction or perforation. One of the main complications is abscess formation. The most specific CT finding is a dilated appendix (> 6 mm) with peripheral fat stranding. Additional findings include thickened appendiceal wall and hyperemia.
- **Infectious colitis:** Infectious colitis is typically long segment. The causative agents include parasites, protozoa, bacteria, and viruses. There are variable imaging features including low attenuating bowel wall thickening, fat stranding, and multiple air-fluid levels from increased fluid/liquid feces. The accordion sign refers to oral contrast between extremely thickened colonic haustra.

■ Additional Diagnostic Considerations

- **Diverticulitis:** Diverticular occlusion can occur in any part of the bowel but is most common distally. The diverticular inflammation may lead to erosion and potentially microperforation. On CT, fat stranding is seen adjacent to a high-density diverticulum. Complications include abscess and fistula.
- **Omental infarct:** Infarction of the greater omentum is a rare cause of abdominal pain and is a result of omental torsion or venous thrombosis/insufficiency. It can be spontaneous; however, predisposing factors are obesity, congestive heart failure, recent abdominal surgery/trauma, or strenuous activity. The omentum infarcts less often than the small bowel or colon because of its rich gastroepiploic collateral vessel supply. Imaging features include a nonenhancing omental fatty mass.

■ Diagnosis

Diverticulitis of right colon.

✓ Pearls

- Diverticulitis has focal fat stranding surrounding a diverticulum.
- Identifying the ileocecal valve first on CT will sometimes help finding the appendix.
- Crohn's disease most commonly involves the terminal ileum and is characterized by skip lesions.

Suggested Readings

Choi SH, Han JK, Kim SH, et al. Intussusception in adults: from stomach to rectum. AJR Am J Roentgenol. 2004; 183(3):691–698

Pereira JM, Sirlin CB, Pinto PS, Jeffrey RB, Stella DL, Casola G. Disproportionate fat stranding: a helpful CT sign in patients with acute abdominal pain. Radiographics. 2004; 24(3):703–715

Thornton E, Mendiratta-Lala M, Siewert B, Eisenberg RL. Patterns of fat stranding. AJR Am J Roentgenol. 2011; 197(1):W1–14

Case 74

Julia J. Hobson

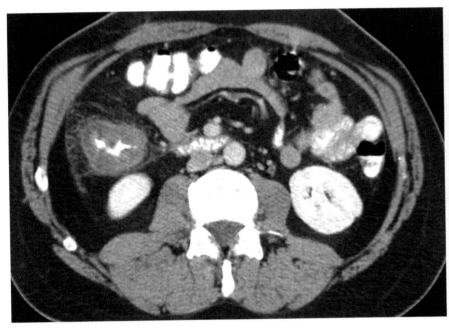

Fig. 74.1 CT axial image with intravenous and oral contrast shows marked circumferential cecal wall thickening, pericolonic fat stranding and luminal narrowing. (Image courtesy of Rocky C. Saenz.)

■ Clinical History

A 36-year-old male with leukemia and abdominal pain (▶ Fig. 74.1).

■ Key Finding

Symmetric cecal wall thickening.

■ Top 3 Differential Diagnoses

- **Inflammatory Bowel disease:** Idiopathic inflammatory diseases of the colon include both Crohn's disease and ulcerative colitis. Common presenting symptoms are abdominal pain and diarrhea, with or without blood. Crohn's disease can occur anywhere along the gastrointestinal tract, but most commonly involves the terminal ileum and proximal large bowel. Ulcerative colitis tends to involve the distal colon, but can involve the proximal colon with "backwash" ileitis, symmetric wall thickening either short or long segment, mesenteric lymphadenopathy, and peripheral fat stranding in active disease. Complications of Crohn's disease include strictures, abscess, fistula, and sinus tract formation. Complications of ulcerative colitis include stricture and toxic megacolon. Chronic ulcerative colitis can lead to loss of haustra resulting in the classic "lead pipe" colon.
- **Adenocarcinoma:** Colon cancer is one of the most commonly diagnosed cancers and is potentially curable if detected early. Approximately one-fourth of colon cancers occur in the cecum. Early cancers are often found on endoscopy; however, barium enema can show plaque-like or pedunculated polyps. On CT, asymmetric bowel wall thickening with luminal narrowing can be seen. Additional findings of pericolonic fat stranding and loss of the fat planes between colon and adjacent structures suggests local tumor extension. PET–CT is also used for staging, which is necessary to determine ideal patient management.
- **Typhlitis:** Also known as neutropenic colitis, typhlitis is a necrotizing enterocolitis that occurs in neutropenic patients, most commonly those receiving chemotherapy for leukemia. Patients present with abdominal pain, bloody diarrhea, and right lower quadrant pain. The diagnostic study of choice is CT, which will show massive symmetric/circumferential wall thickening with mucosal edema (hypoattenuation) involving the cecum (may also involve the proximal colon and terminal ileum) and adjacent inflammatory stranding. In severe cases, bowel wall necrosis and perforation can occur.

■ Additional Diagnostic Considerations

- **Infectious Colitis:** Bowel wall inflammation due to bacterial, viral, fungal, or parasitic infection. *Yersinia*, cytomegalovirus (CMV), *Salmonella*, tuberculosis, histoplasma, and ameba infections commonly involve the cecum and proximal colon. Pan colon involvement is typically seen with CMV and *Clostridium*.
- **Appendicitis:** Acute appendicitis is a common cause of abdominal pain necessitating surgical intervention. Inflammation from acute appendicitis can spread to the cecum resulting in cecal wall thickening. Additionally, wall thickening can occur between the cecal lumen and base of the appendix.

■ Diagnosis

Neutropenic colitis, typhlitis.

✓ Pearls

- Crohn's disease is most commonly seen in the terminal ileum and proximal large bowel.
- One-fourth of colon cancers occur in the cecum.
- Typhlitis is seen in neutropenic patients commonly involving the cecum.

Suggested Readings

Boyd SK, Cameron-Morrison JD, Hobson JJ, et al. CT imaging of large bowel wall thickening. J Am Osteopath Coll Radiol. 2016; 5(2):14–22

Fernandes T, Oliveira MI, Castro R, Araújo B, Viamonte B, Cunha R. Bowel wall thickening at CT: simplifying the diagnosis. Insights Imaging. 2014; 5(2):195–208

Iyer RB, Silverman PM, DuBrow RA, Charnsangavej C. Imaging in the diagnosis, staging, and follow-up of colorectal cancer. AJR Am J Roentgenol. 2002; 179(1):3–13

Case 75

Reehan M. Ali

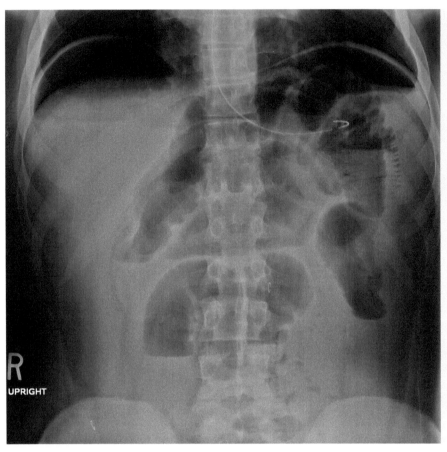

Fig. 75.1 Abdominal X-ray taken in the upright position shows multiple air-fluid levels in non-dilated small bowel loops. Free air is seen under the diaphragm.

■ **Clinical History**

A 63-year-old male with abdominal pain after recent surgery (▶Fig. 75.1).

■ Key Finding

Small bowel air-fluid levels.

■ Top 3 Differential Diagnoses

• **Mechanical obstruction:** Most classic association with air-fluid levels as noted on an upright radiograph. Typically, mechanical obstruction is associated with differential air-fluid levels, meaning levels are seen "stacked" or at different levels when viewed on the frontal upright abdominal film. The positive predictive value of differential air-fluid levels in small bowel obstruction is highest at levels of 20 mm or greater in height. This is seen in conjunction with dilated small bowel loops that are greater than 2.5 cm in diameter when measuring from outer wall to outer wall. The most common causes are overwhelmingly postsurgical adhesions (developed world) and hernias (developing world).

• **Ileus:** A term used to describe aperistaltic bowel not caused by mechanical obstruction. It typically presents with non-colicky abdominal pain that is prolonged and often occurs after surgery. Radiographically it can be difficult to distinguish from mechanical obstruction as many features overlap. In contrast to mechanical obstruction, air-fluid levels are seen at the same level as opposed to "differential" as seen in mechanical obstruction. CT will also demonstrate lack of a transition point and lack of distal decompressed loops of small and large bowel. Medications have also been implicated, most commonly opioids.

• **Sentinel loop:** Sentinel loop refers to a localized dilated loop of small bowel which is adjacent to a site of intra-abdominal inflammation. The sentinel loop often has an associated air-fluid level. This is not diagnostic of an intra-abdominal process but is an associated feature. Therefore, the sentinel loop prompts further evaluation with cross-sectional imaging when seen on abdominal imaging.

■ Additional Diagnostic Considerations

Inflammation: A few air-fluid levels within nondilated loops of small bowel are usually not clinically significant. Occasion-ally, this can be seen in a patient with underlying inflammatory gastroenteritis.

■ Diagnosis

Postoperative ileus.

✓ Pearls

• Differential air-fluid levels are commonly associated with mechanical small bowel obstruction.

• Air-fluid levels seen at the same level on an upright X-ray are likely due to ileus.

• Sentinel loop refers to a dilated loop of small bowel containing air-fluid level adjacent to an inflammatory process.

Suggested Readings

Federle MP, Jeffrey RB, Woodward PJ, Borhani A. Diagnostic Imaging: Abdomen. 2nd ed. Philadelphia, PA: Lippincott Williams & Wilkins; 2009

Harlow CL, Stears RL, Zeligman BE, Archer PG. Diagnosis of bowel obstruction on plain abdominal radiographs: significance of air-fluid levels at different heights in the same loop of bowel. AJR Am J Roentgenol. 1993; 161(2):291–295

Silva AC, Pimenta M, Guimarães LS. Small bowel obstruction: what to look for. Radiographics. 2009; 29(2):423–439

Case 76

Michael L. Schwartz

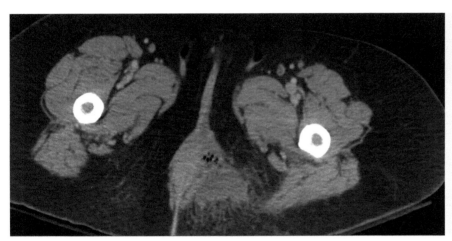

Fig. 76.1 Contrast enhanced axial CT image through the lower pelvis demonstrates a focal fluid attenuated collection with air adjacent to the rectum. In addition, there is perirectal fat stranding. (Image courtesy of Rocky C. Saenz.)

■ **Clinical History**

A 53-year-old female with bright blood per rectum (▶ Fig. 76.1).

■ Key Finding

Perirectal cyst.

■ Top 3 Differential Diagnoses

- **Abscess:** Perirectal abscess is an infected collection in perirectal region often associated with a perianal fistula. These occur most commonly spontaneously secondary to impaired drainage of the anal glands. Approximately 10% of cases are related to pelvic infections, trauma, cancer, inflammatory bowel disease, and radiation therapy. On CT, the classic findings include ring enhancing, fluid attenuated focus with peripheral fat standing. Greater than 80% of patients will develop a fistula chronically. Antibiotic therapy may result in spontaneous resolution while some require surgical reduction.
- **Duplication cyst:** Perirectal cysts are rare congenital lesions from embryonic hindgut. They are also known as tailgut duplication cyst or retrorectal cystic hamartomas. They have a strong female predilection and are often asymptomatic. These cysts are typically posterior to the rectum. Complications include infection and bleeding. Malignant degeneration has been reported. Surgical excision is preferred treatment.
- **Inflammatory bowel disease:** Crohn's disease and ulcerative colitis may both affect the rectum. Crohn's disease currently affects half a million people in North America. Crohn's disease patients typically present in the third decade of life with bloody diarrhea, frequent small bowel movements, abdominal pain, and tenesmus. Imaging is optimally performed with CT or MRI enterography technique that is superior to barium fluoroscopy. Crohn's disease more commonly involves the right colon but can involve any portion of the gastrointestinal tract. Crohn's disease is associated with discontinuous transmural ulceration, which can develop both perirectal abscess and fistula formation. Fistula formation can occur between bowel loops, vagina, urinary bladder or abdominal wall/skin.

■ Additional Diagnostic Considerations

Lymphogranuloma venereum: Lymphogranuloma venereum is a sexually transmitted disease caused by Chlamydia trachomatis and may result in proctitis and or colitis. It is more common in men and is a granulomatous inflammatory response to the infected mucosa. Rectal involvement is common. Lymphogranuloma venereum may lead to perirectal abscess and fistula formation. Tetracycline is used for acute treatment.

■ Diagnosis

Spontaneous perirectal abscess.

✓ Pearls

- The majority of perirectal abscesses occur spontaneous due to impaired drainage of the anal glands.
- A retrorectal cyst without inflammatory changes should be considered a duplication cyst.
- When an abscess is seen carefully evaluate for a fistula.

Suggested Readings

Boyd SK, Cameron-Morrison JD, Hobson JJ, Saenz R. CT imaging of large bowel wall thickening. J Am Osteopath Coll Radiol. 2016; 5(2):14–22

Hayelar M, Griepentrog K. Tailgut cyst: case report and literature review. Int J. Surg Case Rep. 2015; 10:166–168

Khati NJ, Sondel Lewis N, Frazier AA, Obias V, Zeman RK, Hill MC. CT of acute perianal abscesses and infected fistulae: a pictorial essay. Emerg Radiol. 2015; 22(3):329–335

O'Malley RB, Al-Hawary MM, Kaza RK, Wasnik AP, Liu PS, Hussain HK. Rectal imaging: part 2, perianal fistula evaluation on pelvic MRI—what the radiologist needs to know. AJR Am J Roentgenol. 2012; 199(1):W43:W53

Case 77

Jake Figner

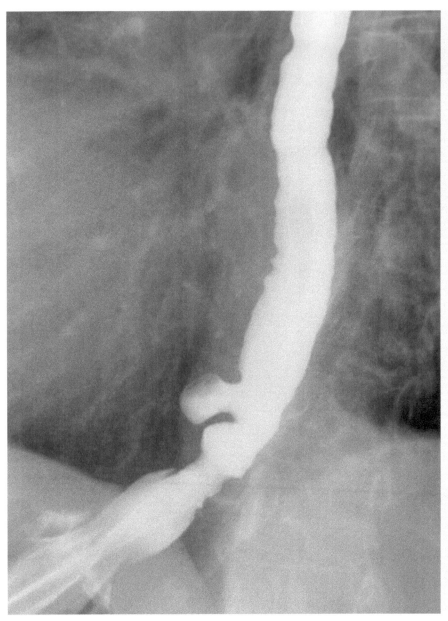

Fig. 77.1 Posterior oblique fluoroscopy image from an upper gastrointestinal image of the distal esophagus shows a focal, well-circumscribed, outpouching of the distal esophagus above the diaphragm. (Image courtesy of Sharon Kreuer.)

■ Clinical History

A 48-year-old female with general abdominal pain (▶ Fig. 77.1).

■ Key Finding

Outpouching of the distal esophagus above the diaphragm.

■ Top 3 Differential Diagnoses

- **Epiphrenic pulsion diverticulum:** Pulsion diverticula typically arise from the right posterior–lateral esophageal wall. These are not "true" diverticula as they are result of mucosal layer herniating through muscular layer. Diverticula are best seen on barium esophagram and appear as a focal luminal outpouching. The diverticula are a result of increased intraluminal pressure causing protrusion of the mucosa through the muscular wall. These are strongly associated with esophageal dysmotility. Epiphrenic diverticulum may present as a retrocardiac mass on a frontal chest X-ray and in this scenario are difficult to distinguish from a hiatal hernia.
- **Hiatal hernia:** Herniation of abdominal contents through the esophageal hiatus. The majority involve superior displacement of gastroesophageal junction above the hiatus (sliding type).

There may also be superior herniation of the gastric fundus which may present as left-sided retrocardiac mass with air-fluid level on chest X-ray. Less commonly the gastroesophageal junction may remain in normal position while the stomach herniates superiorly through the hiatus (paraesophageal type). Hiatal hernias will be seen on barium studies as a pouch above the diaphragm containing gastric rugae.
- **Prominent phrenic ampulla:** Also known as the esophageal vestibule, it is the portion of the esophagus lying between the A and B rings. The phrenic ampulla is a normal structure that may be more prominent in some patients. Distinguishable from other entities on barium studies due to the normal position of the lower esophageal sphincter and its lack of gastric rugae.

■ Additional Diagnostic Considerations

Eosinophilic esophagitis: Inflammation of the esophagus with characteristic infiltration of eosinophils. Most characteristic imaging finding is concentric esophageal strictures on barium swallow (ring esophagus). It can be seen anywhere along the gastrointestinal tract and may manifest as fold thickening and submucosal edema within the bowel. Most of those affected have allergy/food intolerance history. Biopsy of esophagus is required for definitive diagnosis. Eosinophilic esophagitis responds well to steroid treatment.

■ Diagnosis

Epiphrenic diverticulum.

✓ Pearls

- Epiphrenic diverticula typically arise from right posterior–lateral wall.
- Hiatal hernia will typically be left sided on radiograph while epiphrenic diverticulum will typically be right sided.

- Phrenic ampulla is a normal structure, which can be prominent in some patients.

Suggested Readings

Dean C, Etienne D, Carpentier B, Gielecki J, Tubbs RS, Loukas M. Hiatal hernias. Surg Radiol Anat. 2012; 34(4):291–299

Fasano NC, Levine MS, Rubesin SE, Redfern RO, Laufer I. Epiphrenic diverticulum: clinical and radiographic findings in 27 patients. Dysphagia. 2003; 18(1):9–15

Federle MP, Jeffrey RB, Woodward PJ, Borhani A. Diagnostic Imaging: Abdomen. 2nd ed. Philadelphia, PA: Lippincott Williams & Wilkins; 2009

Case 78

Andrew Mizzi

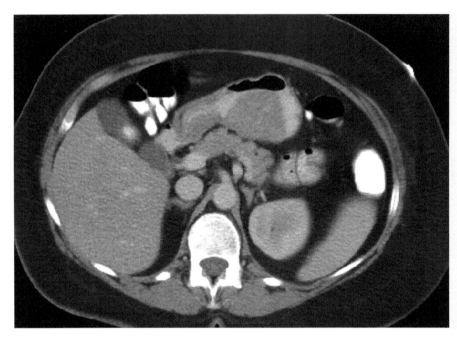

Fig. 78.1 CT image of the upper abdomen shows a focal lesion along the posterior wall of the stomach. (Image courtesy of Rocky C. Saenz.)

■ Clinical History

A 76-year-old male with epigastric pain (▶ Fig. 78.1).

■ Key Finding

Gastric solid mass.

■ Top 3 Differential Diagnoses

- **Gastric adenocarcinoma:** Adenocarcinoma arises from the gastric epithelium and is the most common gastric malignancy accounting for greater than 95% of malignant stomach tumors. Most occur sporadically. There is an important association with *H. pylori* infection and about 10 to 15% have a genetic predisposition. Median age is 70 years for males and 74 years for females. Gastric adenocarcinoma can occur anywhere in the stomach but about half the time it presents in the pyloric region and one fourth of the time in the body and fundus. Distal stomach masses may present with gastric outlet obstruction. It can present as gastric focal wall thickening on CT. Other patterns include polypoid mass, ulcerated mass, or infiltrating lesion with loss of normal rugal fold pattern.
- **Lymphoma:** Primary gastric lymphoma represents 1 to 5% of malignant tumors of the stomach. Lymphoma is the second most common gastric malignancy. Ninety percent of primary gastric lymphoma are mucosa associated lymphoid tissue (MALT) or diffuse large B-cell lymphoma (DLBCL). MALT is often associated with *H. pylori* infection. It is predominately non-Hodgkin's lymphoma (NHL) type. It is frequently found in the antrum. On CT, lymphoma can present as focal or diffuse wall thickening usually greater than 1 cm, ulcerated polypoid lesions or submucosal nodular form.
- **Gastric gastrointestinal stromal tumor (GIST):** Most common mesenchymal origin neoplasm. The majority of these lesions occur in the stomach. It expresses tyrosine kinase growth factor receptor that distinguishes it from leiomyomas, leiomyosarcoma, schwannoma, and neurofibroma. On CT, GIST presents as a large exophytic, hypervascular mass. Calcifications are present in 5 to 10% of cases. Lymphadenopathy is not seen. GIST has an association with neurofibromatosis type I.

■ Additional Diagnostic Considerations

- **Benign gastric polyp:** Usually asymptomatic and found incidentally on barium examinations. In rare cases, it may present with epigastric pain, gastric outlet obstruction, and hematemesis. Incidence increases with age. Fundic gland polyps represent 74% of all gastric polyps in Western countries where prevalence of *H. pylori* is less prevalent. In countries with high prevalence of *H. pylori*, polyps are usually hyperplastic and adenomas. Fundic gland polyps have a low malignant potential. Adenomas are typically seen in atrophic gastric mucosa and may be associated with familial polyposis syndromes.
- **Gastric carcinoids:** Sporadic gastric carcinoid is a subtype of gastric carcinoid that usually presents as a large solitary lesion (the two other sub types present as multiple small lesions). They are usually metastatic upon diagnosis. In total, all types of gastric carcinoids are rare tumors that comprise 1% of all gastric neoplasms.

■ Diagnosis

Gastric adenocarcinoma.

✓ Pearls

- Gastric adenocarcinoma is the most common stomach malignancy.
- Sister Mary Joseph node is an umbilical nodule secondary to metastasis seen in up to 3% of intra-abdominal and pelvic malignancies.
- Gastrointestinal tract is most common extranodal site involved by lymphoma.

Suggested Readings

Federle MP, Jeffrey RB, Woodward PJ, Borhani A. Diagnostic imaging: abdomen. 2nd ed. Lippincott Williams & Wilkins; 2009

Lockhead P, El-Omar E. Gastric tumors: an overview. Atlas Genet Cytogenet in Oncol Haematol. 2009; 13(10):761:767

Shen Y, Kang HK, Jeong YY, et al. Evaluation of early gastric cancer at multidetector CT with multiplanar reformation and virtual endoscopy. Radiographics. 2011; 31(1):189–199

Case 79

Reehan M. Ali

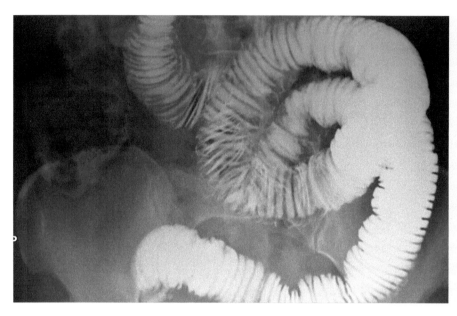

Fig. 79.1 Overhead X-ray from a small bowel barium study reveals diffusely thickened small bowel folds.

■ Clinical History

A 61-year-old male generalized abdominal pain (▶ Fig. 79.1).

■ Key Finding

Diffuse thickened small bowel folds.

■ Top 3 Differential Diagnoses

- **Inflammatory:** Inflammatory processes typically cause irregular fold thickening. The folds become distorted and form angles with adjacent folds. While any inflammatory process can cause this appearance, the key to differentiating them relies on noting the site of disease, provided clinical history and other supportive radiographic findings. For example, Crohn's disease will show involvement of the terminal ileum along with the "string sign," separation of bowel loops, skip lesions, and possible fistula formation. Gastric involvement in addition to small bowel can be seen in eosinophilic gastroenteritis. The presence of a malabsorption syndrome such as fever, arthritis, and lymphadenopathy can be seen in Whipple's disease. Biopsy of the small bowel will show periodic acid–Schiff (PAS)-positive granules in the lamina propria.

- **Hemorrhage:** Hemorrhage causes uniform, regular thickening of the small bowel folds. This can create the classic "picket fence" or "stack of coins" configuration due to the parallel alignment of the small bowel folds. Bowel loops will often show separation as well. This can be caused by multiple reasons including, but not limited to, anticoagulant therapy, connective tissue diseases, coagulation abnormalities, bleeding varices, and hemorrhagic neoplasm.
- **Edema:** Another common cause of regular small bowel thickening. This is most commonly related to hypoproteinemia due to hepatic cirrhosis. Similarly, nephrotic syndrome and protein-losing enteropathies also result in edema. While protein losing diseases typically cause generalized bowel thickening, lymphatic blockage from tumor infiltration and angioneurotic edema will cause a similar fold pattern but typically are more localized.

■ Additional Diagnostic Considerations

- **Lymphoma/leukemia:** Approximately 25% of patients with lymphoma will have small bowel involvement at autopsy. Lymphomatous/leukemic involvement of the small bowel is typically irregular in nature with diffuse distribution. The bowel loops will show separation due to mesenteric involvement of the disease.

- **Infection:** Irregular thickening of small bowel folds that has a multitude of causes. This includes *Giaradiasis* (correlate with history of recent travel to an endemic area), *Yersinia* enterocolitis, *Strongyloidiasis*, and typhoid fever are other possible etiologies.

■ Diagnosis

Small bowel hemorrhage related to coagulopathy.

✓ Pearls

- Regular diffuse small bowel fold thickening is most likely related to hemorrhage or edema.
- Inflammatory conditions are the most common cause of irregular fold thickening.

- Narrowing the differential relies on looking on involvement pattern, clinical signs/symptoms, and associated radiologic findings.

Suggested Readings

Eisenberg RL. Thickening of small bowel folds. AJR Am J Roentgenol. 2009; 193(1):W1:W6

Federle MP, Jeffrey RB, Woodward PJ, Borhani A. Diagnostic Imaging: Abdomen. 2nd ed. Philadelphia, PA: Lippincott Williams & Wilkins; 2009

Rubesin SF, Rubin RA, Herlinger H. Small bowel malabsorption: clinical and radiological perspectives. Radiology. 1992; 184:2973

Case 80

Julia D. Cameron-Morrison

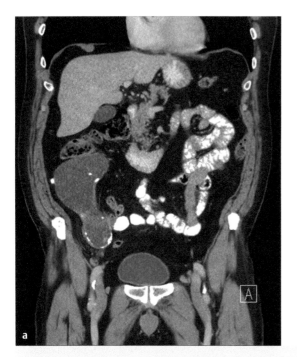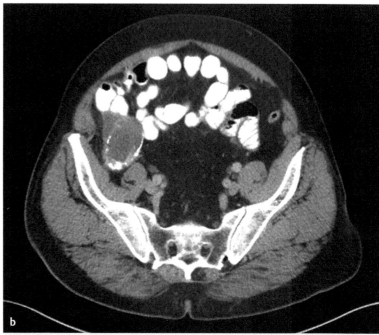

Fig. 80.1 Coronal (**a**) and axial (**b**) images from a CT abdomen and pelvis with intravenous and oral contrast demonstrates a large well-circumscribed blind ending tubular cystic structure within the right lower quadrant with curvilinear mural calcifications along its dependent portion. Subtle hyperattenuated internal debris is present.

■ Clinical History

A 69-year-old male with right lower quadrant pain (▶Fig. 80.1).

■ Key Finding

Right lower quadrant cystic mass with peripheral calcification.

■ Top 3 Differential Diagnoses

- **Appendicitis/appendiceal abscess:** Appendicitis most commonly presents with periumbilical pain eventually localizing to the right lower quadrant. Classic findings in appendicitis include a dilated appendix measuring greater than or equal to 7 mm with surrounding inflammatory fat stranding, with or without associated free fluid and appendicolith. Complications include rupture with abscess formation and pneumoperitoneum.
- **Mucocele of the appendix:** Most commonly asymptomatic, mucocele of the appendix results from chronic cystic dilation by abnormal mucin accumulation. Three histologic subtypes exist including mucosal hyperplasia, mucinous cystadenoma (most common) and mucinous cystadenocarcinoma. On CT, an encapsulated round or oval, thin walled cystic mass is seen in the right lower quadrant. These most commonly measure 3 to 6 cm and approximately 50% have curvilinear mural calcification. Pseudomyxoma peritonei can be seen with rupture.
- **Cecal adenocarcinoma:** Finding of cecal adenocarcinoma is similar to those of colon neoplasms in other portions of the bowel, often presenting due to hematochezia or bowel obstruction. These masses can be large at presentation. On imaging, there may be signs of transmural invasion, adenopathy, or distant metastasis. Associated inflammatory changes are rare.

■ Additional Diagnostic Considerations

Adnexal mass: Right lower quadrant pain in women often stems from ovarian or adnexal origin, with possible etiologies including simple or complex ovarian cysts, tubo-ovarian abscess, endometriomas, and both benign and malignant ovarian neoplasms. When large, it may be difficult to localize to the adnexa and can simulate a cecal/appendiceal cystic mass. On cross-sectional imaging following the gonadal artery and broad ligament to the ovary may be helpful in localizing the lesions origin.

■ Diagnosis

Mucocele of the appendix, mucinous cystadenoma.

✓ Pearls

- Enlarged appendix with inflammatory changes less than 2 cm is considered to be appendicitis.
- Mucoceles of the appendix present as large cystic masses greater than 3 cm with calcifications.
- Pseudomyxoma peritonei is associated with rupture of mucin secreting tumors.

Suggested Readings

Beydoun T, Kreuer S. Cystic right lower quadrant mass. J Am Osteopath Coll Radiol. 2012; 1(4):32–34

Jeong YY, Outwater EK, Kang HK. Imaging evaluation of ovarian masses. Radiographics. 2000; 20(5):1445–1470

Madwed D, Mindelzun R, Jeffrey RB, Jr. Mucocele of the appendix: imaging findings. AJR Am J Roentgenol. 1992; 159(1):69–72

Pickhardt PJ, Levy AD, Rohrmann CA, Jr, Kende AI. Primary neoplasms of the appendix: radiologic spectrum of disease with pathologic correlation. Radiographics. 2003; 23(3):645–662

Case 81

Michael L. Schwartz

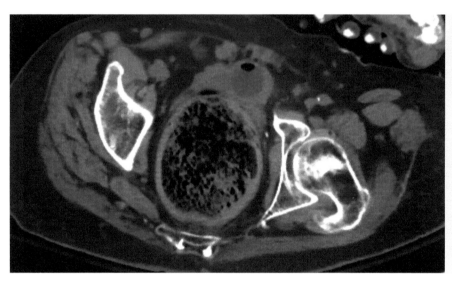

Fig. 81.1 A noncontrast axial CT image through the lower pelvis shows a dilated rectum with abnormal, symmetric wall thickening and posterior fat-stranding. (Image courtesy of Rocky C. Saenz.)

■ Clinical History

A 66-year-old male with bloating and pelvic pain (▶ Fig. 81.1).

■ Key Finding

Marked rectal distention with fecal impaction and wall thickening.

■ Top 3 Differential Diagnoses

- **Stercoral colitis:** This is an inflammatory colitis of the rectal wall secondary to fecal impaction (fecaloma) with increased intraluminal pressure. The fecaloma results in rectal and eventual perirectal hazy fat. The rectal wall is thickened diffusely or focally (if stercoral ulcer is present). Complications include perforation/peritonitis with a high mortality rate. Typically, a disease of elderly, chronically disabled, and/or institutionalized patient. In young patient, etiology is primarily narcotic abuse.
- **Ogilvie syndrome/ileus:** Dilated rectum and colon without an obstructive lesion (tumor, infection, or inflammation). Colonic ileus can dilate the rectum but is most prominent in the cecum. Etiologies include trauma, metabolic imbalance, postoperative, infectious, and cardiac disease. Pseudo-obstruction (Ogilvie syndrome) is a potentially fatal condition of acute colonic distention without an underlying mechanical lesion. CT will show luminal distention without an abrupt transition point.
- **Inflammatory bowel disease:** Crohn's disease and ulcerative colitis both result in bowel wall thickening. Ulcerative colitis is more common in the left colon and Crohn's disease is more common in the right colon. The wall thickening is more prominent in Crohn's disease typically greater than 10 mm. Ulcerative colitis complications include colonic stricture or a fixed and dilated colon (lead pipe). Ulcerative colitis classic findings are concentric wall thickening involving the left colon and rectum.

■ Additional Diagnostic Considerations

- **Adenocarcinoma:** Adenocarcinoma is the most common colorectal malignancy. Typical CT findings are irregular, asymmetric rectal wall thickening, and luminal narrowing. Complications include obstruction proximal to a transition point created by the mass-like wall thickening. It commonly presents with surrounding fat stranding and adenopathy.
- **Proctitis:** An inflammation of the lining of the rectum can be acute or chronic. On cross-sectional imaging, the rectal wall thickening is classically concentric without luminal distention. Etiologies include radiation therapy, sexually transmitted infections, inflammatory diseases, ischemia, and trauma.

■ Diagnosis

Stercoral colitis.

✓ Pearls

- In uncomplicated fecal impaction, rectal wall is thin differentiating this from stercoral colitis.
- The rectal wall is thickened in proctitis but without luminal distention, unlike stercoral colitis.
- Postoperative patients with distention typically are due to an ileus.

Suggested Readings

Boyd SK, Cameron-Morrison JD, Hobson JJ, Saenz R. CT imaging of large bowel wall thickening. J Am Osteopath Coll Radiol. 2016; 5(2):14–22

Choi JS, Lim JS, Kim H, et al. Colonic pseudoobstruction: CT findings. AJR Am J Roentgenol. 2008; 190(6):1521–1526

Heffernan C, Pachter HL, Megibow AJ, Macari M. Stercoral colitis leading to fatal peritonitis: CT findings. AJR Am J Roentgenol. 2005; 184(4):1189–1193

Case 82

Jake Figner

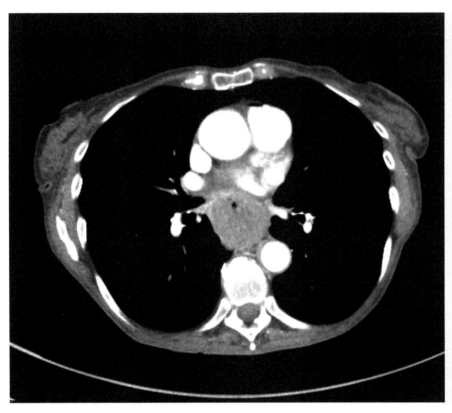

Fig. 82.1 CT with intravenous contrast of the lower chest demonstrates eccentric wall thickening of the distal esophagus which is mass-like.

■ **Clinical History**

An 88-year-old female with dysphagia (▶Fig. 82.1).

■ Key Finding

Eccentric wall thickening of the distal esophagus.

■ Top 3 Differential Diagnoses

- **Esophageal carcinoma:** The most common type of esophageal carcinoma is squamous cell carcinoma (SCC). SCC is typically seen in the proximal two-thirds while adenocarcinoma is more commonly seen in the distal One-thirds. Adenocarcinoma is the second most common type of cancer. Both can present as either circumferential or asymmetric wall thickening. Mediastinal lymphadenopathy suggests localized metastasis. Risk factors for esophageal SCC include tobacco use, alcohol consumption, achalasia, and long standing esophagitis. Adenocarcinoma is more closely related with gastroesophageal reflux and Barrett's metaplasia.
- **Esophagitis:** Inflammation of the esophagus most commonly caused by gastroesophageal reflux but can also be secondary to infection, chemotherapy, caustic ingestion, or radiation. CT may demonstrate wall thickening, submucosal edema (target sign), and thickened folds. Esophagus may demonstrate a "shaggy" appearance on barium studies.
- **Esophageal varices:** Dilated and tortuous collateral veins which may be "uphill" due to increased portal venous pressure or "downhill" due to superior vena cava (SVC) obstruction. Varices may present on CT as wall thickening with a lobular contour. Tortuous radiolucent filling defects can be seen on barium esophagram. Variceal hemorrhage is the most serious complication. Treatment may include blood pressure control or vascular ligation. Transjugular intrahepatic portosystemic shunt (TIPS) can be performed to relieve portal hypertension. Varicoid carcinoma should be considered if the esophagus demonstrates a varicoid appearance and does not distend with contrast administration.

■ Additional Diagnostic Considerations

Lymphoma and metastasis: Metastasis of the esophagus is most commonly by direct spread, although lymphatic or hematogenous spread is also possible. Gastric and lung cancers are most common primaries with esophageal metastasis. Lymphoma involving the esophagus is most commonly due to non-Hodgkin. The esophagus is the least commonly affected portion of the gastrointestinal tract by lymphoma. Primary esophageal lymphoma may be seen in AIDS patients.

■ Diagnosis

Esophageal adenocarcinoma.

✓ Pearls

- SCC is more strongly associated with smoking and alcohol use. SCC is typically seen in proximal two-third of esophagus.
- Adenocarcinoma is more often a result of chronic gastroesophageal reflux disease (GERD) with progression to Barrett's esophagus and adenocarcinoma. It is more often seen in distal one-third of esophagus.
- Esophageal varices may be "downhill" or "uphill" and present as serpiginous filling defects. Varicoid carcinoma should be considered if the esophagus does not distend.
- The esophagus is the portion of the gastrointestinal tract least commonly affected by lymphoma. Direct invasion from lung or gastric carcinoma represent the most common esophageal metastases.

Suggested Readings

Bhalla M, Silver RM, Shepard JA, McLoud TC. Chest CT in patients with scleroderma: prevalence of asymptomatic esophageal dilatation and mediastinal lymphadenopathy. AJR Am J Roentgenol. 1993; 161(2):269–272

Federle MP, Jeffrey RB, Woodward PJ, Borhani A. Diagnostic Imaging: Abdomen. 2nd ed. Philadelphia, PA: Lippincott Williams & Wilkins; 2009

Hong SJ, Kim TJ, Nam KB, et al. New TNM staging system for esophageal cancer: what chest radiologists need to know. Radiographics. 2014; 34(6):1722–1740

Reinig JW, Stanley JH, Schabel SI. CT evaluation of thickened esophageal walls. AJR Am J Roentgenol. 1983; 140(5):931–934

Case 83

Rocky C. Saenz

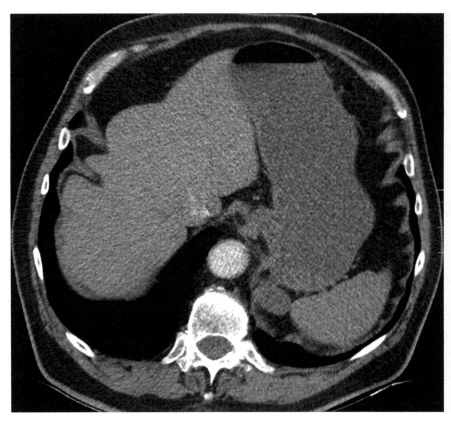

Fig. 83.1 CT abdomen with intravenous contrast shows a well-circumscribed focus posterior to the gastric fundus.

■ Clinical History

A 43-year-old male with abdominal pain (▶Fig. 83.1).

■ Key Finding

Lesion posterior to the stomach.

■ Top 3 Differential Diagnoses

- **Gastric diverticulum:** Gastric diverticulum is not uncommon. The most common location is in the cardiac region. The key to the diagnosis is visualizing the connection of the diverticulum to the stomach. This may be confirmed on CT with oral contrast or barium fluoroscopy. Typically these are true diverticula and extend through all three layers of the stomach wall.
- **Adrenal mass:** The most common mass of the adrenal gland is an adenoma. Adenomas account for greater than 90% of adrenal masses. The second most common cause of adrenal lesions is metastasis. Adrenal pheochromocytomas are hypervascular lesions that are typically greater than 3 cm in size. Adrenal primary carcinomas are usually large lesions greater than 6 cm in size. CT adrenal washout studies have the highest sensitivity for differentiating adenomas from metastasis.
- **Accessory spleen:** It represents benign splenic tissue that is congenital origin. The most common location of it is around the hilum of the spleen. The key to diagnosis is noting the same attenuation on CT or signal intensity on MRI as the native spleen. Approximately 10 to 30% of patients have accessory spleens. An accessory spleen can hypertrophy after splenectomy.

■ Diagnosis

Gastric diverticulum.

✓ Pearls

- Gastric diverticulum can be confirmed on a barium study with contrast filling.
- An air-fluid level in a posterior gastric mass is a diverticulum.
- Adrenal adenomas that are lipid rich are easily diagnosed on MRI chemical shift imaging.

Suggested Readings

Federle MP, Jeffrey RB, Woodward PJ, Borhani A. Diagnostic Imaging: Abdomen. 2nd ed. Philadelphia, PA: Lippincott Williams & Wilkins; 2009

Schwartz AN, Goiney RC, Graney DO. Gastric diverticulum simulating an adrenal mass: CT appearance and embryogenesis. AJR Am J Roentgenol. 1986; 146(3):553–554

Case 84

Reehan M. Ali

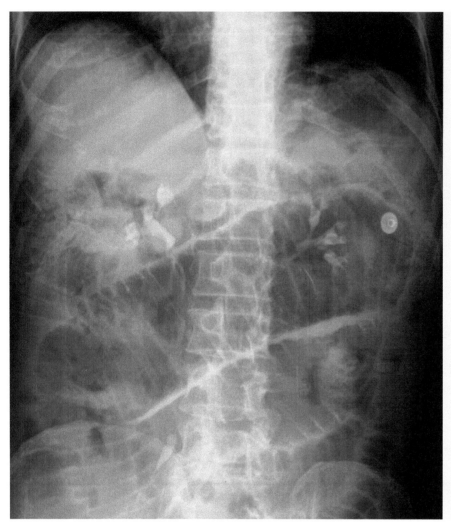

Fig. 84.1 Abdominal X-ray taken in the supine position shows markedly dilated small bowel loop. (Image courtesy of Rocky C. Saenz.)

■ Clinical History

An 83-year-old male with early satiety (▶ Fig. 84.1).

■ Key Finding

Dilated small bowel loops.

■ Top 3 Differential Diagnoses

- **Mechanical obstruction:** Dilated small bowel loops are greater than 2.5 cm in diameter when measuring from outer wall to outer wall. Stacked air-fluid levels are seen on the upright abdominal film. CT is utilized to further characterize the degree of obstruction (low-grade partial, high-grade partial or complete) and to identify a transition point to aid in surgical planning. Small bowel follow-through is typically used to aid in partial versus complete obstruction characterization although delayed CT after the administration of oral contrast has accomplished similar results in the literature. The most common causes are overwhelmingly postsurgical adhesions (developed world) and hernias (developing world).
- **Ileus:** A term used to describe aperistaltic bowel not caused by mechanical obstruction. Radiographically it can be difficult to distinguish from mechanical obstruction as many features overlap. Clinical information can aid in differentiation as patients will typically present with non-colicky abdominal pain, which is prolonged and often occurs after surgery. CT will also demonstrate lack of a transition point and lack of distal decompressed loops of small and large bowel. Medications have been implicated as well, most commonly opioids.
- **Scleroderma:** Results in systemic sclerosis due to the deposition of collagen. In addition to small bowel dilatation, can cause reversal of jejunal/ileal fold pattern that is caused by villous atrophy and crypt hypertrophy leading to chronic fluid overload. Classically it is seen with sacculations along with antimesenteric border. Look for associated imaging findings such as esophageal dilatation and pulmonary fibrosis.

■ Additional Diagnostic Considerations

Sprue: Sprue results in lack of mucosal folds in the jejunum. This leads to a featureless appearance of the jejunum, which then appears as a "cast" of itself which is termed the "Moulage sign."

■ Diagnosis

Small bowel obstruction.

✓ Pearls

- Small bowel is dilated when it is larger than 2.5 cm.
- Look for a transition point and distal decompressed small bowel loops to differential mechanical obstruction from an ileus.
- Inflammatory conditions resulting in small bowel dilatation will have other radiographic signs to aid in the diagnosis.

Suggested Readings

Federle MP, Jeffrey RB, Woodward PJ, Borhani A. Diagnostic Imaging: Abdomen. 2nd ed. Philadelphia, PA: Lippincott Williams & Wilkins; 2009

Lappas JC, Reyes BL, Maglinte DD. Abdominal radiography findings in small-bowel obstruction: relevance to triage for additional diagnostic imaging. AJR Am J Roentgenol. 2001; 176(1):167–174

Silva AC, Pimenta M, Guimarães LS. Small bowel obstruction: what to look for. Radiographics. 2009; 29(2):423–439

Case 85

Kathy M. Borovicka

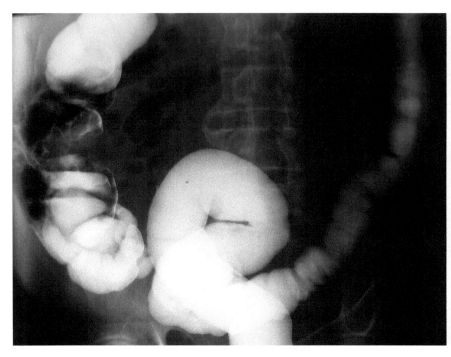

Fig. 85.1 Overhead image from a barium enema demonstrates persistent mucosal irregularity involving the cecum with eccentric wall thickening and luminal narrowing. (Image courtesy of Rocky C. Saenz.)

■ **Clinical History**

A 70-year-old female with pencil stools and abdominal pain (▶Fig. 85.1).

■ Key Finding

Asymmetric cecal wall thickening.

■ Top 3 Differential Diagnoses

• **Adenocarcinoma:** Adenocarcinoma is the most common carcinoma of the colon. The cecum accounts for 25% of all adenocarcinomas within the colon. In the cecum, they can grow to be large without causing obstruction and can serve as lead points for intussusception. CT features include asymmetric wall thickening within a shorter segment of bowel, abrupt change from abnormal to normal bowel wall, and minimal adjacent fatty infiltration. When large, these masses can be bulky and polypoid. In 10% of cases, these cecal masses can extend and involve the terminal ileum and result in congestion and edema of the terminal ileum. On barium evaluations, luminal narrowing is identified.

• **Diverticulitis:** Diverticular disease is most common in the distal colon and less common in the cecum. Identification of cecal diverticuli, asymmetric or circumferential bowel wall thickening, and pericecal inflammatory change are key CT findings. Visualization of a normal appendix and pericolonic inflammation at the site of the cecal diverticula excludes appendicitis. Complications include perforation with pneumoperitoneum and abscess formation.

• **Infectious colitis:** Infections result in focal or diffuse bowel wall thickening with ulcerations. Certain organisms are known to affect the right colon with occasional spread to the terminal ileum and the possibility of affecting the distal colon. These are salmonellosis (typhoid fever), *Yersinia* enterocolitis, tuberculosis, cytomegalovirus (CMV), histoplasmosis, mucormycosis, and amebiasis. CT may show thickened folds and wall thickening, haustral loss from edema or spasm, ulcerations, and narrowing of the lumen. Each organism may cause a slightly different appearance within the segments involved.

■ Additional Diagnostic Considerations

• **Inflammatory disease:** Crohn's disease affects the terminal ileum and the cecum. Skip lesions with wall thickening, wall edema with layered enhancement, mesenteric fat stranding, and lymph nodes are identified within the acute stage of the disease. Complications of fistula formation, sinus tracts, and abscesses are also noted. Ulcerative colitis is a pancolitis involving the entire colon from the rectum to the cecum. Decreased haustrations and ulcerations on barium enema examinations are noted. The risk of colon carcinoma is greater in ulcerative colitis than in Crohn's disease with 25% of ulcerative colitis cases having multiple carcinomas.

• **Lymphoma:** The cecum is the most common location of primary lymphoma in the colon with possible extension to involve the terminal ileum and the appendix. Single or multiple segments of more symmetric circumferential wall thickening with marked wall thickening (1.5–7 cm) is identified. Aneurysmal dilation of the bowel and ulceration with fistulous communication with other bowel loops are potential complications. Significant lymphadenopathy can also be identified.

■ Diagnosis

Adenocarcinoma.

✓ Pearls

• Carcinomas in the cecum when large may be lead points for intussusception.
• Crohn's disease is more common along the right colon while ulcerative colitis is more common along the left colon and rectum.

• Diverticulitis should only be considered when diverticula are present.

Suggested Readings

Boyd SK, Cameron-Morrison JD, Hobson JJ, et al. CT imaging of large bowel wall thickening. J Am Osteopath Coll Radiol. 2016; 5(2):14–22

Federle MP, Jeffrey RB, Woodward PJ, Borhani A. Diagnostic Imaging: Abdomen. 2nd ed. Philadelphia, PA: Lippincott Williams & Wilkins; 2009

Hoeffel C, Crema MD, Belkacem A, et al. Multi-detector row CT: spectrum of diseases involving the ileocecal area. Radiographics. 2006; 26(5):1373–1390

Case 86

Julia D. Cameron-Morrison

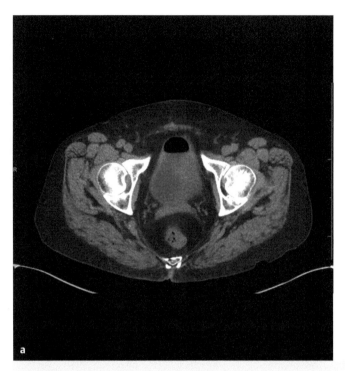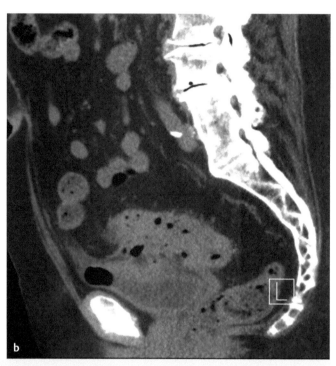

Fig. 86.1 Axial (**a**) and sagittal (**b**) images from a CT pelvis without contrast demonstrate an air-fluid level in urinary bladder and thickening of the superior bladder wall. Sigmoid colon inflammation is present with loss of the fat plane between the urinary bladder and colon.

■ Clinical History

A 74-year-old female with a urinary tract infection with remote history of hysterectomy (▶ Fig. 86.1).

■ Key Finding

Air in the urinary bladder in absence of a catheter.

■ Top 3 Differential Diagnoses

- **Diverticulitis:** Diverticulitis is the most common cause of colovesical fistula formation and is associated with approximately half of cases. While more common in men, overall there is an increased risk in women following hysterectomy. The fistula tract is rarely seen directly. Indirect findings of a colovesical fistula include intravesicular air with focal bladder wall thickening and/or inflammatory changes of the colon with loss of the fat plane between the colon and the urinary bladder. Occasionally, cystography or a contrast enema may demonstrate the fistulous tract.

- **Recent instrumentation:** Air can be introduced into the urinary bladder with instrumentation, most commonly following introduction or removal of a catheter. The presence of a Foley catheter bulb within the bladder lumen accounts for vesicular air. The lack of urinary bladder wall thickening and absence of perivesicular fat stranding excludes inflammation.
- **Cystitis:** When infection of the bladder occurs in the presence of gas forming bacteria, intravesicular air and urinary bladder wall thickening can be seen simulating a fistula. On CT, look for perivesicular fat stranding without involvement of the surrounding bowel.

■ Additional Diagnostic Considerations

- **Inflammatory bowel disease:** Fistula formation is a known complication of Crohn's disease. While it most commonly involves the terminal ileum any portion of bowel can be involved. In addition to secondary signs of colovesical fistula, classic findings of Crohn's disease may be seen including circumferential bowel wall thickening often with skip lesions, mesenteric hyperemia, fatty infiltration of the bowel wall, and strictures.

- **Neoplasm/carcinoma:** Both genitourinary and gastrointestinal neoplasms have been associated with colovesical fistulas. On CT, indirect signs of fistula can be seen including air within the urinary bladder. There will be associated bladder and/or colonic wall thickening in the absence of surrounding inflammatory change. Lymphadenopathy may also be seen.

■ Diagnosis

Colovesical fistula secondary to diverticulitis.

✓ Pearls

- Correlate for history of recent instrumentation when air is seen within the bladder.
- Hysterectomy increases the risk of colovesical fistula formation in women.

- A direct fistulous tract is rarely seen, so secondary signs are helpful.

Suggested Readings

Boyd SK, Cameron-Morrison JD, Hobson JJ, Saenz R. CT imaging of large bowel wall thickening. J Am Osteopath Coll Radiol. 2016; 5(2):14–22

Federle MP, Jeffrey RB, Woodward PJ, Borhani A. Diagnostic Imaging: Abdomen. 2nd ed. Philadelphia, PA: Lippincott Williams & Wilkins; 2009

Yu NC, Raman SS, Patel M, Barbaric Z. Fistulas of the genitourinary tract: a radiologic review. Radiographics. 2004; 24(5):1331–1352

Case 87

Jake Figner

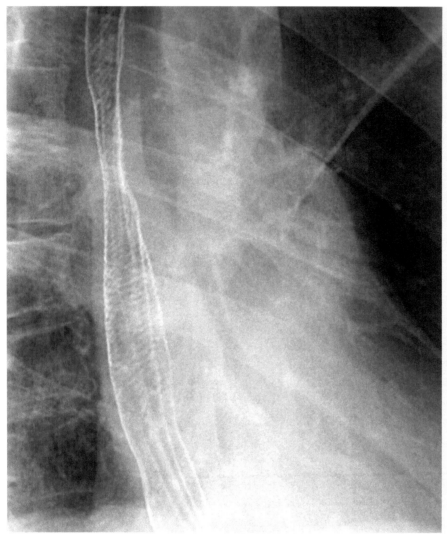

Fig. 87.1 Lateral fluoroscopy image from an upper gastrointestinal image of the distal esophagus. The image demonstrates transverse folds of the esophagus with a normal luminal diameter. (Image courtesy of Rocky C. Saenz.)

■ Clinical History

A 28-year-old female with lower chest pain (▶Fig. 87.1).

■ Key Finding

Transverse esophageal folds/lines.

■ Top 3 Differential Diagnoses

- **Feline esophagus:** Transverse esophageal lines involving the entire circumference of the esophagus. The esophageal markings are transient in nature, thin (1–2 mm), and almost always seen in association with gastroesophageal reflux. Feline esophagus is named after the morphologic similarity to a cat's esophagus. The transverse folds typically resolve during swallowing.
- **Esophageal web:** A mucosal fold resulting in variable degree of esophageal narrowing. It often appears as a thin (1–2 mm wide) shelf-like filling defect but can also appear as a circumferential radiolucent ring. Webs are usually asymptomatic and may be seen anywhere throughout the esophagus. Webs are most common within the upper cervical esophagus. Esophageal webs have several associated conditions including chronic gastroesophageal reflux, Plummer–Vinson syndrome, chronic gastroesophageal reflux, and eosinophilic esophagitis.
- **Diffuse esophageal spasm (DES):** DES results in irregular esophageal motility that can cause noncardiac chest pain or dysphagia. The key imaging features on fluoroscopy include transverse bands and nonperistaltic contractions with both anterograde and retrograde movement of contrast. Transverse bands will be larger in size when compared to the feline esophagus. These can uncommonly result in a classic "corkscrew" or "rosary bead" esophagus.

■ Additional Diagnostic Considerations

Eosinophilic esophagitis: Inflammation of the esophagus with characteristic infiltration of eosinophils. Most characteristic imaging finding is concentric esophageal strictures on barium swallow (ring esophagus). It can be seen anywhere along the gastrointestinal tract and may manifest as fold thickening and submucosal edema within the bowel. Most of those affected have allergy/food intolerance history. Biopsy of esophagus is required for definitive diagnosis. Eosinophilic esophagitis responds well to steroid treatment.

■ Diagnosis

Feline esophagus.

✓ Pearls

- Feline esophagus is almost always associated with gastroesophageal reflux. It is transient and will resolve during swallowing.
- Larger transverse folds with bidirectional movement on contrast suggest DES.
- Esophageal webs are associated with esophagitis, Plummer–Vinson syndrome, and chronic reflux.

Suggested Readings

Levine MS, Goldstein HM. Fixed transverse folds in the esophagus: a sign of reflux esophagitis. AJR Am J Roentgenol. 1984; 143(2):275–278

Picus D, Frank PH. Eosinophilic esophagitis. AJR Am J Roentgenol. 1981; 136(5):1001–1003

Samadi F, Levine MS, Rubesin SE, Katzka DA, Laufer I. Feline esophagus and gastroesophageal reflux. AJR Am J Roentgenol. 2010; 194(4):972–976

Case 88

Vernon F. Williams, Jr.

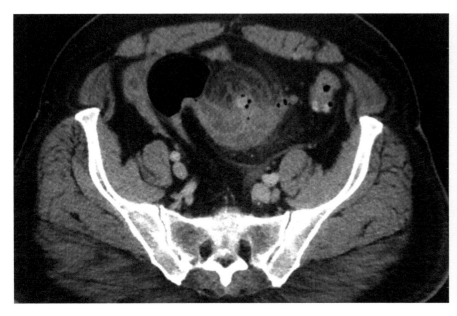

Fig. 88.1 CT axial image with intravenous contrast demonstrates fat stranding adjacent to the sigmoid colon which has a couple diverticula. (Image courtesy of Rocky C. Saenz.)

■ **Clinical History**

A 44-year-old male with lower midabdominal pain (▶Fig. 88.1).

■ Key Finding

Pericolonic fat stranding.

■ Top 3 Differential Diagnoses

- **Diverticulitis:** Diverticular occlusion most commonly occurs in the sigmoid colon and results in inflammation leading to erosion and potentially perforation. The fat stranding is disproportionately greater than the adjacent reactive focal wall thickening. Imaging features include the comma sign (accumulation of fluid on the sigmoid mesentery root) and the centipede sign (mesenteric vessel engorgement). Complications include abscess and fistula. When diverticulitis is complicated intervention may be needed.
- **Epiploic appendagitis:** Epiploic appendages are fat-filled peritoneal pouches that arise from the colonic serosal surface with a vascular stalk (two arteries and one vein). The appendages have limited mobility leaving them prone to torsion. CT demonstrates an oval fatty mass with peripheral fat stranding. This is a self-limiting disease with imaging findings often outlasting symptoms (up to 18 months after initial presentation). The appendages may calcify after an ischemic insult and can result in peritoneal loose bodies.
- **Acute Colitis:** There are many causes of colitis which can result in left lower quadrant fat stranding. Etiologies include ischemia, infection, radiation, neoplasm, inflammatory bowel disease, and fecal impaction. Findings are often variable and clinical history can help clinch the diagnosis. Ischemic bowel is usually a result of atherosclerosis, embolic/thrombotic disease, or hypoperfusion. CT findings in ischemic colitis early phase overlap with other causes of colitis, but in the late phase pneumatosis and portal venous gas are noted.

■ Additional Diagnostic Considerations

- **Adenocarcinoma:** Carcinoma presents as focal wall thickening and pericolonic stranding, mimicking colitis. Regional lymphadenopathy and distant metastasis are secondary findings that suggest carcinoma. Correlation with colonoscopy and carcinoembryonic antigen level should be considered in suspicious patients.
- **Inflammatory disease:** Crohn's disease and ulcerative colitis are idiopathic conditions leading to bowel wall inflammation.

In ulcerative colitis the inflammation is limited to the mucosal layer, and Crohn's disease is transmural. Ulcerative colitis begins in the rectum progressing proximally without skip lesions (vs. Crohn's). Chronic disease will lead to fixed colonic dilation (a "lead pipe" appearance). If ulcerative colitis reaches the terminal ileum, it will result in dilation and is termed "backwash" ileitis. Ulcerative colitis also increases the risk of colon cancer by 10% (while Crohn's does not).

■ Diagnosis

Diverticulitis of sigmoid colon.

✓ Pearls

- Fat stranding around a diverticulum is diverticulitis.
- Epiploic appendagitis most commonly affects the left colon.

- Ulcerative colitis increases the risk of cancer.

Suggested Readings

Boyd SK, Cameron-Morrison JD, Hobson JJ, Saenz R. CT imaging of large bowel wall thickening. J Am Osteopath Coll Radiol. 2016; 5(2):14–22

Pereira JM, Sirlin CB, Pinto PS, Jeffrey RB, Stella DL, Casola G. Disproportionate fat stranding: a helpful CT sign in patients with acute abdominal pain. Radiographics. 2004; 24(3):703–715

Thornton E, Mendiratta-Lala M, Siewert B, Eisenberg RL. Patterns of fat stranding. AJR Am J Roentgenol. 2011; 197(1):W1:W14

Case 89

Andrew Mizzi

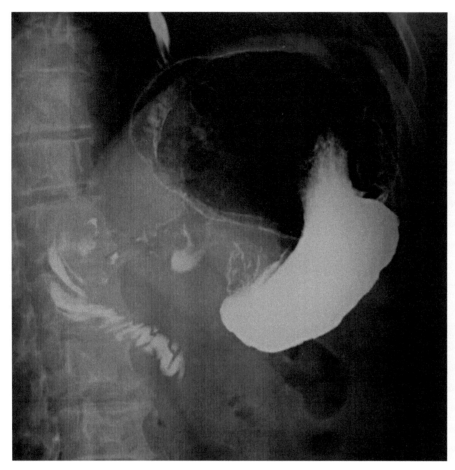

Fig. 89.1 Single Upper gastrointestinal barium frontal image which shows a focal ulcer pit along the greater curve of the distal stomach with mucosal irregularity and duodenal wall thickening. (Image courtesy of Rocky C. Saenz.)

■ Clinical History

A 53-year-old male with epigastric pain (▶Fig. 89.1).

■ Key Finding

Gastric ulcer.

■ Top 3 Differential Diagnoses

- **Peptic ulcer disease:** An ulcer is a focal disruption of the mucosa into the muscularis mucosa and deeper layers of the wall. Gastric and duodenal ulcers most commonly present as epigastric pain usually after meals. Barium studies are more accurate than cross-sectional imaging in visualizing ulcerations. Classic benign ulcers are typically seen as smooth shape pit, straight radiating folds with an ulcer that projects outside the contour of the stomach lumen. When peptic ulcer disease is suspected on barium studies it can be confirmed with endoscopy. *H. pylori* infection is an important test in all patients with peptic ulcers. Peptic ulcer disease complications include gastrointestinal bleeds and hematemesis. Patients are treated for *H. pylori* infection and advised to avoid the use of nonsteroidal anti-inflammatory drugs. Cross-sectional imaging is poor in detecting ulcers but excellent in detection of complications of such as free air and fluid collections related to perforation.
- **Crohn's disease:** Crohn's disease is one form of inflammatory bowel disease. It is the most common inflammatory disease affecting the small bowel. Crohn's disease can affect any part of the alimentary tract from the mouth to anus. Granulomatous inflammation starts along the submucosa and eventually develops to transmural involvement. It causes edema, ulcers, and fibrosis. In chronic phase, it manifests as stenosis and fistulas. It affects mostly young adults but can have a late onset. On imaging, Crohn's disease is most commonly seen in the terminal ileum as stenosis (string sign) and/or fistula formation. Also seen are sacculations associated with the strictures. Aphthoid ulcers are seen in early Crohn's disease from erosions into the mucosa. Larger ulcerations can be seen anywhere in the alimentary canal. Crohn's disease has a high incidence of recurrence in surgically treated patients.
- **Gastric adenocarcinoma:** Gastric adenocarcinoma is the most common malignancy of the stomach (≈ 90%). Primary gastric adenocarcinoma can also result in focal ulcers. Malignant ulcers on barium studies typically have lobulated folds, irregular ulcer pit shape, and nodularity at ulcer margin and may project inside or outside the expected lumen of the stomach. Scirrhous carcinoma accounts for 5 to 15% of cases and presents as linitis plastica. Adenocarcinoma risk factors include nitrites, salted, and smoked foods.

■ Additional Diagnostic Considerations

Gastritis: Acute gastritis encompasses a number of causes of gastric mucosal inflammation. It can be seen incidentally on imaging or found on work up for epigastric pain, nausea/emesis, and loss of appetite. Gastritis can result from infection (*H. pylori* being the most common), systemic illness, or massive trauma, autoimmune, or caustic ingestion. It can also be seen in immunosuppressed states or eosinophilic gastritis.

■ Diagnosis

Gastric ulcer secondary to Crohn disease.

✓ Pearls

- The most common cause of gastritis is *H. pylori*.
- Benign ulcers are typically seen as straight radiating folds with a smooth ulcer that projects outside the contour of the stomach lumen.
- Malignant ulcers have lobulated folds, irregular ulcer pit shape, and nodularity at ulcer margin and can project inside or outside the stomach lumen.

Suggested Readings

Federle MP, Jeffrey RB, Woodward PJ, Borhani A. Diagnostic Imaging: Abdomen. 2nd ed. Philadelphia, PA: Lippincott Williams & Wilkins; 2009

Guniganti P, Bradenham CH, Raptis C, Menias CO, Mellnick VM. CT of gastric emergencies. Radiographics. 2015; 35(7):1909–1921

Rubesin SE, Levine MS, Laufer I. Double-contrast upper gastrointestinal radiography: a pattern approach for diseases of the stomach. Radiology. 2008; 246(1):33–48

Case 90

Vernon F. Williams, Jr.

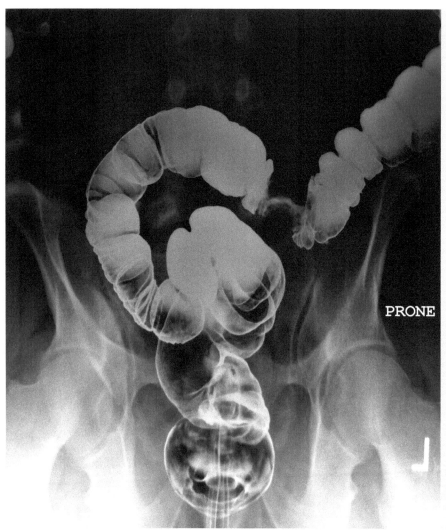

Fig. 90.1 Single frontal barium enema image demonstrating a focal, short segment luminal narrowing of a sigmoid colon.

■ Clinical History

A 69-year-old female with abdominal pain, constipation (▶Fig. 90.1).

■ Key Finding

Colonic short segment luminal narrowing.

■ Top 3 Differential Diagnoses

- **Malignancy:** Colorectal malignancies can be primary or metastatic. The most common primary malignancy is adenocarcinoma. Imaging features include focal irregular/asymmetric soft-tissue wall thickening that narrows the bowel lumen. Apple core lesions can be seen on barium examinations. Calcifications and low-density lymph nodes are involved in the mucinous subtype. Complications include fistula, obstruction, and intussusception. Lymphoma is another rare primary malignancy involving the large bowel and typically affects multiple colonic segments. Primary malignancies that can metastasize to the colon include ovarian carcinoma from direct invasion and gastric carcinoma drop metastases.

- **Inflammatory disease:** Benign inflammatory conditions such as ulcerative colitis and Crohn's disease can mimic neoplasm on imaging. Crohn's disease typically involves the right colon and the terminal ileum. In Crohn's disease, wall thickening preferentially involves the mesenteric side of the bowel wall. Imaging features include discontinuous involvement ("skip lesions"), fistulas, strictures, abscesses (transmural inflammation), and mesenteric fat proliferation.

- **Infectious colitis:** Infectious colitis is the most common cause of focal bowel wall thickening and is frequently the sequela of diverticulitis. Imaging features are colonic air-fluid levels, wall thickening, and increased mucosal enhancement. This may be either long segment of focal. Intestinal tuberculosis is rare and also involves the ileocecal region and has discontinuous involvement similar to Crohn's. Amoebic colitis is caused by *E. histolytica* and it spares the ileum, differentiating it from Crohn's.

■ Additional Diagnostic Considerations

- **Endometriosis:** Endometriosis can locally penetrate organs of the gastrointestinal tract. Endometrial implants to the gastrointestinal tract occur in one-fourth of patients with endometriosis. It most commonly affects the bowel segments in the dependent portion of pelvis and is rarely found proximal to the terminal ileum (rectosigmoid > appendix > cecum > distal ileum). The implants eventually erode through the subserosa and cause thickening and fibrosis of the muscularis propria. Inflammatory response to cyclic hormonal hemorrhage leads to complications, including adhesions, stricture, and obstruction.

- **Postsurgical:** Anastomosis of the colon can result in a focal colonic stricture. Identification of postsurgical changes at the site of the stricture and a surgical history will lead to the correct diagnosis.

■ Diagnosis

Adenocarcinoma.

✓ Pearls

- Colonic malignancy may appear as an "apple core" lesion on barium studies.
- Endometriosis favors the rectosigmoid colon and rarely involves the small bowel.
- Colonoscopy and biopsy can help exclude malignancy in the setting of bowel wall thickening.

Suggested Readings

Boyd SK, Cameron-Morrison JD, Hobson JJ, Saenz R. CT imaging of large bowel wall thickening. JAOCR. 2016; 5(2):14–22

Horton KM, Abrams RA, Fishman EK. Spiral CT of colon cancer: imaging features and role in management. Radiographics. 2000; 20(2):419–430

Macari M, Balthazar EJ. CT of bowel wall thickening: significance and pitfalls of interpretation. AJR Am J Roentgenol. 2001; 176(5):1105–1116

Woodward PJ, Sohaey R, Mezzetti TP, Jr. Endometriosis: radiologic-pathologic correlation. Radiographics. 2001; 21(1):193–216, 288–294

Case 91

Michael L. Schwartz

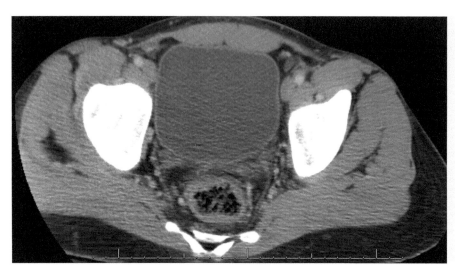

Fig. 91.1 Contrast enhanced axial CT image through the lower pelvis reveals abnormal, symmetric wall thickening of the rectum. (Image courtesy of Rocky C. Saenz.)

■ **Clinical History**

A 27-year-old male with bright blood per rectum (▶ Fig. 91.1).

■ Key Finding

Symmetric rectal wall thickening.

■ Top 3 Differential Diagnoses

- **Proctitis:** An inflammation of the lining of the rectum can be acute or chronic. On cross-sectional imaging, the rectal wall thickening is classically concentric measuring greater than 6 mm with associated perirectal fat stranding. Presenting symptoms include rectal pain, bloody stools, and urgency. Rectal and perirectal abscess are complications of advanced infection, Crohn's, and immunocompromised patients. Etiologies include radiation therapy, sexually transmitted infections, inflammatory diseases, ischemia, and trauma. Ischemic proctitis is rare secondary to rich vascular supply to rectum. Chronic radiation induced proctitis typically has an onset of 9 to 14 months but can occur over decades.
- **Inflammatory bowel disease:** Crohn's disease and ulcerative colitis both result in bowel wall thickening. Ulcerative colitis involves the rectum and extends continuously and proximally to potentially involve the entire colon, whereas Crohn's disease typically does not involve the rectum and is discontinuous. The wall thickening in ulcerative colitis may be symmetric and diffuse. Patients present with gradually worsening episodes of

bloody diarrhea, frequent small bowel movements, urgency, colicky lower abdominal pain, fever, and weight loss. Arthritis is the most common extraintestinal presentation. Ulcerative colitis patients have an increased risk of developing colorectal cancer, which is directly related to the extent and duration of disease. Another common complication is colonic stricture or a fixed and dilated colon (lead pipe). Ulcerative colitis classic finding is concentric wall thickening involving the left colon and rectum.

- **Adenocarcinoma:** Adenocarcinoma is the most common colorectal malignancy and is related to the mucin producing glands. Typical CT findings are heterogeneously enhancing irregular mass with asymmetric rectal wall thickening and luminal narrowing. Complications include obstruction, perforation, and fistula formation. When advanced, it may present with metastatic lesions and adenopathy. Metastatic disease is most commonly seen involving the liver. MRI is the most accurate means of staging. Treatment depends on the stage.

■ Additional Diagnostic Considerations

- **Lymphoma:** Colonic lymphoma is uncommon. It can present as wall thickening but classically is a large lesion with widespread adenopathy. The prognosis of primary colonic lymphoma is poor with the 5-year survival rate only being 50%.
- **Internal Hemorrhoids:** Internal hemorrhoids are large lobulated folds extending greater than 3 cm above anorectal

junction. Contrast CT can demonstrate dilated vessels mimicking a mass or wall thickening but are usually diagnosed by their typical serpiginous appearance. Etiologies include decrease venous return from straining or prolonged sitting on a toilet and pregnancy.

■ Diagnosis

Proctitis.

✓ Pearls

- Rectal wall greater than 6 mm is always abnormal despite nondistention.
- Large rectal mass with extensive adenopathy consider lymphoma.

- Rectal wall thickening extending to the descending colon should be considered to be ulcerative colitis.

Suggested Readings

Boyd SK, Cameron-Morrison JD, Hobson JJ, Saenz R. CT imaging of large bowel wall thickening. J Am Osteopath Coll Radiol. 2016; 5(2):14–22

Federle MP, Jeffrey RB, Woodward PJ, Borhani A. Diagnostic Imaging: Abdomen. 2nd ed. Philadelphia, PA: Lippincott Williams & Wilkins; 2009

Jhaveri KS, Hosseini-Nik H. MRI of rectal cancer: an overview and update on recent advances. AJR Am J Roentgenol. 2015; 205(1):W42:W55

Case 92

Reehan M. Ali

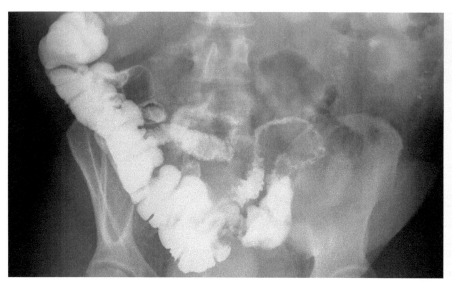

Fig. 92.1 Single image from a barium small bowel antegrade study which shows a long segment of bowel wall thickening involving the ileum in the left pelvis. Second shorter segment of luminal narrowing also noted. (Image courtesy of Rocky C. Saenz.)

■ Clinical History

A 36-year-old male with bloody stools and pain (▶Fig. 92.1).

■ Key Finding

Long segment small bowel wall thickening.

■ Top 3 Differential Diagnoses

- **Ischemic enteritis:** Thickening of the bowel is one of the most common but least specific signs of bowel ischemia. CT appearance depends on pathologic stage of injury to the bowel which can range from mild mural edema to transmural infarction. In addition to bowel wall thickening, other findings include mesenteric edema and ascites. Intestinal pneumatosis and gas in the mesenteric and portal veins are indicative of severe ischemia and the wall is typically thinned when it reaches this stage.
- **Inflammatory bowel disease:** Crohn's disease may affect any portion of the bowel and is most commonly seen involving the right colon and terminal ileum. It is classically described as having a "halo" or "target" appearance of the bowel wall thickening on cross-sectional imaging, with alternative layers of hyperattenuated mucosa, hypoattenuated intramural edema, and hyperattenuated serosa. Mucosal hyperemia is a more sensitive indicator of active disease and is readily diagnosed on CT enterography. Extraenteric findings can aid in diagnosis and include the "comb sign" which relates to engorged vasa recta within the mesentery that run perpendicular to the bowel.
- **Infectious enteritis:** In contrast to infectious colitis, infectious enteritis appears only mildly thickened. The enhancement pattern may be homogeneous or striated due to intramural edema. Certain organisms show characteristic patterns of involvement. Parasitic enteritis caused by *Giardia* and *Strongyloides* involves the proximal small bowel, while bacterial infections such as *Salmonella* and *Yersinia* affect the distal small bowel. Tuberculosis, typhlitis, and amebiasis typically involve the distal ileum and cecum.

■ Diagnosis

Crohn disease.

✓ Pearls

- Be cognizant of the classic signs of Crohn's disease including enteric and extraenteric findings.
- Pneumatosis equals ischemic bowel until proven otherwise.
- Distribution of small bowel involvement can provide a diagnostic clue as to the offending organism in infectious enteritis.

Suggested Readings

Childers BC, Cater SW, Horton KM, Fishman EK, Johnson PT. CT evaluation of acute enteritis and colitis: is it infectious, inflammatory or ischemic? Radiographics. 2015; 35(7):1940–1941

Federle MP, Jeffrey RB, Woodward PJ, Borhani A. Diagnostic Imaging: Abdomen. 2nd ed. Philadelphia, PA: Lippincott Williams & Wilkins; 2009

Wittenberg J, Harisinghani MG, Jhaveri K, Varghese J, Mueller PR. Algorithmic approach to CT diagnosis of the abnormal bowel wall. Radiographics. 2002; 22(5):1093–1107, discussion 1107–1109

Case 93

Rocky C. Saenz

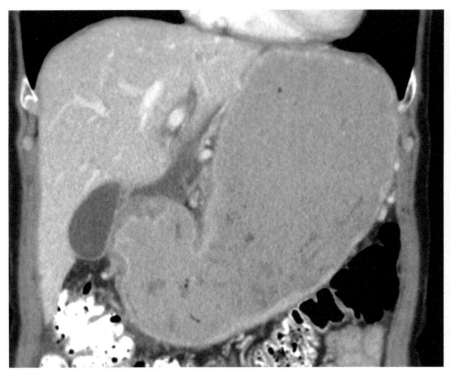

Fig. 93.1 CT coronal image with intravenous and oral contrast shows a dilated stomach with debris and eccentric wall thickening in the antrum.

■ **Clinical History**

A 43-year-old male with abdominal pain (▶Fig. 93.1).

■ Key Finding

Dilated stomach with debris.

■ Top 3 Differential Diagnoses

- **Gastroparesis:** Gastric distention secondary to decreased peristalsis. This leads to retention of food and fluid. On CT, a dilated stomach is seen with debris in lumen which is nonspecific findings. The diagnosis can be confirmed with a nuclear medicine gastric emptying study. Risk factors include neurologic disorders, diabetes (most common etiology), and narcotic use (second most common etiology). Gastroparesis can be treated successfully with medications.
- **Gastric adenocarcinoma:** Gastric adenocarcinoma represents greater than 90% of gastric malignancies. It most commonly occurs in the distal stomach and may present with gastric outlet obstruction. On CT, a dilated stomach is seen with debris in lumen and distal concentric or eccentric focal mass-like wall thickening. Unfortunately, 30% of patients with gastric carcinoma present with incurable, advanced disease. When advanced gastric carcinoma causes outlet obstruction it can be treated with a metallic stent.
- **Gastric bezoar:** It represents benign mass-like appearance to the intraluminal contents of the stomach. This is secondary to chronic ingested but undigested stomach contents. Risk factors are the postoperative stomach, poor mastication, and gastroparesis. On CT, a dilated stomach is seen with mass-like debris in lumen. Bezoars are noted to be mobile on fluoroscopy studies. Bezoars are named according to the contents: pharmacobezoar (medications), phytobezoar (vegetables), lactobzoar (milk products more common in toddlers/infants), and trichobezoar (hair). Treatments include endoscopic lavage and fragmentation and surgical intervention for large obstructing bezoars.

■ Diagnosis

Gastric adenocarcinoma.

✓ Pearls

- Gastric adenocarcinoma will have distal concentric or eccentric focal mass-like wall thickening.
- The gastric wall should be thin and uniform with gastroparesis and bezoar cases.
- Gastroparesis can be confirmed with a nuclear gastric emptying study.

Suggested Readings

Federle MP, Jeffrey RB, Woodward PJ, Borhani A. Diagnostic Imaging: Abdomen. 2nd ed. Philadelphia, PA: Lippincott Williams & Wilkins; 2009

Kim JH, Song HY, Shin JH, et al. Metallic stent placement in the palliative treatment of malignant gastric outlet obstructions: primary gastric carcinoma versus pancreatic carcinoma. AJR Am J Roentgenol. 2009; 193(1):241–247

Ripollés T, García-Aguayo J, Martínez MJ, Gil P. Gastrointestinal bezoars: sonographic and CT characteristics. AJR Am J Roentgenol. 2001; 177(1):65–69

Case 94

Kathy M. Borovicka

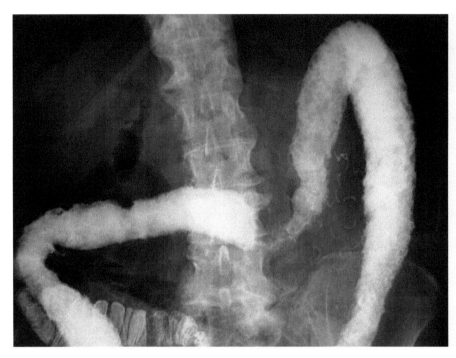

Fig. 94.1 Spot fluoroscopy image of the sigmoid reveals a focal stricture of the colon. Also, note that the visualized colon has an ahaustral appearance. (Image courtesy of Rocky C. Saenz.)

■ Clinical History

A 44-year-old female with left sided abdominal pain (▶Fig. 94.1).

■ Key Finding

Colonic stricture.

■ Top 3 Differential Diagnoses

- **Adenocarcinoma:** Adenocarcinoma is the most common colonic carcinoma. Barium examination can demonstrate the extent of luminal narrowing with the classic description of an apple core lesion with abrupt narrowing, overhanging edges, and shouldering identified. Carcinoma typically involves a shorter segment (less than 10 cm). PET–CT is used for staging, treatment response, and surveillance.
- **Inflammatory disease:** Long-term sequelae of inflammatory conditions such as Crohn's disease and ulcerative colitis can lead to strictures. These are usually more smooth and tapered in comparison to the abrupt narrowing of carcinomas. On barium examinations, other features of chronic inflammatory disease include luminal narrowing, shortened colon, lead pipe colon (ulcerative colitis), loss of haustra, and a widened presacral space (➣ 1.5 cm). Patients with ulcerative colitis are at an increased risk for colon carcinoma with 25% of ulcerative colitis patients having multiple carcinomas.
- **Postischemic:** Ischemic colitis will lead to strictures in approximately 12% of cases. These have a benign appearance with smooth edges and gradual tapering. Hypoperfusion is a predisposing factor such as with hemorrhage, trauma, septic shock, and cardiac issues. Hypoperfusion to the left colon is typically seen in the elderly, and right colon involvement is usually seen in young patients. Imaging in the acute phase may demonstrate hypoattenuation of the bowel wall from edema, hyperattenuation from submucosal hemorrhage, thumbprinting from symmetric circumferential bowel wall thickening, pneumatosis, and portomesenteric venous gas.

■ Additional Diagnostic Considerations

- **Postsurgical:** Anastomosis of the colon can result in a colonic stricture. Identification of postsurgical changes at the site of the stricture and a surgical history will lead to the correct diagnosis. Surgery itself has been used for benign gastrointestinal strictures for patients that do not respond to conservative therapy. Patients that cannot tolerate surgery may be candidates for fluoroscopically guided or endoscopically guided balloon or bougie dilatation. Stent placement of colonic strictures is used in the acute setting.
- **Postradiation:** Pelvic radiation for carcinoma can result in inflammation of the colon and occurs in approximately 50% of patients. Acute inflammation results in colitis with wall thickening and pericolonic inflammation. Chronic radiation changes occur in 6 to 24 months following radiation therapy, secondary to radiation induced endarteritis. Strictures have a benign appearance with smooth tapering noted. An appropriate history is instrumental to the correct diagnosis.

■ Diagnosis

Ulcerative colitis with sigmoid stricture.

✓ Pearls

- An irregular stricture with abrupt narrowing and overhanging edges is usually malignant.
- Pneumatosis is indicative of ischemic colitis.
- Benign appearing strictures with an ahaustral colon are usually ulcerative colitis.

Suggested Readings

Boyd SK, Cameron-Morrison JD, Hobson JJ, et al. CT imaging of large bowel wall thickening. J Am Osteopath Coll Radiol. 2016; 5(2):14–22

Federle MP, Jeffrey RB, Woodward PJ, Borhani A. Diagnostic Imaging: Abdomen. 2nd ed. Philadelphia, PA: Lippincott Williams & Wilkins; 2009

Shin JH, Kim JH, Song HO. Interventional management of benign strictures of the gastrointestinal tract from the stomach to the colon. Gastrointestinal Intervention. 2013; 2(1):7–11

Case 95

Paul B. DiDomenico

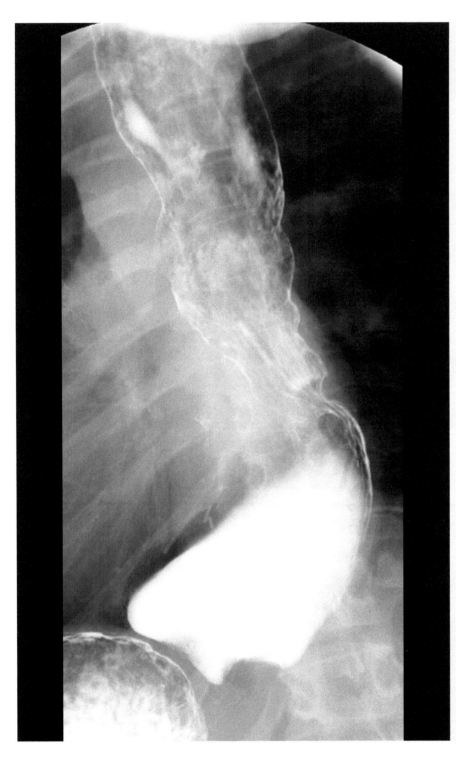

Fig. 95.1 A slightly oblique frontal view from an esophagram reveals a dilated esophagus that tapers to a "bird's beak" appearance distally at the gastroesophageal junction. (Image courtesy of Rocky C. Saenz.)

■ Clinical History

Patient with chronic dysphagia (▶Fig. 95.1).

◼ Key Finding

Esophageal dilatation.

◼ Top 3 Differential Diagnoses

- **Achalasia:** Achalasia is a disease of the myenteric plexus of the esophagus that results in failure of relaxation of the lower esophageal sphincter. Persistent contraction of the lower esophageal sphincter results in smooth distal tapering with a classic "bird's beak" appearance, proximal dilatation on barium esophagram, and diminished or absent peristalsis. Primary (idiopathic) achalasia is thought to be due to degeneration of the myenteric plexus, while secondary achalasia results from destruction of the plexus by infiltrating tumor, or infections such as Chagas' disease or fungal infection. Treatment options include calcium channel blockers, pneumatic dilatation, or Heller myotomy.
- **Scleroderma:** Scleroderma is a collagen vascular disease in which smooth muscle becomes fibrotic. This affects the distal two-thirds of the esophagus, which is lined by smooth muscle, resulting in dysmotility and dilatation. The lower esophageal sphincter becomes incompetent and there is patulous dilation of the gastroesophageal junction, which may help distinguish this disorder from achalasia. The resulting chronic reflux, however, may cause a peptic stricture that may mimic achalasia.
- **Esophageal/gastric carcinoma:** Malignancy of either the distal esophagus or gastric cardia may cause mass effect at the gastroesophageal junction resulting in a tapered narrowing of the lower esophagus with dysmotility and dilatation. Irregularity of the mucosa, "shouldering" mass effect, and correlation with history may suggest malignancy, though final diagnosis would be made via endoscopy and biopsy.

◼ Additional Diagnostic Considerations

- **Esophagitis with stricture:** Long-standing reflux, often with a coexisting hiatal hernia, may result in a peptic stricture at the distal esophagus with narrowing of a short distal segment seen on barium esophagram. Esophageal motility is usually normal, and there is minimal dilatation of the esophagus.
- **Postsurgical changes (vagotomy):** Vagotomy has been reported as a secondary cause of achalasia secondary to neuronal damage or fibrosis at the gastroesophageal junction. These changes result in focal narrowing of the distal esophagus with proximal dilatation.

◼ Diagnosis

Achalasia.

✓ Pearls

- Smooth tapering of the distal esophagus on esophagram ("bird's beak") is a key finding in achalasia.
- Scleroderma often scars the distal esophagus, resulting in a patulous gastroesophageal junction and chronic reflux.
- Irregular tapering of the distal esophagus on esophagram is a concerning finding for carcinoma.

Suggested Readings

Federle MP, Jeffrey RB, Woodward PJ, Borhani A. Diagnostic Imaging: Abdomen. 2nd ed. Philadelphia, PA: Lippincott Williams & Wilkins; 2009

Levine MS, Rubesin SE. Diseases of the esophagus: diagnosis with esophagography. Radiology. 2005; 237(2):414–427

Woodfield CA, Levine MS, Rubesin SE, Langlotz CP, Laufer I. Diagnosis of primary versus secondary achalasia: reassessment of clinical and radiographic criteria. AJR Am J Roentgenol. 2000; 175(3):727–731

Case 96

Andrew Mizzi

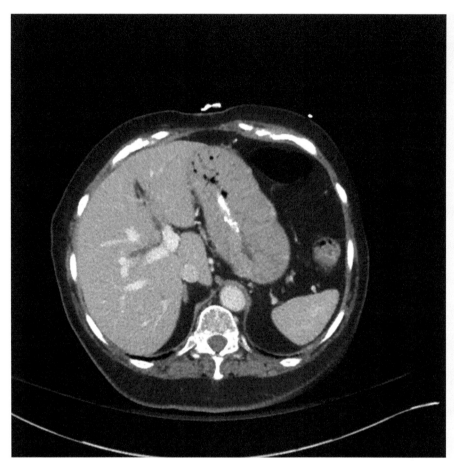

Fig. 96.1 CT axial image of the upper abdomen with intravenous and oral contrast shows marked thickening of the stomach with poor distention.

■ **Clinical History**

A 73-year-old female with epigastric pain (▶ Fig. 96.1).

■ Key Finding

Marked gastric wall thickening.

■ Top 3 Differential Diagnoses

- **Gastric adenocarcinoma:** Gastric adenocarcinoma is the most common malignancy of the stomach. It can mimic esophageal or other adjacent organs carcinomas with direct stomach spread when the interface of their borders is effaced. *H. pylori* infection has an association with gastric carcinoma. Gastric carcinoma has a predilection for involvement of the distal stomach and may present as gastric outlet obstruction.
- **Lymphoma:** Infiltrative gastric lymphoma causes enlargement of gastric folds. Multiple ulcerated lesions can occur, and polypoid gastric lymphoma can present as multiple intraluminal masses. Homogeneous wall thickening with less pronounced enhancement helps to favor lymphoma from gastric carcinoma. Perigastric fat planes are usually preserved in lymphoma. Significant abdominal adenopathy may also be seen with lymphoma.

- **Menetrier's disease:** Menetrier's disease is a rare form of hypertrophic gastropathy. It should be noted that unlike other conditions causing gastritis, Menetrier's is not an inflammatory condition of the stomach. It is characterized by stomach wall thickening secondary to overgrowth of the mucous membrane lining of the stomach. It results in thick rugal folds. Menetrier's disease decreases acid forming cells in the stomach. It is associated with excessive mucous production in the stomach and hypoproteinemia. Ascites may result of protein loss. It has a bimodal distribution with children affected at under 10 years of age and adults incidence peak at 55 years. In the younger population it may be linked to cytomegalovirus (CMV) infection. In the adult form it is related to activation of epidermal growth factor receptor and may be related to *H. pylori* infection while some may have a genetic etiology component.

■ Additional Diagnostic Considerations

- **Gastritis:** Acute gastritis encompasses a number of causes of gastric mucosal inflammation. It can be seen incidentally on imaging or found on work up for epigastric pain, nausea/emesis and loss of appetite. Gastritis can result from infection (*H. pylori*), systemic illness or, massive trauma, autoimmune or caustic ingestion. It can also be seen in immunosuppressed states or eosinophilic gastritis.
- **Zollinger–Ellison syndrome:** Zollinger–Ellison syndrome results from pancreatic gastrin secreting tumors that

stimulate acid secreting cells in the stomach. It results in gastrointestinal mucosal ulcerations. It can occur sporadically or as autosomal dominant familial multiple endocrine neoplasia type 1 syndrome. Patients present with multiple gastrointestinal ulcerations most common involving the duodenum and small bowel. On CT, it presents with thickened rugal folds or multiple gastric masses.

■ Diagnosis

Menetrier disease.

✓ Pearls

- Distinguishing characteristics of Menetrier's disease from inflammatory conditions include decreased acid formation and hyponatremia.

- Gastric adenocarcinoma is the most common malignancy.

Suggested Readings

Federle MP, Jeffrey RB, Woodward PJ, Borhani A. Diagnostic Imaging: Abdomen. 2nd ed. Philadelphia, PA: Lippincott Williams & Wilkins; 2009

Friedman J, Platnick J, Farruggia S, Khilko N, Mody K, Tyshkov M. Ménétrier disease. Radiographics. 2009; 29(1):297–301

Horton KM, Hruban RH, Yeo C, Fishman EK. Multi-detector row CT of pancreatic islet cell tumors. Radiographics. 2006; 26(2):453–464

Case 97

Julia J. Hobson

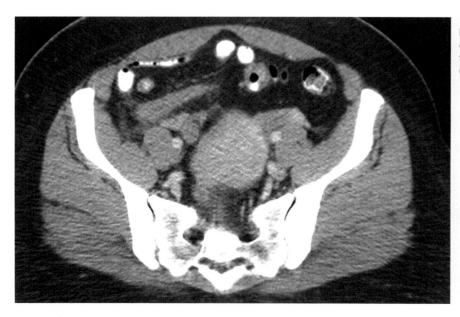

Fig. 97.1 CT axial image with intravenous and oral contrast shows circumferential appendix wall thickening and periappendiceal fat stranding. (Image courtesy of Rocky C. Saenz.)

■ Clinical History

A 24-year-old female with right lower quadrant pain (▶ Fig. 97.1).

■ Key Finding

Appendiceal wall thickening.

■ Top 3 Differential Diagnoses

• **Appendicitis:** Appendicitis is a common cause of acute abdominal pain requiring emergent surgery, with approximately 12% and men and 25% of women experiencing acute appendicitis in their lifetime. Symptoms include anorexia with abdominal pain that starts periumbilically and migrates to the right lower quadrant. Laboratory studies will show an elevated white blood cell count. CT findings suggesting acute appendicitis include an appendix greater than 6 mm in diameter with thickened, hyperenhancing walls and adjacent inflammatory stranding. Complications include perforation and abscess formation. Treatment is surgical removal of the appendix.

• **Appendiceal neoplasm:** Appendiceal neoplasms are uncommon and only seen in approximately 1% of appendectomy specimens. Of primary malignant neoplasms of the appendix, mucinous tumors are the most common, with adenocarcinoma and carcinoid tumors the next commonly seen. On CT, mucinous neoplasms will present as a cystic mass in the appendix with irregular walls. If a curvilinear mural calcification is seen, this is highly suggestive of mucinous neoplasm, but is only seen in approximately 50% of cases. If rupture occurs, the gelatinous material with accumulate in the peritoneum resulting in pseudomyxoma peritonei with characteristic imaging findings of peripheral scalloping of solid organs. Adenocarcinoma will be seen as a soft-tissue mass with adjacent inflammation and loss of fat planes suggesting local invasion. Carcinoid of the appendix is usually found incidentally on appendectomy.

• **Colon carcinoma:** Colonic adenocarcinoma is the most common gastrointestinal malignancy in Western societies. Wall thickening in the cecum from adenocarcinoma can cause obstruction of the appendiceal lumen and result in dilation of the appendix, with or without wall thickening or inflammation adjacent to the appendix. Signs of distant disease including mesenteric lymph nodes and liver metastasis may be seen at time of imaging. Confirmation of adenocarcinoma can be done with endoscopy and biopsy.

■ Additional Diagnostic Considerations

Inflammatory bowel disease: The appendix can be involved in inflammatory bowel disease, although it is not very common. Patients can have signs and symptoms similar to acute appendicitis with acute right lower quadrant abdominal pain or they can present with more chronic and intermittent right lower quadrant pain. Imaging findings are also similar with appendiceal wall thickening and adjacent inflammation.

■ Diagnosis

Acute appendicitis.

✓ Pearls

• Acute appendicitis is a common cause of right lower quadrant pain and appendiceal wall thickening.
• Mucinous tumors are the most common primary malignancies of the appendix.

• Inflammatory bowel disease may involve the appendix and can mimic acute appendicitis.

Suggested Readings

Beydoun T, Kreuer S. Cystic right lower quadrant mass. J Am Osteopath Coll Radiol. 2012; 1(4):32–34

Boyd SK, Cameron-Morrison JD, Hobson JJ, Saenz R. CT imaging of large bowel wall thickening. J Am Osteopath Coll Radiol. 2016; 5(2):14–22

Pickhardt PJ, Levy AD, Rohrmann CA, Jr, Kende AI. Primary neoplasms of the appendix: radiologic spectrum of disease with pathologic correlation. Radiographics. 2003; 23(3):645–662

Case 98

Reehan M. Ali

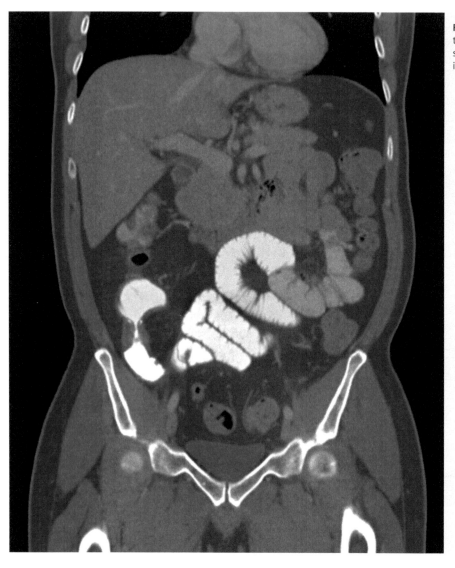

Fig. 98.1 Contrast enhanced coronal CT image through the lower abdomen with oral contrast shows a short segment stricture involving the ileum.

■ Clinical History

A 41-year-old male with right lower quadrant pain (▶ Fig. 98.1).

■ Key Finding

Short segment small bowel wall thickening.

■ Top 3 Differential Diagnoses

• **Adenocarcinoma:** Most commonly occurring in the duodenum, followed by the proximal jejunum. Typical CT appearance is of a focal segment of asymmetric bowel-wall thickening. The bowel wall demonstrates areas of heterogeneous enhancement with regions of ulceration more readily apparent on CT enterography studies. Often, these can occlude or narrow the bowel lumen which can lead to small bowel obstruction.

• **Crohn's disease:** Crohn's disease should be included in the differential with any region of small bowel thickening. It is classically described as having a "halo" or "target" appearance of the bowel wall, with alternative layers of hyperattenuated mucosa, hypoattenuated intramural edema, and hyperattenuated serosa. Mucosal hyperemia is a more sensitive indicator of active disease and is readily diagnosed on CT enterography. Extraenteric findings can aid in diagnosis and include the "comb sign" which relates to engorged vasa recta within the mesentery that run perpendicular to the bowel.

• **Ischemic enteritis:** Can be acute or chronic with acute being far more common. Acute ischemic enteritis has a high mortality rate making the diagnosis an important one. CT appearance depends on pathologic stage of injury to the bowel which can range from mild mural edema to transmural infarction. In addition to bowel wall thickening, other findings include mesenteric edema and ascites. Closed-loop small bowel obstructions are a special case which can also lead to ischemic enteritis.

■ Diagnosis

Crohn disease.

✓ Pearls

• Be cognizant of the classic signs of Crohn's disease including enteric and extraenteric findings.

• CT enterography can aid in differentiating various causes.

• When suspecting an acute ischemic etiology make sure to review imaging to find a possible occlusive thrombus.

Suggested Readings

Federle MP, Jeffrey RB, Woodward PJ, Borhani A. Diagnostic Imaging: Abdomen. 2nd ed. Philadelphia, PA: Lippincott Williams & Wilkins; 2009

Macari M, et al. A pattern approach to the abnormal small bowel: a multitechnique imaging approach. AJR. 2007; 188:1344–1355

Wittenberg J, Harisinghani MG, Jhaveri K, Varghese J, Mueller PR. Algorithmic approach to CT diagnosis of the abnormal bowel wall. Radiographics. 2002; 22(5):1093–1107, discussion 1107–1109

Case 99

Sharon Kreuer

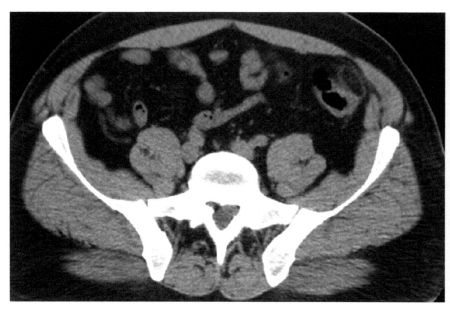

Fig. 99.1 CT axial image without contrast of the lower abdomen demonstrates left lower quadrant pericolonic fat stranding which is surrounding an ovoid fat density adjacent to the sigmoid colon. (Image courtesy of Rocky C. Saenz.)

■ Clinical History

A 36-year-old male with left lower quadrant pain (▶ Fig. 99.1).

■ Key Finding

Pericolonic fat stranding surrounding a fat density.

■ Top 3 Differential Diagnoses

- **Epiploic appendagitis:** Epiploic appendages are fatty projections from the serosal surface of the colon. Epiploic appendages have a vascular stalk that can torse, resulting in necrosis and inflammation. These are most numerous at the sigmoid colon. Epiploic appendages are arranged in two rows along the colon extending from the cecum to the rectosigmoid junction (the rectum has no epiploic appendages). The classic CT appearance of appendagitis is that of pericolonic inflammation with central fat density. Epiploic appendagitis is a self-limiting disease and treatment is targeted at pain management.
- **Diverticulitis:** Diverticulitis describes the inflammation, erosion, and microperforation of colonic pseudodiverticuli, most commonly involving the sigmoid colon. Short segment wall thickening with pericolonic inflammation and loculated small amounts of extraluminal air (pneumoperitoneum) are findings of uncomplicated diverticulitis. These patients are treated conservatively with antibiotics. When more extensive pneumoperitoneum, pericolonic abscess, fistula, or portal vein thrombophlebitis with liver abscess occur; these may require surgical intervention or percutaneous drainage.
- **Ulcerative Colitis:** Ulcerative colitis is an inflammatory bowel disease that may involves the entirety of the colon including the rectum and also the terminal ileum. Shallow, nontransmural ulcers are not readily seen on CT with the imaging diagnosis suggested from secondary findings. These include a pseudopolyp appearance of colonic wall thickening resulting from confluent ulcerations and intervening islands of normal mucosa, ahaustral fold pattern, target or stratified mucosal enhancement, and occasional strictures. These patients are at a higher risk for developing colorectal carcinoma and toxic megacolon. Definitive therapy is total colectomy.

■ Additional Diagnostic Considerations

Pseudomembranous colitis: Pseudomembranous colitis typically is a pancolitis that results from overgrowth of *Clostridium difficile* after antibiotic therapy. Its appearance on CT is that of markedly thickened colonic wall secondary to mucosal edema with minimal associated mesenteric inflammation. Wall thickening is commonly described as accordion-like, polypoid, or "thumb printing" appearance. Most severe complications include toxic megacolon and perforation. Supportive and antibiotic therapy is the first-line treatment.

■ Diagnosis

Epiploic appendagitis.

✓ Pearls

- Epiploic appendagitis presents with pericolonic inflammation with central fat attenuation and is self-limiting.
- Diverticulitis is a mimicker of epiploic appendagitis, both seen most often in the sigmoid colon.
- Ulcerative and pseudomembranous colitis more commonly present with pancolonic inflammation.

Suggested Readings

Boyd SK, Cameron-Morrison JD, Hobson JJ, Saenz R. CT imaging of large bowel wall thickening. J Am Osteopath Coll Radiol. 2016; 5(2):14–22

Dalrymple NC, Leyendecker JR, Oliphant M. Problem Solving in Abdominal Imaging. 1st ed. Philadelphia, PA: Mosby Elsevier; 2009

Sing AK, Gervais, D, A, Hahn, PF. Acute epiploic appendagitis and its mimicks. Radiographics. 2005; 25(6):1521–1534

Case 100

Andrew Mizzi

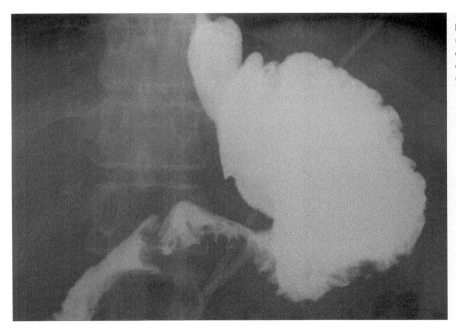

Fig. 100.1 Single image from a single contrast upper gastrointestinal with oral contrast demonstrates two large defects along the greater curvature of the stomach with poor distention. (Image courtesy of Rocky C. Saenz.)

■ Clinical History

A 73-year-old female with epigastric pain (▶Fig. 100.1).

■ Key Finding

Multiple gastric lesions.

■ Top 3 Differential Diagnoses

- **Gastric adenocarcinoma:** Gastric adenocarcinoma is the most common malignancy of the stomach. It can mimic esophageal or other adjacent organs carcinomas with direct stomach spread when the interface of their borders is effaced. Gastric carcinoma tends to affect the more elderly population. *H. pylori* infection has an association with gastric carcinoma. Gastric carcinoma has a predilection for involvement of the distal stomach and can present as gastric outlet obstruction.
- **Lymphoma:** Infiltrative gastric lymphoma causes enlargement of gastric folds. Multiple ulcerated lesions can occur, and polypoid gastric lymphoma can present as multiple intraluminal masses. Homogeneous wall thickening with less pronounced enhancement helps to favor lymphoma from gastric carcinoma. Perigastric fat planes are usually preserved in lymphoma. Significant abdominal adenopathy may also be seen with lymphoma. Menetrier's disease can mimic lymphoma of the stomach due to rugal fold thickening.

- **Metastasis:** Metastatic disease to the stomach is relatively rare. It is usually a sign of advanced disease with poor prognosis. Most common primary sites that lead to stomach metastases are esophagus, malignant melanoma, lung, cervix, breast (most common), colon, and testicular cancers. Metastasis can be solitary or multiple. CT appearance depends on the origin of the primary such as direct invasion from the esophagus presenting as a polypoid or lobulated mass of proximal stomach. Omental caking from ovarian origin can present as displacing and/or indentation on the stomach wall. Invasive lobular carcinoma has a greater tendency to metastasize to the stomach than invasive ductal carcinoma of the breast. Breast metastasis can present as multiple small lesions or linitis plastica (leather bottle) appearance. Malignant melanoma can present as "Bull's eye" target lesions or nodular caveating ones. Metastatic gastric lesions are uncommon and only seen in 2% of cancer patients.

■ Additional Diagnostic Considerations

Gastric gastrointestinal stromal tumor (GIST): GIST is the most common mesenchymal tumor of the GI tract. Up to 70% of GIST tumors affect the stomach. On CT, the typical presentation is a large exophytic mass. The large size can affect the majority of the stomach. Often it appears heterogeneous due to necrosis and hemorrhage. Ulcerations can occur in up to 50% of cases. Calcifications are less common but can be seen in up to 10% of cases.

■ Diagnosis

Gastric metastasis from breast carcinoma.

✓ Pearls

- Gastric adenocarcinoma is the most common malignancy.
- Only consider gastric metastasis in patients with disseminated carcinoma.

- Breast carcinoma is the most common cause of gastric metastasis.

Suggested Readings

Federle MP, Jeffrey RB, Woodward PJ, Borhani A. Diagnostic Imaging: Abdomen. 2nd ed. Philadelphia, PA: Lippincott Williams & Wilkins; 2009

Horton KM, Fishman EK. Current role of CT in imaging of the stomach. Radiographics. 2003; 23(1):75–87

Lo Re G, Federica V, Midiri F, et al. Radiological Features of Gastrointestinal Lymphoma. Gastroenterol Res Pract. 2016;2016:2498143

Case 101

Michael L. Schwartz

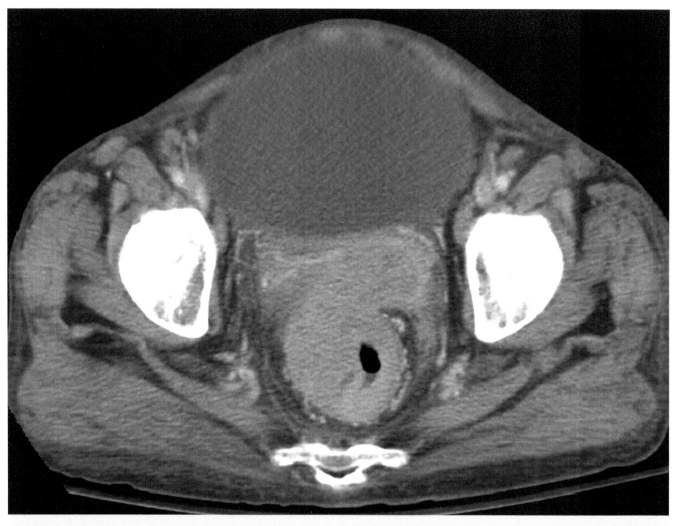

Fig. 101.1 IV contrast enhanced axial CT image through the lower pelvis reveals abnormal, eccentric wall thickening of the rectum. Also, there is loss of the fat plane between the anterior rectum and lower uterine segment. (Image courtesy of Rocky C. Saenz.)

■ **Clinical History**

A 53-year-old female with bright blood per rectum (▶ Fig. 101.1).

■ Key Finding

Asymmetric rectal wall thickening.

■ Top 3 Differential Diagnoses

• **Adenocarcinoma:** Adenocarcinoma is the most common rectal malignancy and is related to the mucin producing glands. Incidence increases with age. Greater than 90% of these cancers arise from adenomatous polyps. Typical CT findings are heterogeneously enhancing irregular mass with asymmetric rectal wall thickening and luminal narrowing. Complications include obstruction, perforation, and fistula formation. When advanced it may present as a saddle, apple core, or carpet type lesion. Treatment is mesorectal excision, neoadjuvant radiation therapy and chemotherapy.

• **Polyps:** Polyps are intraluminal lesions and are divided into neoplastic and nonneoplastic. Polyps are the most common benign tumor of the colon. The most common location is sigmoid followed by the rectum. Generally, the larger the polyp, the higher the chance are of neoplasia. Polyps 1 to 2 cm in size have a 10 to 20% chance of malignant degeneration while polyps less than 1 cm have a 1% chance. Therefore, polyps greater than 1 cm are usually removed via colonoscopy.

• **Intramural mass:** These tumors include intramural leiomyomas, lipoma, and schwannomas. These are typically smooth margin masses. Endometriosis can also result in an extramural mass (third most common benign tumor). Trauma may produce an intramural hematoma. The most common intramural mass is a lipoma and is the second most common benign tumor. On CT, it is diagnosed by noting its fat attenuation.

■ Additional Diagnostic Considerations

• **Lymphoma:** Gastrointestinal lymphoma in the colon is the third most common site after stomach and small bowel respectfully. Non-Hodgkin's lymphoma (NHL) is the most common. The lesions are classically large lesions with associated luminal distention and regional or widespread adenopathy. There is usually no evidence for colon obstruction. Unfortunately, the prognosis of primary colonic lymphoma is poor with the 5 year survival rate only being only 50%.

• **Colitis:** Colitis or proctitis can mimic a mass. On cross-sectional imaging, rectal wall thickening of 3 to 6 mm is considered indeterminate with nondistention, but when greater than 6 mm is abnormal. Rectal and perirectal abscess are complications of Crohn's and immunocompromised patients. Rectosigmoid isolated infectious colitis is more commonly associated with actinomycosis, gonorrhea, chlamydia (lymphogranuloma venereum), tuberculosis, herpes, and syphilis.

■ Diagnosis

Adenocarcinoma.

✓ Pearls

• Rectal wall thickening greater than 6 mm is always abnormal.
• Consider lymphoma with a large rectal mass and adenopathy.

• Consider familial polyposis with innumerable colonic lesions.

Suggested Readings

Federle MP, Jeffrey RB, Woodward PJ, Borhani A. Diagnostic Imaging: Abdomen. 2nd ed. Philadelphia, PA: Lippincott Williams & Wilkins; 2009

Jaffe T, Thompson WM. Large-bowel obstruction in the adult: classic radiographic and CT findings, etiology, and mimics. Radiology. 2015; 275(3):651–663

Jhaveri KS, Hosseini-Nik H. MRI of rectal cancer: an overview and update on recent advances. AJR Am J Roentgenol. 2015; 205(1):W42–55

Case 102

Kathy M. Borovicka

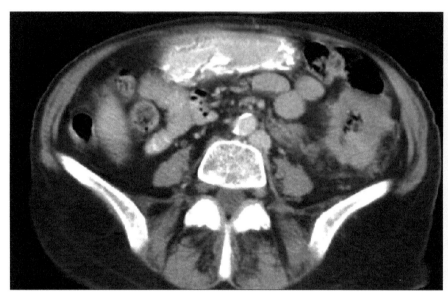

Fig. 102.1 CT axial image with intravenous and oral contrast through the lower pelvis reveals abnormal, eccentric wall thickening of the sigmoid colon. Also, there is pericolonic fat stranding. (Image courtesy of Rocky C. Saenz.)

■ Clinical History

A 73-year-old male with bright blood per rectum (▶Fig. 102.1).

■ **Key Finding**

Asymmetric sigmoid wall thickening.

■ **Top 3 Differential Diagnoses**

• **Adenocarcinoma:** Adenocarcinoma is the most common carcinoma of the colon and most commonly occurring in the sigmoid. CT features of sigmoid carcinoma include focal soft-tissue mass, focal, asymmetric wall thickening, and narrowing of the colonic lumen. Asymmetric nodular wall thickening, absence of diverticula in the thickened segment, and the presence of shouldering are highly suggestive of carcinoma over the diagnosis of diverticulitis. If the tumor wall involvement has resulted in infiltration of the pericolic fat, this can mimic diverticulitis. CT can demonstrate the length of the segment involved, regional involvement, and distant metastasis (liver is the most common site).

• **Diverticulitis:** Diverticular disease is much more common in the Western world with the sigmoid colon being the most common location. These small herniations of the mucosa and submucosa through the muscular layers may result in muscular hypertrophy. CT findings include segmental wall thickening, hyperemia, and adjacent pericolonic fat stranding. Complications include perforation with pneumoperitoneum, abscess, and fistula. The presence of fluid in the root of the mesentery and engorgement of the sigmoid mesenteric vessels is more common with diverticulitis than with a carcinoma.

• **Polyps:** Polyps are intraluminal lesions that may be neoplastic or nonneoplastic. Polyps are the most common benign tumor of the colon. The most common location is the sigmoid followed by the rectum. The most common type of polyp is the adenomatous, and the most common subtype is tubular adenoma. Polyps less than 1 cm have a 1% chance of malignancy. On CT, polyps may appear as eccentric wall thickening or mass-like.

■ **Additional Diagnostic Considerations**

• **Colitis:** Colitis can be a mimicker of a mass. On CT, the colon wall is abnormal when it is thicker than 3 mm. Colitis has many causes including infection, inflammatory, trauma, radiation, and ischemia. Infections with chlamydia, gonorrhea, and herpes involve the rectosigmoid colon. Other infectious agents usually involve the right colon over the sigmoid colon. Radiation of pelvic organs may result in colitis of the sigmoid and rectum. The rectosigmoid along with the splenic flexure are watershed areas of the colon. These watershed areas are susceptible to hypovolemia, especially in the elderly patients. In severe cases, pneumatosis related to necrosis may be seen, requiring surgical intervention.

• **Lymphoma:** Gastrointestinal lymphoma of the colon is uncommon. The most common location in the colon is the cecum. The lesions may have focal wall thickening averaging 5 cm with adenopathy.

■ **Diagnosis**

Adenocarcinoma.

✓ **Pearls**

• Colitis is usually long segment (> 10 cm) whereas carcinoma is usually short segment.
• When diverticulitis is the diagnosis a follow-up colonoscopy should be performed to exclude an underlying carcinoma.

• Colitis typically has concentric bowel wall thickening versus carcinoma, which has eccentric thickening.

Suggested Readings

Boyd SK, Cameron-Morrison JD, Hobson JJ, et al. CT Imaging of Large Bowel Wall Thickening. J Am Osteopath Coll Radiol. 2016; 5(2):14–22

Horton KM, Corl FM, Fishman EK. CT evaluation of the colon: inflammatory disease. Radiographics. 2000; 20(2):399–418

Horton KM, Abrams RA, Fishman EK. Spiral CT of colon cancer: imaging features and role in management. Radiographics. 2000; 20(2):419–430

Lips LMJ, Cremers PTJ, Pickhardt PJ, et al. Sigmoid cancer versus chronic diverticular disease: differentiating features at CT colonography. Radiology. 2015; 275(1):127–135

Case 103

Shaun Loh

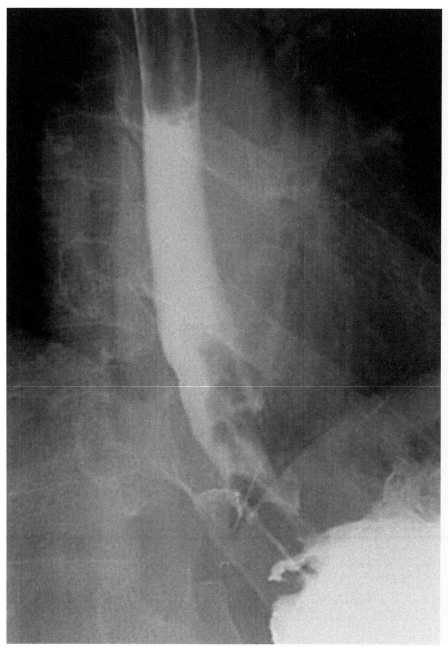

Fig. 103.1 Esophagram demonstrates tortuous longitudinal submucosal filling defects in the distal esophagus.

■ Clinical History

A 40-year-old male with a 2-week history of "food sticking" in his throat (▶ Fig. 103.1).

■ Key Finding

Esophageal submucosal thickened folds.

■ Top 3 Differential Diagnoses

- **Varices:** Varices are a common sequela of portal hypertension, often secondary to chronic liver disease. They are classified according their pathophysiology as either uphill or downhill varices. Uphill varices are more common and involve the distal portion of the esophagus. They form as a result of portal hypertension, where increased pressures cause upward flow of blood from the portal vein through collateral flow through the azygous vein to the superior vena cava (SVC). Uphill varices commonly cause gastrointestinal bleeding. Downhill varices, on the other hand, are rarer and involve the proximal esophagus. An obstruction of the SVC results in downward flow through the azygous vein to the inferior vena cava (IVC) and portal vein. Common causes of SVC obstruction include lung cancer, mediastinitis, retrosternal goiters, or thymomas. Downhill varices may present with symptoms of SVC syndrome, including facial, periorbital, or neck swelling. In an esophagram, varices typically appear as longitudinal, serpentine, radiolucent filling defects that vary in size with changes in patient positioning and phase of respiration.

- **Reflux esophagitis:** The inflammatory changes and submucosal edema in esophagitis may appear as thickened, tortuous folds, much like varices. The thickened folds in the setting of esophagitis, however, will remain fixed in appearance. An adequate clinical history combined with endoscopy will readily differentiate between the two.
- **Varicoid esophageal carcinoma:** Esophageal carcinoma is a common malignancy of the gastrointestinal tract. Advanced esophageal carcinomas may present as infiltrating, polypoid, ulcerative, or varicoid lesions. The varicoid type lesion is the least common subtype and appears on esophagrams as thickened, rigid, serpentine, longitudinal filling defects due to the submucosal spread of tumor. They are frequently confused for varices but differ in that varicoid tumors have fixed configurations and do not change their appearance in response to esophageal peristalsis, respiratory maneuvers, or repositioning of the patient. Diagnosis is confirmed with endoscopic biopsy.

■ Additional Diagnostic Consideration

Lymphoma: Lymphoma rarely involves the esophagus but when it does, signs of lymphoma are seen in other parts of the body. Most cases of esophageal lymphoma are from contiguous spread from the gastric cardia or fundus. When lymphoma infiltrates in a submucosal fashion, it produces fixed, tortuous, longitudinal folds. Endoscopic biopsy will help aid in the diagnosis.

■ Diagnosis

Esophageal varices.

✓ Pearls

- Portal hypertension causes uphill esophageal varices while SVC obstruction causes downhill varices.
- Esophageal varices will vary in size and appearance with patient positioning; they enhance avidly.

- Reflux esophagitis may present with mucosal abnormalities and thickened folds.
- Varicoid esophageal carcinoma is the least common tumor subtype.

Suggested Readings

Federle MP, Jeffrey RB, Woodward PJ, Borhani A. Diagnostic Imaging: Abdomen. 2nd ed. Philadelphia, PA: Lippincott Williams & Wilkins; 2009

Kim YJ, Raman SS, Yu NC, To'o KJ, Jutabha R, Lu DS. Esophageal varices in cirrhotic patients: evaluation with liver CT. AJR Am J Roentgenol. 2007; 188(1):139–144

Matsumoto A, Kitamoto M, Imamura M, et al. Three-dimensional portography using multislice helical CT is clinically useful for management of gastric fundic varices. AJR Am J Roentgenol. 2001; 176(4):899–905

Case 104

Reehan M. Ali

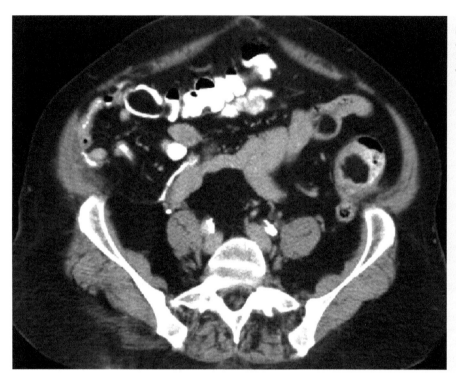

Fig. 104.1 CT of the lower abdominal demonstrates two fat density lesions in the small bowel and another in the sigmoid colon. (Image courtesy of Rocky C. Saenz.)

■ **Clinical History**

A 55-year-old male with general abdominal pain (▶Fig. 104.1).

■ Key Finding

Fatty intraluminal mass.

■ Top 3 Differential Diagnoses

- **Lipoma:** Lipomas are the most common fat-containing intraluminal mass in the small bowel but overall are still a rare entity. They present as a well-circumscribed intraluminal mass measuring fat attenuation on CT. Lesions will follow fat signal on all MR sequences. Important to note on CT as they may become the lead point for an intussusception. CT enterography is the gold standard for imaging diagnosis.
- **Intussusception:** Intussusception refers to "telescoping" of a bowel loop into itself. This is caused by a lead point typically a mass or inflamed bowel. An intussusception may contain invaginated mesenteric fat, which can mimic a small bowel lipoma. Utilizing reformatted multiplane CT is valuable for differentiating between these two entities. Small bowel intussusception is usually self-limited.
- **Angiomyolipoma:** Exceedingly rare with only a few case reports present. These will typically present in the ileum and will share imaging characteristics with renal angiomyolipomas. Patients can present with intussusception and hemorrhage. Imaging key is to identify different tissue types from blood vessels, smooth muscle, and adipose cells.

■ Diagnosis

Lipoma.

✓ Pearls

- The key to diagnosing a small bowel lipoma is noting its fat content.
- CT enterography is the gold standard for imaging diagnosis.
- Small bowel lipomas are benign and require no further workup.

Suggested Readings

Fang SH, Dong DJ, Chen FH, Jin M, Zhong BS. Small intestinal lipomas: diagnostic value of multi-slice CT enterography. World J Gastroenterol. 2010; 16(21):2677–2681

Federle MP, Jeffrey RB, Woodward PJ, Borhani A. Diagnostic Imaging: Abdomen. 2nd ed. Philadelphia, PA: Lippincott Williams & Wilkins; 2009

Macari M, et al. A pattern approach to the abnormal small bowel: a multitechnique imaging approach. AJR. 2007; 188:1344–1355

Case 105

Julia D. Cameron-Morrison

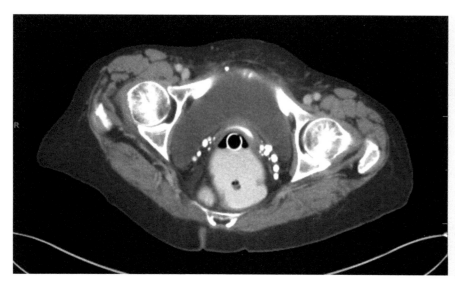

Fig. 105.1 CT axial image through the pelvis with intravenous and rectal contrast demonstrates rectal contrast within the vagina.

■ **Clinical History**

An 81-year-old female with pelvic pain (▶Fig. 105.1).

■ Key Finding

Rectal contrast within the vagina.

■ Top 3 Differential Diagnoses

• **Post hysterectomy complication:** Postsurgical complication following hysterectomy is the most common etiology of colovaginal fistulas, typically from extension of postsurgical inflammatory changes. Fecal discharge from the vagina, which can sometimes be confused with fecaluria, is the most common presentation. Other common presentations include pelvic/abdominal pain, flatus, and mucus per vagina. On cross-sectional imaging, the vaginal cuff will often give the appearance of an inflammatory mass between the colon and urinary bladder. Administration of rectal contrast as part of a barium enema or pelvic CT can demonstrate the fistulous tract.

• **Diverticulitis:** Diverticulitis is the second most common cause of colovaginal fistulas. There is an increased risk in women fol-

lowing hysterectomy, even when remote due to the proximity of the colon to the vaginal cuff. The fistula tract is rarely seen directly and typically only following administration of rectal contrast. An associated abscess may be seen between the vagina and colon. Additionally, there will be classic findings of diverticulitis, such as colonic wall thickening and surrounding inflammatory changes with loss of the fat plane between the colon and vagina.

• **Neoplasm/carcinoma:** Both genitourinary and gastrointestinal neoplasms have been associated with colovaginal fistulas. Findings of neoplasm, such as localized bladder or colonic wall thickening in the absence of surrounding inflammatory change, may be present. Associated lymphadenopathy may be seen.

■ Additional Diagnostic Considerations

Inflammatory bowel disease: Fistula formation is a known complication of Crohn's disease. While it most commonly involves the terminal ileum any portion of bowel can be involved. Classic findings in Crohn's disease include circumferential bowel wall thickening often with skip lesions, mesenteric hyperemia, fatty infiltration of the bowel wall, and strictures.

■ Diagnosis

Colovaginal fistula secondary to diverticulitis.

✓ Pearls

• Rectal contrast for barium enema and pelvic CT may demonstrate the fistulous tract.
• Increased risk of colovaginal fistula with hysterectomy, even when remote.

• Look for abscess formation between the colon and vagina with loss of normal fat planes.

Suggested Readings

Boyd SK, Cameron-Morrison JD, Hobson JJ, Saenz R. CT Imaging of Large Bowel Wall Thickening. J Am Osteopath Coll Radiol. 2016; 5(2):14–22
Federle MP, Jeffrey RB, Woodward PJ, Borhani A. Diagnostic Imaging: Abdomen. 2nd ed. Philadelphia, PA: Lippincott Williams & Wilkins; 2009

Yu NC, Raman SS, Patel M, Barbaric Z. Fistulas of the genitourinary tract: a radiologic review. Radiographics. 2004; 24(5):1331–1352

Case 106

Reehan M. Ali

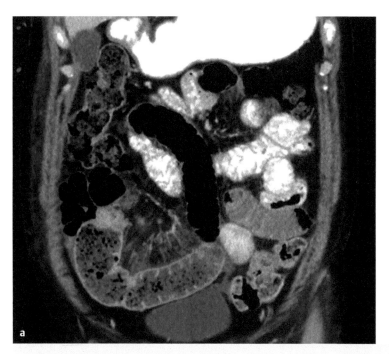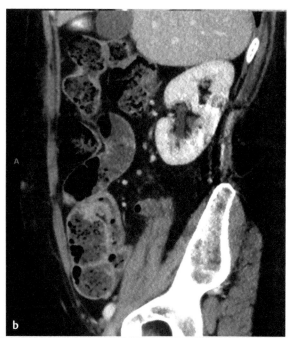

Fig. 106.1 Contrast enhanced coronal **(a)** and sagittal **(b)** CT images through the abdomen reveal a briskly enhancing mass involving the ileum with a resulting ileus. (Image courtesy of Rocky C. Saenz.)

■ Clinical History

A 61-year-old male asymptomatic with elevated serum chromogranin-A (▶Fig. 106.1).

■ Key Finding

Solid small bowel mass.

■ Top 3 Differential Diagnoses

- **Metastases:** Metastases represent the most common small bowel malignancy, far more common than primary malignancies. Tumor can spread via direct extension, lymphatic, intraperitoneal, or hematogenous methods. Intraperitoneal seeding is the most common method of spread. Most common primary malignancies to spread to the small bowel are colon, ovarian, and appendiceal. Complications can be seen with these lesions, including intussusception, as these lesions typically are polypoid in shape and implant on the mesenteric border of the small bowel.
- **Carcinoid:** Tumor whose incidence has been increasing over the past several decades and has now surpassed adenocarcinoma as the most common small bowel neoplasm. Distal ileum is the second most common location of carcinoid overall (appendix being first). Increasingly they are being found in the duodenum. Typically presents as a large mesenteric mass with desmoplastic reaction and retraction of adjacent small bowel loops. Calcification may be present in up to 70% of cases. More likely to see hepatic metastases from carcinoid when compared to other small bowel primary neoplasms.
- **Adenocarcinoma:** Now surpassed by carcinoid as the most common primary small bowel neoplasm, this still represents roughly 25 to 40% of all small bowel neoplasms. The majority occurs in the duodenum and most are discovered via endoscopy. The jejunum is the second most common site. Typically presents as a focal circumferential mass with shouldering at the margins and can present with small bowel obstruction. Less frequently presents as a polypoid mass that leads to intussusception. Often shows moderate enhancement and will metastasize to the liver and peritoneum. Fat stranding due to mesenteric fat infiltration and lymph node metastases favor adenocarcinoma over lymphoma.

■ Additional Diagnostic Considerations

- **Lymphoma:** Lymphoma makes up approximately 20% of all small bowel tumors. Most commonly found in the distal ileum. On imaging, typically presents as a thick walled infiltrating mass. It can cause dilatation of the small bowel without obstruction. Less commonly presents as an intraluminal polypoid mass. Large adenocarcinomas and lymphoma have overlapping imaging characteristics. Bulky mesenteric or retroperitoneal lymphadenopathy and splenomegaly are supporting findings to suggest lymphoma.
- **Gastric gastrointestinal stromal tumors (GISTs):** They represent 9% of all small bowel tumors. Most frequently they occur in the stomach followed by jejunum and ileum. Size is an important factor as tumors smaller than 2 cm are usually benign and those larger than 5 cm are often malignant. These are typically a well-defined exophytic mass with clear differentiation from the mesentery.

■ Diagnosis

Carcinoid tumor.

✓ Pearls

- Metastases are the most common malignancy of the small bowel.
- Carcinoid is the most common primary small bowel malignancy.
- A small bowel mass with splenomegaly and bulky lymphadenopathy favors lymphoma.

Suggested Readings

Federle MP, Jeffrey RB, Woodward PJ, Borhani A. Diagnostic Imaging: Abdomen. 2nd ed. Philadelphia, PA: Lippincott Williams & Wilkins; 2009

Macari M, et al. A pattern approach to the abnormal small bowel: a multitechnique imaging approach. AJR. 2007; 188:1344–1355

McLaughlin PD, Maher MM. Primary malignant diseases of the small intestine. AJR Am J Roentgenol. 2013; 201(1):W9–14

Case 107

Julia D. Cameron-Morrison

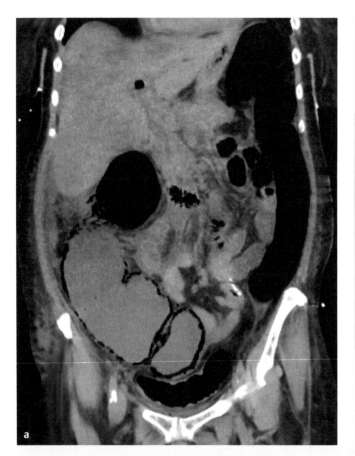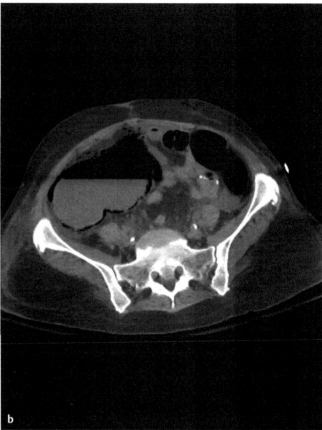

Fig. 107.1 CT coronal **(a)** and axial **(b)** images through the abdomen and pelvis without contrast demonstrate air within the right colonic wall. Multiple punctate foci of free air are seen anterior to the cecum. Trace free fluid is present.

■ Clinical History

A 67-year-old female with abdominal pain and distention (▶Fig. 107.1).

■ Key Finding

Pneumatosis intestinalis.

■ Top 3 Differential Diagnoses

- **Bowel necrosis:** There are multiple etiologies of pneumatosis intestinalis some of which can lead to serious morbidity/mortality if not recognized early. The most common is bowel necrosis, which can result from ischemia/infarction, infection, and caustic ingestion. Imaging findings depend on the underlying cause, of which ischemia is the most common. When secondary to bowel necrosis, the pneumatosis will often appear more linear within the bowel wall. Associated imaging features that can help lead to diagnosis of bowel necrosis include bowel wall thickening, pneumoperitoneum, portal venous gas, occlusion of vasculature on CT angiography, and absence of mucosal enhancement or intense mucosal enhancement.
- **Iatrogenic:** Iatrogenic causes of pneumatosis intestinalis include post-endoscopy, postoperative, and medication induced. These tend to be more benign in their course. Both endoscopy and postoperative changes are thought to result from mucosal disruption and increased intraluminal air, while medications are thought to increase mucosal permeability and decrease immune response leading to bacterial gas formation in the wall. Correlation with patient history and recent surgical procedures are invaluable in determining the etiology.
- **Pseudopneumatosis:** Air trapped against the mucosal surface by intraluminal contents can result in an appearance similar to that of pneumatosis intestinalis. This is most commonly seen in the ascending colon. On CT, the air will typically be in the nondependent colon with no air seen on the dependent side, which can help differentiate this entity from true pneumatosis.

■ Additional Diagnostic Considerations

Primary pneumatosis intestinalis: Primary pneumatosis intestinalis accounts for approximately 15% of cases. While most commonly idiopathic, it has also been associated with familial polyposis syndromes. On CT, multiple thin-walled, noncommunicating gas-filled cysts are seen within the subserosal or submucosal layer of the wall. The muscularis and mucosa will appear normal. No other associated findings suggesting a secondary cause will be seen. Clinically these patients will be asymptomatic.

■ Diagnosis

Pneumatosis intestinalis resulting from bowel necrosis.

✓ Pearls

- Pneumatosis intestinalis is a radiologic finding and not a diagnosis.
- The underlying etiology and patient's clinical status determine patient prognosis.
- Lactic acid levels are often elevated with bowel ischemia/necrosis.
- Look for air within the dependent bowel wall to confirm that it isn't pseudopneumatosis.

Suggested Readings

Boyd SK, Cameron-Morrison JD, Hobson JJ, Saenz R. CT imaging of large bowel wall thickening. J Am Osteopath Coll Radiol. 2016; 5(2):14–22

Horton KM, Corl FM, Fishman EK. CT evaluation of the colon: inflammatory disease. Radiographics. 2000; 20(2):399–418

Ho LM, Paulson EK, Thompson WM. Pneumatosis intestinalis in the adult: benign to life-threatening causes. AJR Am J Roentgenol. 2007; 188(6):1604–1613

Case 108

Reehan M. Ali

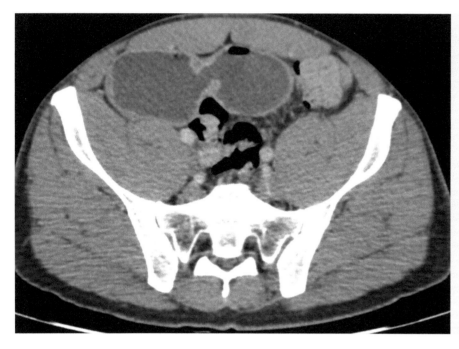

Fig. 108.1 Axial CT enterography image through the lower abdomen with intravenous and oral contrast shows a short segment stricture involving the ileum. (Image courtesy of Rocky C. Saenz.)

■ Clinical History

A 29-year-old male being evaluated for appendicitis (▶ Fig. 108.1).

■ Key Finding

Small bowel stricture.

■ Top 3 Differential Diagnoses

- **Crohn's disease:** CT enterography can be used to differentiate active inflammatory strictures from fibrotic strictures. CT features of active Crohn's disease include alternative layers of hyperattenuated mucosa, hypoattenuated intramural edema, and hyperattenuated serosa (target sign). Mucosal hyperemia is a more sensitive indicator of active disease and is readily diagnosed on CT enterography. Extraenteric findings can aid in diagnosis and include the "comb sign" that relates to engorged vasa recta within the mesentery that run perpendicular to the bowel. Active strictures are thought to be reversible while those that do not enhance are thought to be irreversible.
- **Postinfectious stricture:** Imaging is not very definitive in differentiating between different etiologies of stricture and much of the delineation depends on the total clinical scenario and patient history. *Mycobacterium tuberculosis* is one of the most common organisms implicated in small bowel stricture and also typically will involve the terminal ileum. Looking for extraintestinal signs of Crohn's disease or other systemic involvement of *M. tuberculosis* could aid in differentiation.
- **Postradiation stricture:** CT enterography is the most reliable examination to diagnose the presence of a stricture. History will play a large role in the inclusion of postradiation stricture into the differential. Strictures are typically painless unless they progress to the point of luminal narrowing that could lead to a partial or complete obstruction.

■ Additional Diagnostic Considerations

Metastases: Metastases represent the most common small bowel malignancy. Intraperitoneal seeding is the most common method of spread. Most common primary malignancies to spread to the small bowel are colon, ovarian, and appendiceal. These lesions typically are mass-like and implant on the mesenteric border of the small bowel. However, they can present as focal circumferential wall thickening with luminal narrowing mimicking a stricture.

■ Diagnosis

Crohn's disease.

✓ Pearls

- Crohn's disease is the most common etiology for small bowel stricture.
- CT enterography plays a vital role in determining reversible versus nonreversible stricture.
- History plays a large role in the inclusion of other differential possibilities such as infection and radiation.

Suggested Readings

Chang CW, Wong JM, Tung CC, Shih IL, Wang HY, Wei SC. Intestinal stricture in Crohn's disease. Intest Res. 2015; 13(1):19–26

Federle MP, Jeffrey RB, Woodward PJ, Borhani A. Diagnostic Imaging: Abdomen. 2nd ed. Philadelphia, PA: Lippincott Williams & Wilkins; 2009

Jayanthi V, Girija R, Mayberry JF. Terminal ileal stricture. Postgrad Med J. 2002; 78(924):627–, 631

Case 109

Julia J. Hobson

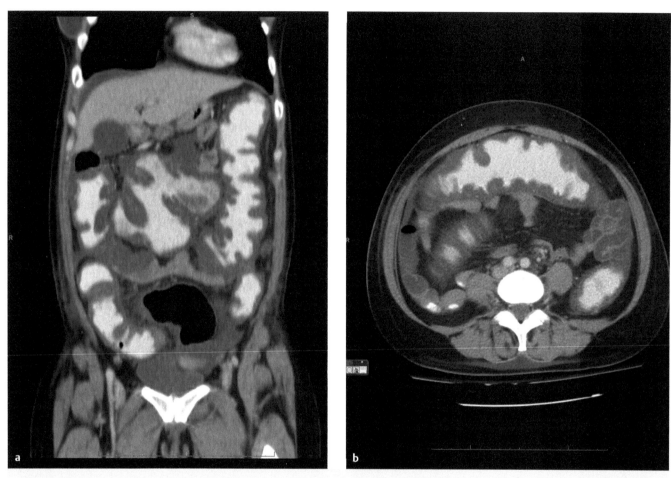

Fig. 109.1 CT coronal image of the abdomen with intravenous and oral contrast **(a)** shows a long segment of right and left colon wall thickening. CT axial image **(b)** also demonstrates wall thickening of the transverse colon and left colon. Free fluid is also noted. (Image courtesy of Rocky C. Saenz.)

■ **Clinical History**

A 56-year-old female with bloody stools and abdominal pain
(▶Fig. 109.1).

■ Key Finding

Colon wall thickening long segment.

■ Top 3 Differential Diagnoses

- **Inflammatory bowel disease:** Inflammatory bowel disease includes Crohn's disease and ulcerative colitis. Common symptoms include abdominal pain, diarrhea, bloody stools, and malabsorption. CT and MR show wall thickening and inflammatory changes in acute disease, and complications including abscess and fistula formation. Barium studies can show mucosal abnormalities, strictures, and fistula formation.
- **Infectious colitis:** Infectious colitis is inflammation of the colon due to a pathogen (bacterial, viral, fungal, or parasitic). Imaging findings of segmental colonic wall thickening with adjacent inflammatory stranding are suggestive of infectious colitis. Causative organism can be suggested based on the affected region of colon. Predominantly right-sided colitis can be seen in *Yersinia*, *salmonella*, cytomegalovirus (CMV),

tuberculosis, and amebiasis, while predominantly left-sided colitis is seen with Shigella or Schistosoma. Pan colitis often occurs with *C. difficile*, *E. coli*, and *Campylobacter*. Laboratory studies are needed for definitive diagnosis.
- **Ischemic colitis:** Often occurring in older patients, ischemic colitis occurs when blood supply to the colon is compromised, and is the leading cause of bowel ischemia. Causes include thromboembolic disease, venous thrombosis, and hypoperfusion states. Symptoms include abdominal pain and bloody diarrhea. Imaging findings will show circumferential wall thickening of large bowel in a vascular distribution. Complications include infarction of the bowel and perforation, both of which require surgical management.

■ Additional Diagnostic Considerations

Diverticulitis: Diverticula are small outpouchings of the colonic mucosa and submucosa, which protrude through the muscular layer. Diverticulosis is common in developed countries, occurring in approximately 50% of people over 50 years of age. Diverticulitis occurs when a single diverticulum becomes occluded, resulting in increased pressure and microperforation. Imaging findings of a colonic segment with diverticula, wall thickening, and pericolonic inflammatory stranding suggests diverticulitis. Complications include abscess formation, fistula formation (commonly to the bladder), and perforation. Barium enema can show long segment stricture in chronic disease.

■ Diagnosis

Infectious colitis, *C. difficile*.

✓ Pearls

- Pan colitis involvement is usually infection.
- Advanced ischemia colitis has intramural air.

- If bowel wall thickening is in a vascular distribution, consider ischemic colitis.

Suggested Readings

Boyd SK, Cameron-Morrison JD, Hobson JJ, Saenz R. CT Imaging of large bowel wall thickening. J Am Osteopath Coll Radiol. 2016; 5(2):14–22

Horton KM, Corl FM, Fishman EK. CT evaluation of the colon: inflammatory disease. Radiographics. 2000; 20(2):399–418

Sheiman L, Levine MS, Levin AA, et al. Chronic diverticulitis: clinical, radiographic, and pathologic findings. AJR Am J Roentgenol. 2008; 191(2):522–528

Case 110

Eleanor L. Ormsby

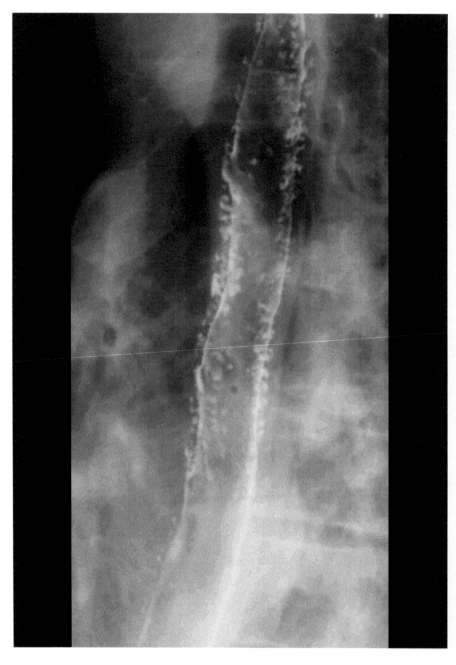

Fig. 110.1 Oblique image from an esophagram demonstrates multiple contrast outpouchings along the midesophageal wall, consistent with intramural pseudodiverticula. (Image courtesy of the Department of Radiology, University of Cincinnati, OH.)

■ Clinical History

A 42-year-old male with odynodysphagia (▶ Fig. 110.1).

■ Key Finding

Esophageal pseudodiverticula.

■ Top 3 Differential Diagnoses

- **Reflux esophagitis:** Pseudodiverticula are flask-shaped out-pouchings of contrast filling dilated mucous glands in the esophageal wall. They are the sequela of chronic irritation and esophagitis. Reflux esophagitis usually affects the distal esophagus as a result of irritation of esophageal mucosa by gastric acid. Esophagram demonstrates thickened distal folds, ulcers (which are usually linear), benign strictures (which classically begin immediately above the gastroesophageal junction), and/or intramural pseudodiverticula. Hiatal hernias are commonly associated with gastroesophageal reflux.
- **Candida esophagitis:** Candida is often cultured in esophageal pseudodiverticulosis, likely due to chronic esophagitis.

It is most commonly seen in immunosuppressed patients, especially in the setting of AIDS. Patients with esophageal stasis, such as those with achalasia or scleroderma, are also at risk for developing Candida esophagitis. Esophagram may demonstrate diffuse mucosal nodularity and ulceration, longitudinally oriented plaques, and pseudodiverticula.
- **Superficial spreading carcinoma:** Superficial spreading carcinoma is an unusual form of squamous cell carcinoma (SCC), which is characterized by small plaque-like mucosal nodularities on esophagram. Focal necrosis and ulceration can also be seen, as can pseudodiverticula. Endoscopic biopsy confirms the diagnosis.

■ Additional Diagnostic Consideration

Drug-induced esophagitis: In most patients with drug-induced esophagitis, there is no underlying esophageal disease. A wide range of drugs can cause esophagitis, including tetracycline, ascorbic acid, and iron-sulfate. Esophagram may show single or multiple shallow ulcerations with possible associated fold

thickening at the level of the aortic arch or the distal esophagus where a transient delay in the passage of bolus occurs. Occasionally, pseudodiverticula may occur. Repeat esophagrams usually demonstrate complete healing, following withdrawal of the medication.

■ Diagnosis

Candida esophagitis.

✓ Pearls

- Transmural inflammation in the esophagus may dilate mural glands and result in pseudodiverticula.
- Candidiasis presents in immunosuppressed patients with mucosal plaques and pseudodiverticula.

- Endoscopy is performed to exclude superficial spreading carcinoma in the setting of pseudodiverticulosis.

Suggested Readings

Lee SS, Ha HK, Byun JH, et al. Superficial esophageal cancer: esophagographic findings correlated with histopathologic findings. Radiology. 2005; 236(2):535–544

Levine MS, Moolten DN, Herlinger H, Laufer I. Esophageal intramural pseudodiverticulosis: a reevaluation. AJR Am J Roentgenol. 1986; 147(6):1165–1170

McGettigan MJ, Menias CO, Gao ZJ, Mellnick VM, Hara AK. Imaging of drug-induced complications in the gastrointestinal system. Radiographics. 2016; 36(1):71–87

Case 111

Alex R. Martin

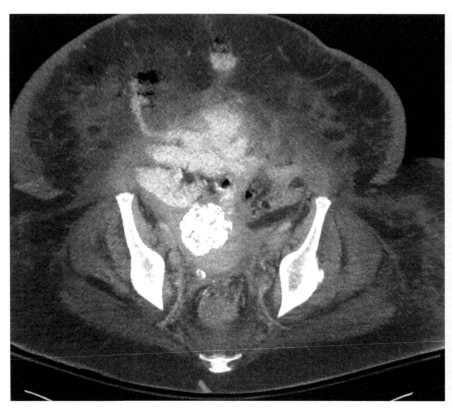

Fig. 111.1 Thick slab image from an oral and intravenous contrast enhanced axial CT image through the pelvis demonstrates enteric contrast tracking through the abdominal wall into the subcutaneous fat in multiple locations with associated subcutaneous emphysema. Calcified uterine fibroid is also noted.

■ Clinical History

A 36-year-old female with draining abdominal wound following surgery (▶ Fig. 111.1).

■ **Key Finding**

Enteric contrast tracking into the subcutaneous fat.

■ **Top 3 Differential Diagnoses**

- **Postsurgical:** This is the most common cause of enterocutaneous fistula (ECF) representing greater than three-fourths of cases. The highest rates of occurrence are with oncologic surgeries. The fistula tract often extends to an incision site and can manifest within the first postoperative week.
- **Inflammatory bowel disease:** Inflammatory bowel disease ECFs can occur spontaneously or be postoperative. They are almost always seen with Crohn's resulting from the characteristic transmural inflammation. Crohn's fistulas most commonly involve the terminal ileum.
- **Malignancy:** Tumor-related ECF ran result from direct extension or secondary infection. This is becoming increasingly rare as colorectal tumors are being diagnosed and treated earlier. If a malignancy presents with ECF, it is likely to be advanced disease (most commonly seen with adenocarcinoma) with high mortality.

■ **Additional Diagnostic Considerations**

Other inflammatory processes: ECF can occur as a result from any inflammatory process such as diverticulitis, radiation therapy, or advanced infection. High associated morbidity results from sepsis, malnutrition, and metabolic disturbances.

Fistulography can easily show communication with bowel. CT/MRI can provide information on underlying disease. ECF will resolve with conservative management in one-thirds to two-thirds of cases, otherwise treatment is surgical.

■ **Diagnosis**

Enterocutaneous fistula, postsurgical.

✓ **Pearls**

- In postsurgical ECF, sequela of prior surgery is usually evident.
- In an otherwise healthy young patient with ECF, inflammatory bowel disease should be considered.
- In an adult patient with ECF and no history of inflammatory bowel disease or prior surgery, malignancy should be excluded.

Suggested Readings

Lee JK, Stein SL. Radiographic and endoscopic diagnosis and treatment of enterocutaneous fistulas. Clin Colon Rectal Surg. 2010; 23(3):149–160

Rahman FN, Stavas JM. Interventional radiologic management and treatment of enterocutaneous fistulae. J Vasc Interv Radiol. 2015; 26(1):7–19, quiz 20

Tonolini M, Magistrelli P. Enterocutaneous fistulas: a primer for radiologists with emphasis on CT and MRI. Insights Imaging. 2017; 8(6):537–548

Case 112

Andrew Mizzi

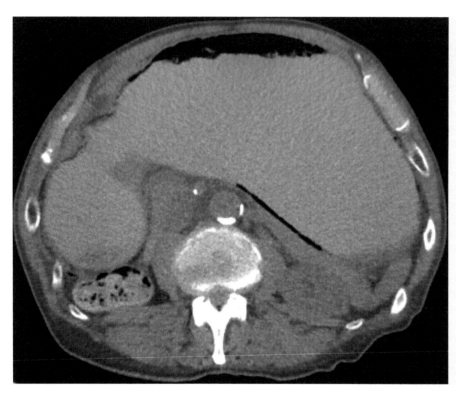

Fig. 112.1 CT image of the upper abdomen with oral contrast shows distention of the stomach with air along its nondependent wall and anterior right wall. (Image courtesy of Rocky C. Saenz.)

■ Clinical History

A 53-year-old male with septic shock in intensive care unit (▶Fig. 112.1).

■ Key Finding

Gastric wall air (emphysema).

■ Top 3 Differential Diagnoses

- **Emphysematous gastritis:** Emphysematous gastritis is a rare entity resulting from infectious pathogens producing gas in the wall (a life-threatening condition). Infectious agents include gas-forming organisms such as *E. coli* and *Clostridium perfringens*. Other organisms implicated include hemolytic streptococci, *Staphylococcus aureus*, and *Clostridium welchii*. Emphysematous gastritis is diagnosed by confirming air in the gastric wall. In addition, air may also be seen in the portal venous system. There is high mortality with fatality ranging from 60 to 80%. Therefore, patients with emphysematous gastritis are gravely ill. Surgical treatment is typically not successful and antibiotic therapy of the infectious etiology usually has a better outcome.
- **Iatrogenic/traumatic injury:** Mechanical trauma to the stomach is a more common source of intramural stomach air than emphysematous gastritis. Etiologies include gastric decompression tube placement, endoscopy procedures including over distention of the stomach lumen, gastric band erosion from bariatric procedures, and trauma from motor vehicle crashes involving the chest or abdomen (trauma with gas dissecting into stomach wall). Clinically, these patients are not severely ill as compared with emphysematous gastritis. On CT, it manifests as linear gas within the gastric wall along either the dependent or nondependent walls (nondependent wall is more sensitive).
- **Caustic:** Ingestion of caustic substances disrupts the gastric mucosal allowing gas to infiltrate the wall. Caustic substances include strong acids and bases. The damaged mucosal lining will often lead to infection and emphysematous gastritis complication. The history and clinical presentation will help to narrow down the etiology and the need for treatment.

■ Diagnosis

Emphysematous gastritis.

✓ Pearls

- Emphysematous gastritis should be the diagnosis of exclusion with air in gastric wall and portal veins.
- Gastric emphysema may also be caused by ischemia and obstruction.
- On CT, gastric emphysema is most accurately diagnosed using the nondependent wall.

Suggested Readings

Federle MP, Jeffrey RB, Woodward PJ, Borhani A. Diagnostic Imaging: Abdomen. 2nd ed. Philadelphia, PA: Lippincott Williams & Wilkins; 2009

Johnson PT, Horton KM, Edil BH, Fishman EK, Scott WW. Gastric pneumatosis: the role of CT in diagnosis and patient management. Emerg Radiol. 2011; 18(1):65–73

Wong YY, Chu WCW. Emphysematous gastritis associated with gastric infarction in a patient with adult polycystic renal disease: CT diagnosis. AJR Am J Roentgenol. 2002; 178(5):1291

Case 113

Robert A. Jesinger

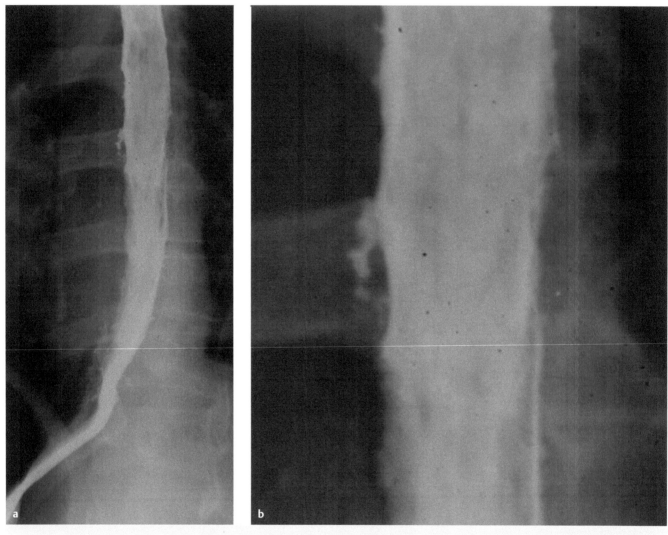

Fig. 113.1 Single-contrast fluoroscopic image **(a)** and coned-down view **(b)** of the esophagus from a barium swallow examination demonstrate a large midesophageal ulcer, as well as additional smaller ulcerations and thickening of the longitudinal folds. (Images courtesy of the Department of Radiology, University of Cincinnati, OH.)

■ Clinical History

A 35-year-old man with chest pain and odynodysphagia
(▶Fig. 113.1).

■ Key Finding

Esophageal ulcers.

■ Top 3 Differential Diagnoses

- **Reflux esophagitis:** Erosions and ulcerations can form in the distal esophagus as a result of irritation of esophageal mucosa from gastric acid. Key imaging findings of esophageal inflammation include longitudinal fold thickening, pooling of contrast in mucosal erosions or ulcers, poor peristalsis, and poor esophageal distension in the region of inflammation. Midesophageal strictures may be seen in severe chronic reflux. Careful visual assessment for Barrett's metaplasia, hiatal hernia, and reflux on fluoroscopy can aid in assessment.
- **Viral esophagitis (cytomegalovirus [CMV], human immunodeficiency virus [HIV], herpes simplex virus [HSV]):** Discrete ulcers against otherwise normal background mucosa are the hallmark of viral esophagitis. Viral esophagitis typically occurs in immunosuppressed patients, especially in the setting of HIV. HSV ulcers tend to be multiple, small, discrete, and focal, while ulcers caused by CMV and HIV are typically large. Although imaging characteristics may suggest the underlying source of ulceration, serology or biopsy is often used for definitive diagnosis and treatment.
- **Drug-induced esophagitis:** Esophageal injury and ulceration may occur from ingested medications if the tablets become trapped in the esophageal lumen. Typically, esophageal dysmotility or an obstructing lesion is present with subsequent ulcer formation from prolonged direct contact with the esophageal mucosa. Common medications that can cause mucosal injury include antimicrobial medications (doxycycline, tetracycline, clindamycin), anti-inflammatory medications, and supplements (potassium chloride, vitamin C).

■ Additional Diagnostic Considerations

- **Caustic esophagitis:** Caustic esophagitis is the consequence of contact injury usually with an alkaline substance. Numerous household and garden chemicals (alkalis), when ingested, can cause both superficial and deep liquefaction necrosis in the esophagus, leading to ulceration and long segment scarring. Acid burns are less frequently encountered and typically lead to less severe superficial mucosal burns.
- **Esophageal carcinoma:** Malignancy should always be considered in the differential diagnosis of mucosal irregularity and ulceration. Both primary squamous cell carcinoma (SCC) and adenocarcinoma in the setting of Barrett's metaplasia can ulcerate. Aggressive midesophageal malignancies can erode into the tracheobronchial tree, resulting in fistula formation.

■ Diagnosis

Viral esophagitis (HSV).

✓ Pearls

- Mucosal ulcers, fold thickening, poor peristalsis, and poor distensibility are key findings in esophagitis.
- HSV typically causes multiple small ulcers; CMV and HIV commonly present as large ulcers.
- Contact injury from prolonged retention of potassium chloride in the esophagus can cause a focal ulcer.
- Esophageal carcinoma and lymphoma should always be considered as a potential cause for an ulcer.

Suggested Readings

McGettigan MJ, Menias CO, Gao ZJ, Mellnick VM, Hara AK. Imaging of drug-induced complications in the gastrointestinal system. Radiographics. 2016; 36(1):71–87

Young CA, Menias CO, Bhalla S, Prasad SR. CT features of esophageal emergencies. Radiographics. 2008; 28(6):1541–1553

Case 114

Brian J. Lewis

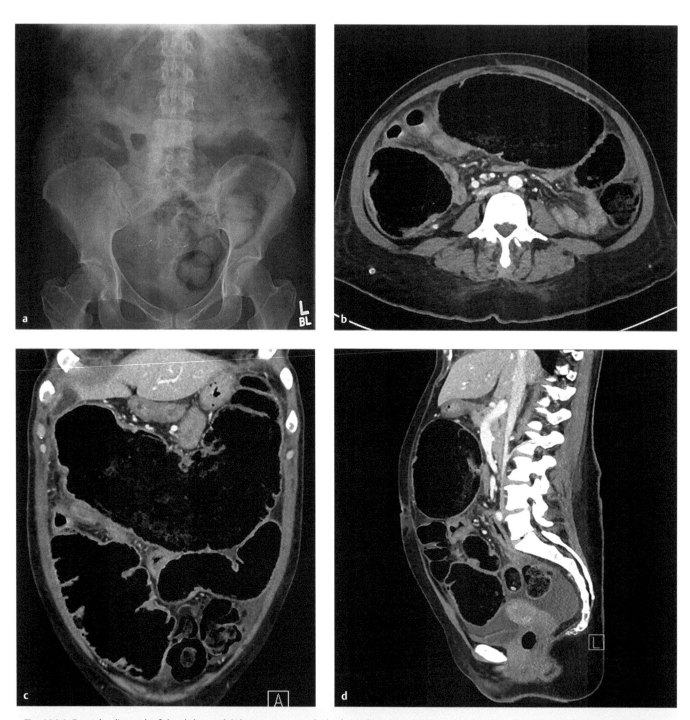

Fig. 114.1 Frontal radiograph of the abdomen (**a**) demonstrates marked colonic distention, most prominent within the transverse colon, with formed stool throughout. Axial (**b**), coronal (**c**), and sagittal (**d**) contrast-enhanced CT images of the abdomen and pelvis reveal marked colonic distention with mucosal irregularity and wall thinning, adjacent fat stranding and thickened bowel loops, and free fluid within the pelvis (**d**). Incidental tubal ligation post-procedural changes are visualized within the pelvis (**a**). (Images courtesy of Dell Dunn, M.D.)

■ Clinical History

A 50-year-old woman with abdominal pain and distension
(▶Fig. 114.1).

■ **Key Finding**

Large bowel dilatation.

■ **Top 3 Differential Diagnoses**

- **Large bowel obstruction:** Colon cancer is the most common cause of large bowel obstruction, accounting for over half of cases. The sigmoid colon and splenic flexure are the most common tumor locations that result in obstruction. Masses large enough to cause luminal obstruction may demonstrate shouldering and central necrosis with infiltration of pericolonic fat, which can mimic diverticulitis with abscess. Pericolonic lymph nodes measuring greater or equal to 1 cm in short axis are suspicious for metastases. Recurrent bouts of diverticulitis with stricture formation are a less common cause of colonic obstruction. Adhesions, which are a common cause of small bowel obstruction, are an additional infrequent cause of large bowel obstruction. Regardless of the underlying etiology, perforation is an uncommon but emergent complication, typically occurring in the setting of a severely dilated cecum.
- **Volvulus:** Volvulus refers to the twisting of bowel with resultant obstruction and dilatation of the affected large bowel. Sigmoid volvulus is most common in elderly patients with a redundant and mobile colon, while cecal and transverse colon volvuli are more likely to occur secondary to a congenital defect in the mesentery, resulting in increased mobility. The "coffee bean" sign is seen in both cecal and sigmoid volvuli radiographically and refers to an apposed loop of dilated bowel likened to the appearance of a coffee bean. The "bird's beak" sign results from smooth tapering of bowel at the point of obstruction, reminiscent of a bird's beak. Specific to sigmoid volvulus, the "inverted U" sign refers to a dilated loop of sigmoid colon pointing to the right upper quadrant. CT often demonstrates the whirl sign with spiraling of collapsed bowel and vessels at the point of obstruction.
- **Colonic pseudo-obstruction (Ogilvie syndrome):** Colonic pseudo-obstruction refers to large bowel dilatation without a mechanical cause or abrupt transition. It most often affects older patients who are fairly ill with a wide range of underlying medical conditions. While the exact etiology remains uncertain, it is thought to result from decreased parasympathetic activity. Gradual transition near the splenic flexure may be seen. Cecal ischemia and perforation are the most feared complications.

■ **Additional Diagnostic Considerations**

Toxic megacolon: Toxic megacolon refers to severe and potentially life-threatening dilatation of the colon resulting from underlying colitis, most commonly pseudomembranous colitis or inflammatory bowel disease. CT demonstrates large bowel dilatation (transverse colon > 6 cm), mucosal irregularity, wall thickening with thumb printing, or thinning with an ahaustral pattern. The risk of perforation increases significantly with greater than 12 cm of cecal dilatation. When suspected, barium enema should be avoided in the setting of toxic megacolon due to increased risk of perforation.

■ **Diagnosis**

Toxic megacolon (as a complication of inflammatory bowel disease).

✓ **Pearls**

- Colon cancer is the most common cause of large bowel obstruction.
- The coffee bean (cecal or sigmoid) or inverted U (sigmoid) signs are seen radiographically with volvuli.
- Toxic megacolon results from an underlying colitis; when suspected, barium enema should be avoided.

Suggested Readings

Jaffe T, Thompson WM. Large bowel obstruction in the adult: classic radiographic and CT findings, etiology, and mimics. Radiology. 2015; 275(3):651–663

Thoeni RF, Cello JP. CT imaging of colitis. Radiology. 2006; 240(3):623–638

Case 115

Shaun Loh

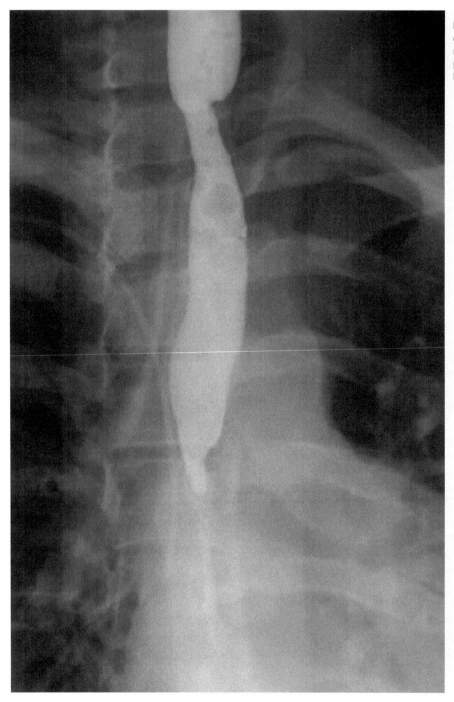

Fig. 115.1 Single contrast anteroposterior esophagram image demonstrates abrupt narrowing involving the midesophagus (which persisted on further imaging). (Image courtesy of Rocky C. Saenz.)

■ Clinical History

A 24-year-old man with dysphagia (▶ Fig. 115.1).

■ Key Finding

Esophageal stricture.

■ Top 3 Differential Diagnoses for Short Segment Strictures

- **Reflux esophagitis:** Reflux esophagitis is one of the most common causes of esophageal strictures. The stricture typically appears as an area of smooth, tapered narrowing in the distal esophagus. Asymmetric scarring can occur, resulting in a more eccentric stricture. Sacculations may be present between multiple strictures.
- **Drug-induced stricture:** The two most common agents implicated in drug-induced esophagitis, tetracycline and doxycycline, typically cause superficial ulceration that heals without stricture formation. Other drugs such as quinidine, potassium chloride, alendronate, and nonsteroidal anti-inflammatory drugs (NSAIDs) may cause larger ulcerations and strictures in the proximal to midesophagus. Tablet medications may lodge in the esophagus due to extrinsic compression from adjacent structures such as the aortic arch or left mainstem bronchus.
- **Esophageal carcinoma:** Squamous cell carcinoma (SCC) accounts for the vast majority of esophageal cancer cases. Risk factors include smoking, alcohol, caustic ingestions, achalasia, and Plummer–Vinson syndrome. Adenocarcinoma from Barrett's esophagitis comprises the majority of the remaining cases. The most common finding is a fixed narrowing of the esophageal lumen. The tumor may also appear as an annular constricting lesion causing a long segment stricture with prominent shoulders. Another pattern is that of a polypoid intraluminal filling defect. Prognosis is poor with a 5% 5-year survival rate.

■ Top 3 Differential Diagnoses for Long Segment Strictures

- **Iatrogenic (nasogastric tube, NGT):** NGTs prevent the lower esophageal sphincter from closing, allowing the acidic gastric contents to bathe the lumen of the distal esophagus. Mucosal injury and stricture formation can ensue. Strictures are most commonly seen with prolonged NGT placement.
- **Caustic ingestion:** Ingestion of strong acids or more commonly bases causes long, symmetric esophageal strictures, usually months to years after the initial injury. The stricture may appear "thread-like" with a diffuse long segmental narrowing, irregular contours, and ulcerations. Treatment entails either esophageal dilation or esophagectomy. There is an increased risk of malignancy after the initial injury.
- **Radiation changes:** Radiation changes occur within the radiotherapy field during the treatment of thoracic and cervical neoplasms. The strictures are often long, smooth, concentric, and tapered.

■ Diagnosis

Stricture from lye ingestion.

✓ Pearls

- Strictures from reflux esophagitis commonly are seen as smooth areas of narrowing in the esophagus.
- Tablet medications may lodge in the esophagus and incite ulceration and stricture formation.
- Irregular areas of esophageal stricturing are concerning for esophageal carcinoma.
- Prolonged NGT placement can result in mucosal injury to the esophagus and stricture formation.

Suggested Reading

Luedtke P, Levine MS, Rubesin SE, Weinstein DS, Laufer I. Radiologic diagnosis of benign esophageal strictures: a pattern approach. Radiographics. 2003; 23(4):897–909

Case 116

Paul B. DiDomenico

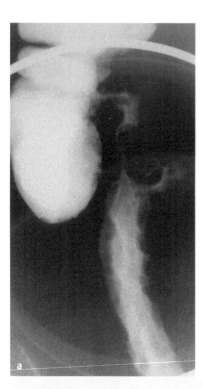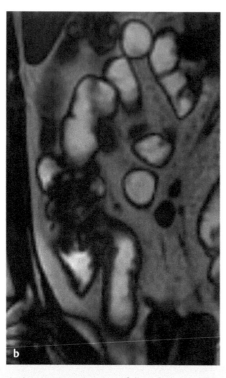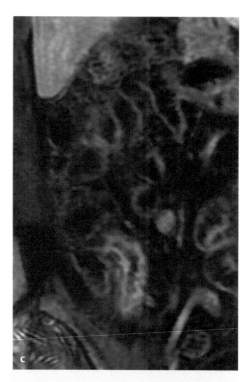

Fig. 116.1 Two patients with the same diagnosis. Spot compression view of the right lower quadrant from a small bowel follow-through study in patient A **(a)** demonstrates irregularity and thickening of the terminal ileum with stricture formation. Coned-down coronal high-resolution T2 MR image (FIESTA) in patient B **(b)** shows bowel wall thickening involving the terminal ileum with luminal narrowing. Coned-down coronal post-contrast T1 image with fat suppression in patient B **(c)** shows abnormal bowel wall thickening and enhancement of the terminal ileum. (Images B & C courtesy of Dell Dunn, M.D.)

■ **Clinical History**

Diarrhea and abdominal pain (▶ Fig. 116.1).

■ Key Finding

Terminal ileal wall thickening.

■ Top 3 Differential Diagnoses

- **Inflammatory bowel disease:** Of the two main types of idiopathic inflammatory bowel disease (ulcerative colitis and Crohn's disease), Crohn's disease characteristically involves the terminal ileum, causing transmural inflammation, thickening, and deep fissuring ulcers. Proliferation of mesenteric fat ("creeping fat") may cause the bowel loops to appear separated on a small bowel follow-through study. Fistulas and sinus tracts are a hallmark of the disease secondary to transmural involvement, and skip (discontinuous) lesions are characteristic. These findings are in contrast to those of ulcerative colitis, which is characterized by continuous involvement of the colon beginning distally and progressing proximally. Ulcerative colitis may cause dilatation of the distal ileum, termed "backwash" ileitis, in approximately 25% of cases.

- **Infection:** Certain infections have a predilection for the terminal ileum, among them *Salmonella*, *Campylobacter*, *Yersinia*, and *M. tuberculosis*. Immunosuppressed patients (HIV/AIDS [human immunodeficiency virus/acquired immunodeficiency syndrome]) are also at increased risk for opportunistic infection from *Cryptosporidium* and cytomegalovirus (CMV). Imaging features of these infections are generally nonspecific, and the diagnosis is usually made through stool analysis, mucosal biopsy, and/or response to empiric antimicrobial therapy.

- **Lymphoma:** Non-Hodgkin's lymphoma (NHL) affects the small bowel in approximately one-third of cases with the ileum being the most common site of involvement. Imaging appearance is variable; however, lymphoma typically manifests as nodular/polypoid or diffuse infiltrative small bowel wall thickening. When the terminal ileum is involved, the bowel wall may be thickened with a narrow lumen, resembling Crohn's disease.

■ Additional Diagnostic Considerations

- **Ischemia:** Ischemia of the superior mesenteric artery (SMA) territory can result in bowel wall thickening due to edema and occasionally hemorrhage. There may be gas in the bowel wall (pneumatosis), which may also be seen in the mesenteric and portal venous system on CT imaging. Intravenous contrast material may aid in visualization of the site of occlusion due to clot or atherosclerotic disease (ASD).

- **Metastatic disease:** Metastatic spread of carcinoma can involve the terminal ileum through direct spread or peritoneal spread (gastrointestinal or genitourinary primary neoplasms), and hematogenous dissemination (malignant melanoma, lung, or breast carcinoma).

■ Diagnosis

Crohn's disease.

✓ Pearls

- Crohn's disease classically involves the distal ileum, with chronic inflammation leading to strictures/fistulae.
- CMV or cryptosporidium involvement of the terminal ileum should prompt an evaluation for HIV.

- Nodular ileal wall thickening is concerning for malignancy, including lymphoma and metastatic disease.

Suggested Readings

Furukawa A, Saotome T, Yamasaki M, et al. Cross-sectional imaging in Crohn disease. Radiographics. 2004; 24(3):689–702

Thoeni RF, Cello JP. CT imaging of colitis. Radiology. 2006; 240(3):623–638

Case 117

Grant E. Lattin, Jr.

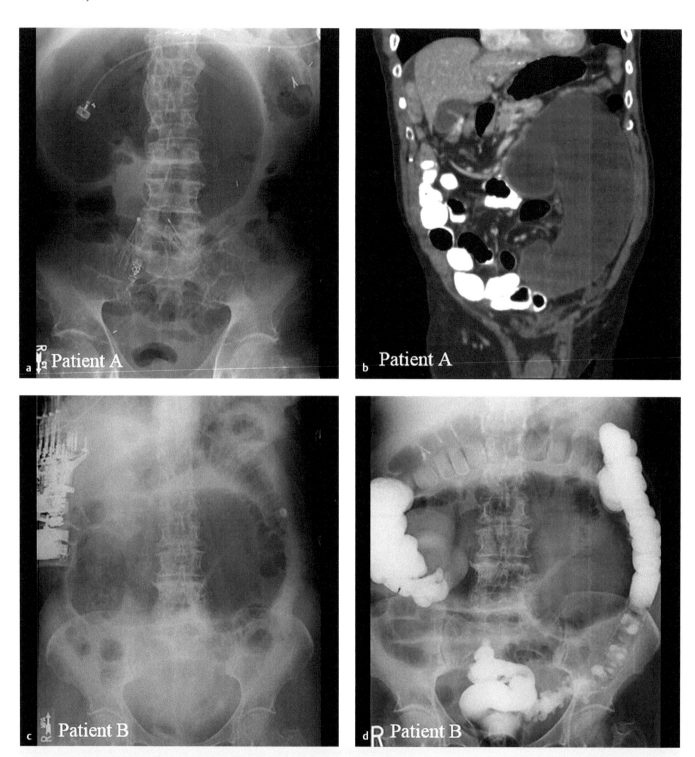

Fig. 117.1 Plain radiograph of the abdomen **(a)** demonstrates a coffee bean-shaped, dilated, loop of bowel which points toward the left upper quadrant. Reformatted coronal CT image **(b)** confirms a dilated cecum that has twisted on the axis of the right colon. Plain radiograph **(c)** and barium enema **(d)** in another patient with the same disease process displays a gas-filled, dilated cecum with "beaking" of contrast within the midascending colon.

■ Clinical History

A 63-year-old man with severe abdominal pain (►Fig. 117.1).

■ Key Finding

Dilated, gas-filled cecum pointing toward the left upper quadrant of the abdomen.

■ Discussion

Cecal volvulus occurs less commonly than sigmoid volvulus but has increased in incidence, now accounting for approximately one-third of all cases of colonic volvulus. Seen usually in younger women, cecal volvulus is due to rotation about the axis of the right colon, often due to a redundant mesentery with narrow fixation, related to incomplete fusion of the right colon to the posterior parietal peritoneum.

Plain film radiographs demonstrate a dilated, gas-filled cecum directed toward the left upper quadrant of the abdomen. Often referred to as having a "kidney bean" or "coffee bean" appearance, cecal volvulus may contain only one air-fluid level, rather than two, as can be observed in sigmoid volvulus. Contrast enema will show "beaking" of the contrast column at the midascending colon. CT will show tapering of the ends of the dilated cecum with "whirling" of adjacent mesenteric vessels.

Although cecal volvulus may present classically with an acute abdomen, an initial differential diagnosis may include cecal bascule, acute ileus, Ogilvie syndrome (mechanical pseudo-obstruction), or toxic megacolon, in addition to sigmoid volvulus. Anatomic distribution of the dilated bowel as well as patient history may assist in making the diagnosis.

Treatment options may include reduction via colonoscopy or surgery, depending on the patient's condition, with surgical management occurring in the majority of cases. Mortality rates for isolated cecal volvulus are reported at 6.6%. Delayed diagnosis and treatment may lead to bowel necrosis, sepsis, bowel perforation, and subsequent death. Prognosis, therefore, depends on the degree of complications associated with the volvulus.

■ Diagnosis

Cecal volvulus.

✓ Pearls

- Cecal volvulus appears as a "coffee bean" configuration of a dilated cecum oriented in the left upper quadrant.
- On barium enema, there is "beaking" of the contrast column within the midascending colon.

- On CT, there is tapering of the ends of the dilated cecum with "whirling" of adjacent mesenteric vessels.

Suggested Readings

Delabrousse E, Sarliève P, Sailley N, Aubry S, Kastler BA. Cecal volvulus: CT findings and correlation with pathophysiology. Emerg Radiol. 2007; 14(6):411–415

Feldman D. The coffee bean sign. Radiology. 2000; 216(1):178–179

Halabi WJ, Jafari MD, Kang CY, et al. Colonic volvulus in the United States: trends, outcomes, and predictors of mortality. Ann Surg. 2014; 259(2):293–301

Case 118

William T. O'Brien, Sr.

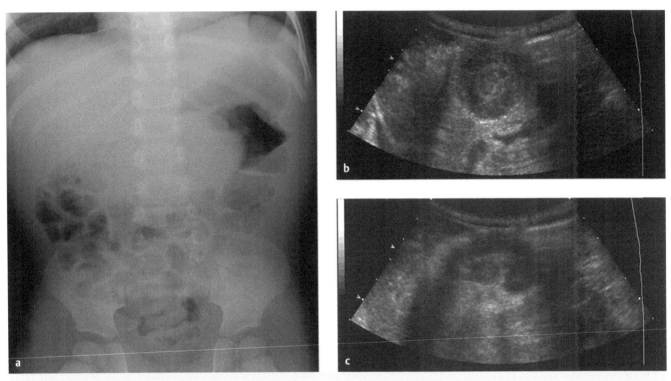

Fig. 118.1 Plain radiograph of the abdomen demonstrates a meniscus of soft tissue projecting distally into the bowel lumen of the transverse colon within the left upper abdomen **(a)**. Sonographic evaluation through this region in the transverse plane reveals bowel wall signature with central concentric rings of increased and decreased echotexture **(b)**. Longitudinal sonographic evaluation reveals circumferential hypoechoic bowel wall with a central region of increased echotexture and distal bowel wall shadowing, an appearance referred to as the "pseudokidney" sign **(c)**.

■ **Clinical History**

A 3-year-old boy with severe intermittent abdominal pain and diarrhea (▶ Fig. 118.1).

■ Key Finding

Intraluminal mass with bowel signature on ultrasound.

■ Discussion

Intussusception is a common and important cause of intestinal obstruction in children. The peak incidence occurs between 5 and 9 months of age will nearly all idiopathic cases occurring before 3 years of age. More than 90% of cases are idiopathic with an antecedent viral infection. If intussusception occurs in a child older than 3 years of age, a pathologic lead point from entities such as lymphoma, Meckel's diverticulum, bowel hemorrhage (Henoch–Schönlein purpura), etc. should be investigated.

With regards to location, 90% of cases of intussusception are ileocolic, with the remainder either ileoileal or colocolic. The clinical symptoms include abdominal pain, vomiting, blood per rectum, palpable abdominal mass, fever, and "currant jelly" stools. Differential diagnosis includes appendicitis and Meckel's diverticulum.

Plain radiographs demonstrate a meniscus of soft tissue protruding into the distal bowel lumen with the location dependent on the type of intussusception. Most cases involve the cecum or ascending colon. On ultrasound, transverse images demonstrate alternating concentric rings of increased and decreased echotexture in a typical target appearance. Longitudinal scanning reveals peripheral hypoechoic bowel wall with a central region of increased echotexture referred to as the "pseudokidney" sign.

When intussusception is suspected based on imaging findings, a diagnostic and therapeutic examination such as an air enema may be performed. Air insufflation is performed via the rectum with a tight seal under fluoroscopic guidance, maintaining a pressure of less than 120 mm of mercury. Once reduced, air will reflux into the small bowel through the ileocecal valve. A follow-up film should demonstrate intraluminal bowel gas without free intraperitoneal air. Similarly, hydrostatic enema under fluoroscopic or ultrasound guidance is another technique used with success. Pediatric surgery should be readily available in the event of an adverse outcome during reduction, such as perforation, which occurs in less than 0.5% of cases. Contraindications to reduction include peritoneal signs on physical examination or free intraperitoneal air on imaging studies.

■ Diagnosis

Intussusception.

✓ Pearls

- Over 90% of cases of intussusception occur before 3 years of age and are idiopathic in nature.
- A pathologic lead point should be suspected in patients older than 3 years of age.

- Imaging findings include a meniscus of soft tissue on plain films and target and pseudokidney sign on the ultrasound.
- When using air reduction technique, pressures should not exceed 120 mm of mercury.

Suggested Readings

Applegate KE. Clinically suspected intussusception in children: evidence-based review and self-assessment module. AJR Am J Roentgenol. 2005; 185 (3, Suppl):S175–S183

Bouali O, Mouttalib S, Vial J, Galinier P. Intussusception in infancy and childhood: radiological and surgical management Arch Pediatr. 2015; 22(12):1312–1317

Donnelly LF. Fundamentals of Pediatric Radiology. Philadelphia, PA: WB Saunders; 2001

Case 119

Cam Chau and Rebecca Stein-Wexler

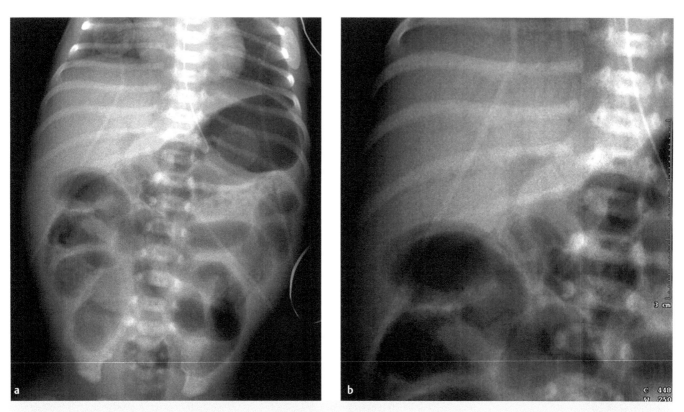

Fig. 119.1 Supine anteroposterior abdominal radiograph **(a)** demonstrates generalized bowel distention, along with linear and rounded lucencies along the bowel wall. Branching lucencies are also seen over the liver. A coned-down view over the right upper quadrant **(b)** better depicts the pneumatosis within gas-distended loops of bowel, as well as the portal venous gas over the liver.

■ Clinical History

A 7-day-old premature infant with respiratory distress, abdominal distention, and bloody diarrhea (▶ Fig. 119.1).

■ Key Finding

Pneumatosis and portal venous gas in a premature infant.

■ Discussion

Necrotizing enterocolitis is the most common gastrointestinal emergency in premature infants. It usually occurs in infants in the neonatal intensive care unit weighing less than 1,000 g at birth, although about 10% of neonates with necrotizing enterocolitis are born at term (cardiac disease or maternal cocaine use is often present). The peak incidence is during the first or second week of life, although necrotizing enterocolitis may occur later in extremely premature infants. The etiology of necrotizing enterocolitis is multifactorial and is associated with prematurity, intestinal ischemia/mucosal damage caused by bacterial colonization, inflammatory mediators, and early feeding. Bowel wall coagulative and hemorrhagic necrosis and inflammation result.

Necrotizing enterocolitis may occur anywhere in the gastrointestinal tract but is found most often in the right colon and terminal ileum. Clinical symptoms include feeding intolerance, vomiting, diarrhea, bloody stools, and abdominal distention. Respiratory distress, acidosis, sepsis, shock, and temperature instability are associated sequela.

Infants with clinical suspicion of necrotizing enterocolitis are followed with serial supine and often also left lateral decubitus radiographs of the abdomen. The earliest finding is fixed bowel distension. Bowel wall pneumatosis constitutes definitive radiographic evidence of necrotizing enterocolitis and is seen in 50 to 70% of patients with this disease. The pneumatosis appears as bubbly or curvilinear lucencies within the bowel wall, depending on whether the gas is submucosal or subserosal. Portal venous gas may be seen as branching lucencies over the liver, with more peripheral extension than occurs with biliary gas. Free intraperitoneal air most often occurs due to perforation of the distal ileum or proximal colon and is the only universally accepted indication for surgical intervention. Radiographic findings of free air include increased lucency over the liver, gas outlining the falciform ligament, and gas on both sides of the bowel wall (Rigler sign) on supine radiographs; additional findings on left lateral decubitus views include triangular lucencies at the nondependent portion of the abdomen, along with larger collections of extraluminal gas.

When there is strong clinical suspicion of necrotizing enterocolitis, or if the diagnosis has been established radiographically, infants are monitored with serial abdominal radiographs. Treatment includes bowel rest and decompression, broad spectrum antibiotics, parenteral nutrition, oxygen, and intravenous fluids. Long-term sequelae include intestinal strictures, malabsorption, fistulae formation, and short gut syndrome. Overall mortality for necrotizing enterocolitis is approximately 20 to 30%.

■ Diagnosis

Necrotizing enterocolitis.

✓ Pearls

- Necrotizing enterocolitis most commonly occurs in premature infants weighing less than 1,000 g at birth.
- Pneumatosis most commonly occurs in the right lower quadrant.
- Portal venous gas is depicted as linear branching lucencies over the peripheral margin of the liver.
- Free intraperitoneal air necessitates surgical intervention.

Suggested Readings

Donnelly LF. Diagnostic Imaging Pediatrics. Salt Lake City, UT: Amirsys; 2005

Epelman M, Daneman A, Navarro OM, et al. Necrotizing enterocolitis: review of state-of-the-art imaging findings with pathologic correlation. Radiographics. 2007; 27(2):285–305

Moss RL, Dimmitt RA, Barnhart DC, et al. Laparotomy versus peritoneal drainage for necrotizing enterocolitis and perforation. N Engl J Med. 2006; 354(21):2225–2234

Case 120

Eleanor L. Ormsby

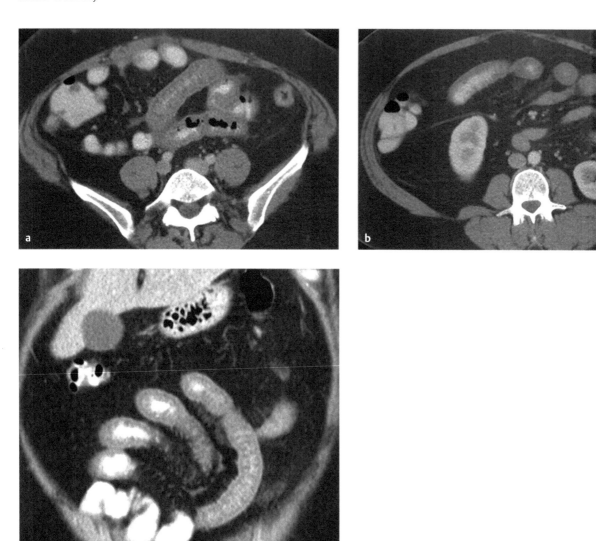

Fig. 120.1 Axial **(a, b)** and coronal reformatted **(c)** contrast-enhanced (oral and intravenous) CT images show several small bowel loops with marked wall thickening and enhancement along the mucosal and serosal surfaces with relative decreased central bowel wall attenuation.

■ Clinical History

Abdominal pain (▶ Fig. 120.1).

■ Key Finding

Small bowel wall thickening.

■ Top 3 Differential Diagnoses

- **Crohn's disease:** Crohn's disease presents with irregularly thickened folds associated with mucosal ulceration (early) and strictures (late). The findings are usually seen in the terminal ileum. The "string sign" has been used to describe marked segmental narrowing of bowel loops. In contrast to ulcerative colitis, lesions in Crohn's disease can be scattered in the small bowel ("skip lesions"), with normal bowel interposed between involved segments. On CT, bowel wall thickening and mesenteric stranding are the most common findings. The fibrofatty proliferation seen in the mesentery is referred to as "creeping fat."
- **Lymphoma:** Small bowel lymphoma can occur with or without predisposing factors, such as immunodeficiency syndromes, celiac sprue, or Crohn's disease. There are different types of imaging findings, including nodular bowel wall thickening, bowel wall infiltration with loss of bowel markings, or intraluminal polypoid masses. There may be associated luminal narrowing or characteristic aneurismal dilatation, which is more common with diffuse infiltration.
- **Bowel wall edema:** Bowel wall edema may result from a variety of etiologies, to include ischemia, vasculopathy, hypoproteinemia, and angioedema. Ischemia may be due to decreased arterial flow or venous congestion or associated with inflammatory processes as is seen with radiation enteritis. Hypoproteinemia results from liver or kidney disease with hypoalbuminemia. Angioedema may be inherited, acquired, or drug-induced due to angiotensin-converting enzyme (ACE) inhibitor or nonsteroidal anti-inflammatory drug (NSAID) therapy. Imaging studies demonstrate bowel wall and fold thickening most often involving the small bowel. Mural stratification may be seen with enhancing mucosal and serosal layers with interposed edematous bowel wall.

■ Additional Diagnostic Considerations

- **Small bowel hemorrhage:** Small bowel is the most common site of intramural hemorrhage and may be due to trauma, mesenteric ischemia, vasculitis, coagulopathy, anticoagulant medication, or Henoch–Schönlein purpura. Short segment uniformly thickened small bowel folds with "stack-of-coins" appearance is the typical finding. Appropriate clinical history helps to differentiate the underlying cause.
- **Metastases:** Metastases to the small bowel commonly present as multiple masses with nodular bowel wall thickening, which may result in fold tethering or ulceration. Metastases can be from intraperitoneal seeding, hematogenous spread, lymphatic spread, or direct extension from a contiguous neoplasm.
- **Whipple's disease:** Whipple's disease is a rare, chronic, systemic disease caused by a bacterial infection (gram-positive bacilli with PAS stain). Patients present with chronic diarrhea, arthralgias, and malabsorption. Thickened proximal small bowel folds with micronodularity (1–2 mm) and low-density mesenteric lymphadenopathy are characteristic findings.

■ Diagnosis

Bowel wall edema (angioedema secondary to ACE inhibitor).

✓ Pearls

- Mucosal ulceration, mesenteric fibrofatty proliferation, and strictures are key findings in Crohn's disease.
- In the setting of trauma, small bowel wall thickening is concerning for hemorrhage.
- Bowel wall edema may be seen with ischemia, vasculopathy, hypoproteinemia, or angioedema.

Suggested Readings

Ishigami K, Averill SL, Pollard JH, McDonald JM, Sato Y. Radiologic manifestations of angioedema. Insights Imaging. 2014; 5(3):365–374

Macari M, Balthazar EJ. CT of bowel wall thickening: significance and pitfalls of interpretation. AJR Am J Roentgenol. 2001; 176(5):1105–1116

Case 121

Cam Chau and Rebecca Stein-Wexler

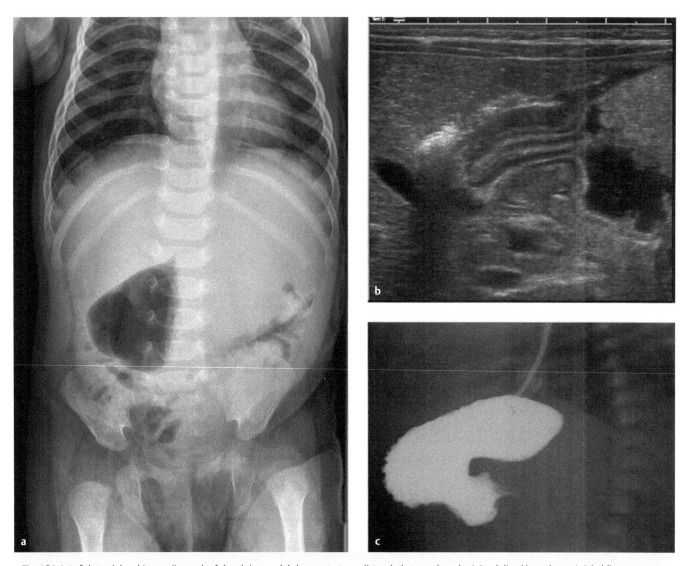

Fig. 121.1 Left lateral decubitus radiograph of the abdomen **(a)** demonstrates a distended stomach and minimal distal bowel gas. Axial oblique ultrasound image **(b)** shows elongation of the pyloric channel and thickening of the hypoechoic muscular wall. A lateral view from an upper gastrointestinal examination **(c)** shows shouldering of the gastric antrum and partial visualization of the elongated and narrowed pyloric channel, resulting in the "string sign." (Images courtesy of Children's Hospital and Research Center Oakland, CA.)

■ Clinical History
....

A 6-week-old infant with a 4-day history of nonbilious vomiting after feeds (▶Fig. 121.1).

■ Key Finding

Gastric outlet obstruction with enlarged pyloris.

■ Discussion

Hypertrophic pyloric stenosis (HPS) develops in early infancy, presenting in infants between 2 and 12 weeks of age. It occurs in 2 to 5 per 1,000 births per year, and the male to female ratio is 4:1 to 5:1. Most common among first-born Caucasians, HPS is not truly inherited but does have a familial link. Its true etiology remains unclear.

Clinical symptoms include nonbilious vomiting that begins as occasional regurgitation but may progress to projectile vomiting after most feedings. Examiners may palpate an olive-shaped mass in the midepigastrium; if found, this sign is 97% specific. Other presentations include hypochloremic, hypokalemic metabolic alkalosis, and weight loss, though this is encountered infrequently due to relatively early diagnosis.

Ultrasound is the examination of choice when HPS is suspected. The patient is positioned supine or right lateral decubitus, and glucose water may be administered to facilitate identification of the pylorus and assess gastric emptying. Peristaltic waves are absent from the thickened, elongated circular pyloric muscle, and the pyloric channel does not open to allow passage of gastric contents. When the pylorus is viewed in cross-section, single wall thickness of greater than 3 mm is generally considered abnormal, as is length greater than 14 mm (these standards do vary slightly among researchers). Pylorospasm may mimic HPS and is diagnosed when the configuration of the pylorus alters, allowing fluid to traverse the channel. Occasionally, HPS is identified on an upper gastrointestinal examination. Exaggerated gastric motility results in a "caterpillar" appearance of the stomach. Barium within the elongated and narrowed pyloric channel results in the "string sign." Mass effect from the hypertrophied muscle causes "shouldering" of the antrum and a "mushroom" appearance of the duodenum.

Nonsurgical treatment of HPS includes administration of atropine and frequent small feedings. Pyloromyotomy is the surgical management of choice, whether open or laparoscopic. The thickened muscle is split longitudinally and the edges closed transversely, relieving the stricture.

■ Diagnosis

HPS.

✓ Pearls

• HPS is most common among first-born Caucasian males and occurs between 2 and 12 weeks of age.
• Ultrasound demonstrates a thickened and elongated pyloris (≥ 3 mm single wall thickness; ≥ 14 mm length).

• Upper gastrointestinal examination demonstrates the "string sign" and shouldering at the gastric antrum.

Suggested Readings

Donnelly LF. Diagnostic Imaging Pediatrics. Salt Lake City, UT: Amirsys; 2005

Hernanz-Schulman M. Infantile hypertrophic pyloric stenosis. Radiology. 2003; 227(2):319–331

Hernanz-Schulman M, Lowe LH, Johnson J, et al. In vivo visualization of pyloric mucosal hypertrophy in infants with hypertrophic pyloric stenosis: is there an etiologic role? AJR Am J Roentgenol. 2001; 177(4):843–848

van der Bilt JD, Kramer WL, van der Zee DC, Bax NM. Laparoscopic pyloromyotomy for hypertrophic pyloric stenosis: impact of experience on the results in 182 cases. Surg Endosc. 2004; 18(6):907–909

Case 122

Robert A. Jesinger

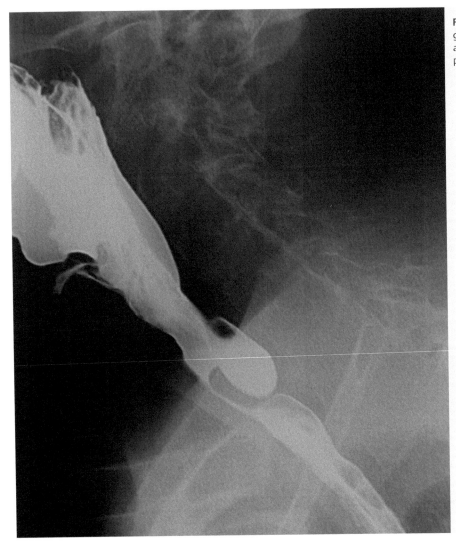

Fig. 122.1 Lateral view from an upper gastrointestinal examination demonstrates a large contrast-filled outpouching along the posterior aspect of the cervical esophagus.

■ **Clinical History**

A 75-year-old female with difficulty swallowing (▶ Fig. 122.1).

■ Key Finding

Esophageal diverticulum.

■ Top 3 Differential Diagnoses

• **Proximal esophageal pulsion diverticulum:** Pulsion (laterally pushing outward) diverticula of the esophagus are thought to develop due to increased intraluminal pressures combined with focal areas of weakness in the esophageal wall. The more common Zenker's diverticulum is a midline defect that occurs in the posterior cervical esophagus above the level of the cricopharyngeal muscle (upper esophageal sphincter). Zenker's diverticulum occurs through Killian's dehiscence, which is at the junction of the cricopharyngeal and inferior pharyngeal constrictor muscles. A Killian–Jamison diverticulum is a lateral defect that occurs in the cervical esophagus at the level of the cricopharyngeal muscle. Both typically occur in older patients, and presenting complaints include dysphagia, halitosis, and intermittent coughing from aspiration. An additional proximal pulsion diverticulum is the lateral hypopharyngeal diverticulum, which occurs more cephalad within the hypopharynx.

These are commonly seen in older patients with COPD, as well as at a younger age in occupations such as glassblowers and wind instrument musicians. They are associated with laryngoceles.

• **Distal esophageal pulsion diverticulum:** Diverticula in the distal esophagus (lower 6–10 cm), termed epiphrenic diverticula, usually occur in the setting of an underlying esophageal motility disorder (achalasia, DES, etc.). Most patients have minimal symptoms, but surgical diverticulectomy is indicated in severely symptomatic patients.

• **Midesophageal traction diverticulum:** Diverticula of the midesophagus commonly develop by "traction" effects from an inflammatory process within the adjacent mediastinum (tuberculosis, histoplasmosis, etc.). Midesophageal diverticula can also be seen in the spectrum of foregut duplications/malformations or in the postsurgical setting after tracheoesophageal fistula repair.

■ Additional Diagnostic Consideration

Intramural pseudodiverticulosis: Intramural pseudodiverticulosis is a rare condition in which numerous 1 to 4 mm saccular outpouchings form within the esophageal wall secondary to inflammatory dilatation of esophageal submucosal glands. Most patients have an associated motility disorder or underlying esophageal strictures.

■ Diagnosis

Proximal esophageal pulsion diverticulum (Zenker's diverticulum).

✓ Pearls

• Zenker is a posterior midline defect that occurs above the level of the cricopharyngeal muscle.
• Killian–Jameson is a lateral defect that occurs at the level of the cricopharyngeal muscle.

• Mediastinal inflammatory processes that scar can create an esophageal traction diverticulum.

Suggested Readings

Duda M, Serý Z, Vojáček K, Rocek V, Rehulka M. Etiopathogenesis and classification of esophageal diverticula. Int Surg. 1985; 70(4):291–295

Federle MP, Jeffrey RB, Woodward PJ, Borhani A. Diagnostic Imaging: Abdomen. 2nd ed. Philadelphia, PA: Lippincott Williams & Wilkins; 2009

Sydow BD, Levine MS, Rubesin SE, Laufer I. Radiographic findings and complications after surgical or endoscopic repair of Zenker's diverticulum in 16 patients. AJR Am J Roentgenol. 2001; 177(5):1067–1071

Part 4

Mesentery and Vascular

4

Case 123

Rocky C. Saenz

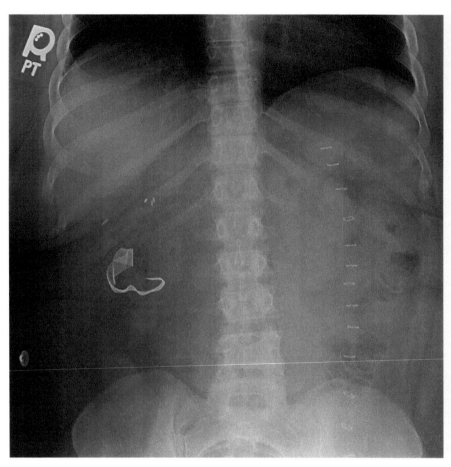

Fig. 123.1 Abdominal X-ray demonstrates irregular linear high density in the right upper quadrant. Surgical staples are noted.

■ **Clinical History**

A 52-year-old female with general abdominal pain, 1 week after surgery (▶Fig. 123.1).

■ Key Finding

Curvilinear high density.

■ Top 3 Differential Diagnoses

- **Textiloma:** Textiloma is also known as gossypiboma and refers to a cotton-based mass left in the body after a surgical procedure. The true incidence is not known, but estimated to be 1 in 1,000 to 1,500 abdominal surgeries. Textilomas account for 50% of malpractice claims for retained foreign bodies. On X-ray, the radiopaque marker strip of the surgical sponge is easily seen as a high density within the mass, whereas the remaining cotton sponge is not well seen. This radiopaque marker strip appears "ribbon-like" in shape. Complications result from the exudative and aseptic fibrotic body response leading to abscess, fistula formation, bowel obstruction, mal-

absorption, and gastrointestinal hemorrhage. Delays in diagnosis may increase mortality and morbidity. Surgical removal is the definitive treatment.
- **Ingested pills/foreign bodies:** The key to diagnosis is noting the irregular and nonanatomical morphologies. Swallowed pills/objects will most likely move location on repeat studies. Metallic objects will be more radiopaque compared to bones and calcific densities.
- **Atherosclerosis:** Atherosclerosis typically appears as curvilinear parallel lines of calcification in the expected location of arteries.

■ Diagnosis

Textiloma, retained surgical sponge.

✓ Pearls

- Retained surgical sponges are identified by noting their radiopaque marker strip.
- Gossypiboma can be seen in any part of the body.

- Calcified vessels are not as dense as metal or high density foreign bodies.

Suggested Readings

Guelfguat M, Kaplinskiy V, Reddy SH, DiPoce J. Clinical guidelines for imaging and reporting ingested foreign bodies. AJR Am J Roentgenol. 2014; 203(1):37–53

Manzella A, Filho PB, Albuquerque E, Farias F, Kaercher J. Imaging of gossypibomas: pictorial review. AJR Am J Roentgenol. 2009; 193(6, Suppl):S94–S101

Case 124

Daniel E. Knapp

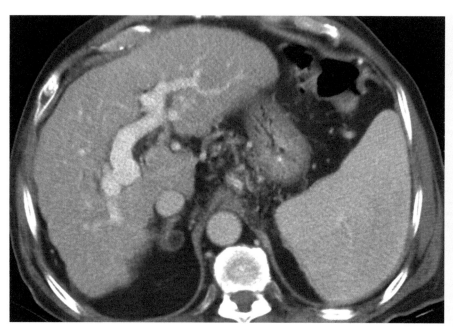

Fig. 124.1 CT axial images of the abdomen with intravenous contrast show enlarged portal veins, nodular liver contours, and enlarged spleen. Also noted is a right adrenal gland adenoma. (Image courtesy of Rocky C. Saenz.)

■ Clinical History

A 57-year-old male with abdominal fullness (▶Fig. 124.1).

■ Key Finding

Portal vein enlargement.

■ Top 3 Differential Diagnoses

- **Portal hypertension:** Elevated portal pressure is due to increased resistance to portal blood flow, most commonly from liver cirrhosis. Defined as absolute portal venous pressure of more than 10 mm Hg or a gradient between portal and systemic veins of greater than 5 mm Hg. Portal hypertension is classified into three categories: presinusoidal from a portal vein or splenic vein thrombus, sinusoidal from liver disease (cirrhosis being the most common, hepatocellular disorder, or hepatic tumor), and postsinusoidal from right heart failure or constrictive pericarditis. Cross-sectional imaging features include portal vein dilation of more than 13 mm (a direct finding), ascites, splenomegaly, varices, recanalization of paraumbilical vein, mesenteric edema, and gallbladder wall thickening. Ultrasound findings include slow (< 15 cm/s) or reversed (hepatofugal) blood flow in the portal vein. There is a high risk of variceal bleeding with portosystemic gradient of more than 12 mm Hg.

- **Cavernous transformation of portal vein:** This process occurs as the sequelae of chronic/persistent portal vein thrombus. It is the replacement of a normal single portal channel into the porta hepatis with numerous tortuous venous channels from dilated collateral veins (thought to be paracholedochal veins). The transformation process takes a variable amount of time, from 1 week to a year. Ultimately, cavernous transformation results in presinusoidal portal hypertension.
- **Superior vena cava (SVC) obstruction:** There are many etiologies of SVC obstruction with the most common being tumor invasion (lymphoma) and thrombosis (commonly related to indwelling lines and tubes). SVC obstruction can result in "downhill" varices from collateralization to redirect the return of blood to the inferior vena cava (IVC) and liver.

■ Diagnosis

Portal hypertension, sinusoidal due to cirrhosis.

✓ Pearls

- Transjugular intrahepatic portosystemic shunt (TIPS) is used to reduce portal pressure in patient with intractable ascites or variceal bleeding.
- Remember hepatopetal flow is toward liver, hepatofugal flow is away from the liver (think of a fugitive running away from the liver).

- The most common cause of portal hypertension is cirrhosis, and the most common cause of cirrhosis is EtOH abuse. The most serious complication is esophageal or gastric variceal bleeding.

Suggested Readings

Gerstenmaier JF, Gibson RN. Ultrasound in chronic liver disease. Insights Imaging. 2014; 5(4):441–455

Lee JY, Kim TY, Jeong WK, et al. Clinically severe portal hypertension: role of multi-detector row CT features in diagnosis. Dig Dis Sci. 2014; 59(9):2333–2343

Liu CH, Hsu SJ, Liang CC, et al. Esophageal varices: noninvasive diagnosis with duplex Doppler US in patients with compensated cirrhosis. Radiology. 2008; 248(1):132–139

Case 125

Kristin Kamienecki

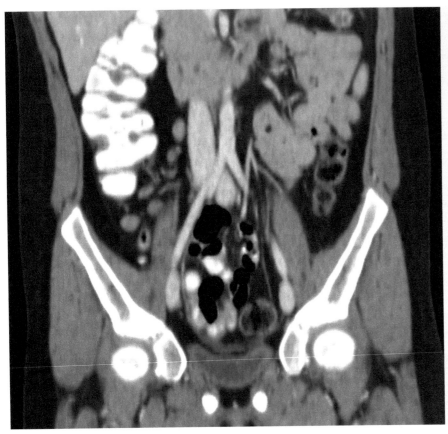

Fig. 125.1 CT coronal image with intravenous and oral contrast demonstrates multiple prominent lymph nodes without peripheral fat-stranding in the right lower quadrant. (Image courtesy of Rocky C. Saenz.)

■ Clinical History

A 22-year-old female with acute right lower quadrant pain (▶Fig. 125.1).

■ Key Finding

Right lower quadrant lymph nodes.

■ Top 3 Differential Diagnoses

- **Mesenteric adenitis:** Typical presentation is a cluster of three or more lymph nodes (5 mm or larger short axis) in the right lower quadrant. The nodes are homogenous in attenuation and classically seen anterior to the right psoas but may be in the root of the mesentery. Primary mesenteric adenitis is defined as having no identifiable inflammatory cause. Secondary mesenteric adenitis is characterized by the concomitant intra-abdominal inflammatory process.
- **Lymphoma:** Lymphoma may result in lymphadenopathy anywhere in the body. Early in the disease course, the nodes may be small, scattered, and discrete. As the disease progresses, the lymph nodes coalesce into soft-tissue masses. The attenuation of the nodes tends to match soft tissue and enhance homogenously.
- **Inflammatory bowel disease:** Mesenteric adenopathy is frequently seen with both Crohn's disease and ulcerative colitis. Crohn's disease is more common. Inflammatory changes of the small or large bowel are usually present but not necessary. Nodes can be seen in the mesenteric root, the mesentery periphery, and the right lower quadrant. The nodes are described as enlarged but not massive. On CT, the nodes are typically soft-tissue attenuation and enhance homogenously.

■ Additional Diagnostic Considerations

Inflammation: Common causes of inflammatory mesenteric lymphadenopathy are appendicitis, diverticulitis, and pancreatitis. In appendicitis, the presence of enlarged right lower quadrant nodes with an abnormal appendix is diagnostic. Appendiceal carcinoma is rare but can mimic appendicitis, especially if perforated (associated adenopathy is larger). Lymphadenopathy related to diverticulitis is usually localized to the area of inflamed colon. Nodes tend to be reactive and small. Perforated colon carcinoma can also mimic diverticulitis and the presence of enlarged nodes may be a clue. Finally, pancreatitis usually results in retroperitoneal and peripancreatic adenopathy. However, as the inflammatory changes of pancreatitis can be extensive any location of abnormal lymph nodes in the abdomen or pelvis is possible.

■ Diagnosis

Mesenteric adenitis.

✓ Pearls

- Lymph node number, size, and distribution are all important indicators of etiology.
- Mesenteric adenopathy in a patient with lymphoma does not always indicate active disease.
- Incidence of primary mesenteric adenitis is considered low.

Suggested Readings

Johnson CD, Schmit G. Mayo Clinic Gastrointestinal Imaging Review. Rochester, MN: Mayo Clinic Scientific Press; 2005

Lucey BC, Stuhlfaut JW, Soto JA. Mesenteric lymph nodes seen at imaging: causes and significance. Radiographics. 2005; 25(2):351–365

Macari M, Hines J, Balthazar E, Megibow A. Mesenteric adenitis: CT diagnosis of primary versus secondary causes, incidence, and clinical significance in pediatric and adult patients. AJR Am J Roentgenol. 2002; 178(4):853–858

Case 126

Gregory D. Puthoff

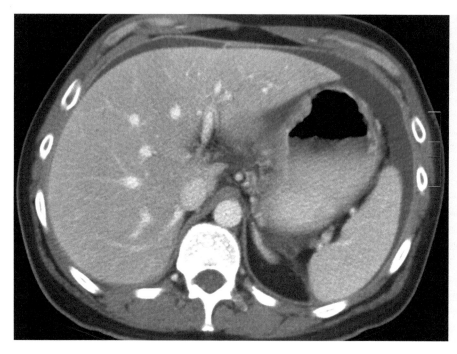

Fig. 126.1 CT with intravenous and oral contrast of the abdomen shows fine, linear enhancement of the peritoneum anteriorly with ascites. (Image courtesy of Rocky C. Saenz.)

■ **Clinical History**

A 56-year-old male diabetic with generalized abdominal pain (▶Fig. 126.1).

■ Key Finding

Peritoneal linear enhancement.

■ Top 3 Differential Diagnoses

- **Peritonitis:** Any inflammatory process within the abdomen can cause abnormal peritoneal enhancement including perforated abdominal viscus, appendicitis, or inflammatory bowel disease. Other infections/inflammatory conditions to consider include spontaneous bacterial peritonitis and pelvic inflammatory disease. Abnormal peritoneal enhancement from an adjacent inflammatory process or infection typically causes smooth enhancement without nodularity.
- **Peritoneal carcinomatosis:** Irregular enhancement of the peritoneum with nodularity is the typical presentation of peritoneal carcinomatosis. Peritoneal carcinomatosis is classically considered with gastrointestinal and ovarian malignancies but can be seen with many other types of tumors including the appendix, breast, or gallbladder. Ascites typically occurs in the setting of peritoneal carcinomatosis and should prompt close evaluation of the peritoneum, especially if it is a new finding in a patient with a known malignancy.
- **Pseudomyxoma peritonei:** Also known as "jelly belly," pseudomyxoma peritonei occurs when the peritoneal cavity is coated with thickened gelatinous material and is classically associated with mucinous carcinomas secreting mucous into the peritoneal cavity. The most common mucinous neoplasm that causes pseudomyxoma peritonei is mucinous adenocarcinoma of the appendix. Radiographic findings overlap large abdominal ascites, although pseudomyxoma peritonei causes more displacement of peritoneal organs and may demonstrate curvilinear calcifications.

■ Additional Diagnostic Considerations

Sclerosing encapsulating peritonitis: It is an inflammatory condition seen in patients undergoing peritoneal dialysis, but it can also occur with idiopathic fibrosis of the peritoneum. Imaging findings typically manifest as thin abnormal enhancing peritoneum with loculated fluid collections.

■ Diagnosis

Peritonitis secondary spontaneous bacterial peritonitis.

✓ Pearls

- Any abdominal inflammatory or infectious process may cause abnormal peritoneal enhancement.
- Malignant or metastatic involvement demonstrates nodular enhancement of the peritoneum.
- Pseudomyxoma peritonei is classically associated with mucinous adenocarcinoma of the appendix.
- New onset abdominal ascites, especially in a patient with a known malignancy should prompt detailed evaluation of the peritoneum to evaluate for peritoneal carcinomatosis.

Suggested Readings

Federle MP, Jeffrey RB, Woodward PJ, Borhani A. Diagnostic Imaging: Abdomen. 2nd ed. Philadelphia, PA: Lippincott Williams & Wilkins; 2009

Filippone A, Cianci R, Delli Pizzi A, et al. CT findings in acute peritonitis: a pattern-based approach. Diagn Interv Radiol. 2015; 21(6):435–440

Levy AD, Shaw JC, Sobin LH. Secondary tumors and tumor-like lesions of the peritoneal cavity: imaging features with pathologic correlation. Radiographics. 2009; 29(2):347–373

Case 127

Elias Antypas

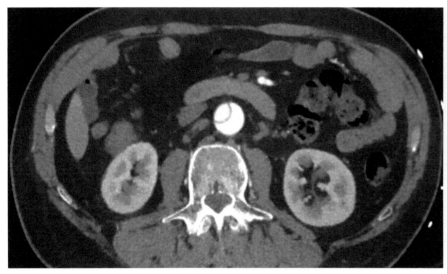

Fig. 127.1 CT axial image with intravenous and oral contrast demonstrates an intimal flap traversing the abdominal aorta. (Image courtesy of Rocky C. Saenz.)

■ **Clinical History**

A 54-year-old male with abdominal pain radiating to his back (▶Fig. 127.1).

■ Key Finding

Abdominal aortic cleft.

■ Top 3 Differential Diagnoses

• **Aortic dissection:** Aortic dissection occurs when blood enters the media layer of the aortic wall though an intimal defect. CT is the best imaging modality and demonstrates an intimal flap resulting in a true and false lumen. The true lumen is contiguous with the normal portion of aorta while the false lumen may be thrombosed or demonstrate delayed flow. Radiographs may demonstrate displaced intimal calcifications. Type A dissection always involves the thoracic ascending aorta only and is treated surgically. If left untreated, there is a 50% mortality rate within 48 hours. A type B dissection involves the descending thoracic aorta and/or arch and is treated medically. It is important to delineate the relationship between the true lumen and the origins of the abdominal aortic branches.

• **Intramural hematoma:** This is caused by arterial bleeding from the vasa vasorum into the media layer resulting in hemorrhage deposition within the wall. There is no appreciable intimal flap or false lumen.
• **Penetrating aortic ulcer (PAU):** PAU occurs when an atheromatous plaque ulcerates and disrupts the internal elastic lamina and extends into the aortic media. On CT, it appears as a contrast filled protrusion into an intramural hematoma, which is isoattenuated to the aorta. There is no appreciable intimal flap or false lumen. This is most commonly seen in the thoracic aorta.

■ Additional Diagnostic Considerations

Pseudodissection: The aortic pulsation can create artifact that mimics an intimal flap and typically involves the left anterior and the right posterior aspects of the ascending aorta.

■ Diagnosis

Aortic dissection.

✓ Pearls

• Aortic dissection demonstrates an intimal flap with a true and false lumen.
• Type A dissection is surgical due to involvement of the aortic root and possibly the coronaries.

• Marfan's syndrome, Ehlers–Danlos syndrome, and other connective tissue diseases are often associated with aortic dissection.
• PAU is focal and isoattenuated to the aorta.

Suggested Readings

Bailkousis NG, Apostolakis EE. Penetrating atherosclerotic ulcer of the thoracic aorta: diagnosis and treatment. Hellenic J Cardiol. 2010; 51(2):153–157

Macura KJ, Corl FM, Fishman EK, Bluemke DA. Pathogenesis in acute aortic syndromes: aortic dissection, intramural hematoma, and penetrating atherosclerotic aortic ulcer. AJR Am J Roentgenol. 2003; 181(2):309–316

Sebastià C, Pallisa E, Quiroga S, Alvarez-Castells A, Dominguez R, Evangelista A. Aortic dissection: diagnosis and follow-up with helical CT. Radiographics. 1999; 19(1):45–60, quiz 149–150

Case 128

Kristin Kamienecki

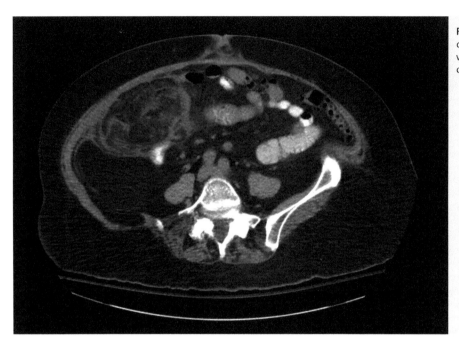

Fig. 128.1 CT axial image with oral contrast demonstrates a large oval shaped fatty focus with peripheral fat-stranding in the right lower quadrant. (Image courtesy of Rocky C. Saenz.)

■ Clinical History

A 67-year-old female with acute right lower quadrant pain (▶Fig. 128.1).

■ Key Finding

Focal mesenteric fat stranding.

■ Top 3 Differential Diagnoses

- **Omental infarct:** Typical presentation is a fatty mass with inflammatory fat-stranding within the right colon. Larger areas of fatty mass may demonstrate gas or fat fluid levels. The adjacent colon should be normal. This is a benign self-limited condition that is treated conservatively with analgesics only. The presentation can be clinically confusing as patients usually present with right lower quadrant pain and fever. Therefore, exclusion of surgically treated etiologies (appendicitis, cholecystitis) or etiologies requiring antibiotics (uncomplicated diverticulitis) is needed. The abnormal CT findings usually resolve in 1 to 2 months.
- **Diverticulitis:** Mesenteric fat stranding is present in a pericolonic distribution. Colonic diverticula are present with associated segmental bowel wall thickening. The sigmoid colon is the most common location. Trace extraluminal fluid and small foci of gas may be seen. Acute complications include abscess formation and perforation. Fistulas may result as a chronic complication.
- **Epiploic appendagitis:** Epiploic appendages are protrusions of fat from the surface of the colon. Torsion of these appendages with secondary ischemia leads to the condition. Classic imaging findings are focal fat stranding with peripheral rim centered away from the colon and absence of or minimal bowel wall thickening. The sigmoid colon is the most commonly affected segment of colon and the inflammation is usually seen anteriorly. A central hyperattenuating dot may be present representing the thrombosed vascular pedicle.

■ Additional Diagnostic Considerations

Mesenteric panniculitis: It is of an unknown etiology with hazy fat stranding usually at the root of the mesentery. This location is the most useful characteristic when differentiating from other etiologies. Lymph nodes may be present. Other imaging features of mesenteric panniculitis include tumoral pseudocapsule and fat halo sign.

■ Diagnosis

Omental infarct.

✓ Pearls

- An omental infarct resulting from prior surgery or trauma may be atypical in location.
- Colon cancer may mimic diverticulitis and follow-up CT may be needed to document resolution.
- A fatty lesion with inflammatory changes in the right lower quadrant is considered to be omental infarct.

Suggested Readings

Johnson CD, Schmit G. Mayo Clinic Gastrointestinal Imaging Review. Rochester, MN: Mayo Clinic Scientific Press; 2005

Kamaya A, Federle MP, Desser TS. Imaging manifestations of abdominal fat necrosis and its mimics. Radiographics. 2011; 31(7):2021–2034

Singh AK, Gervais DA, Hahn PF, Sagar P, Mueller PR, Novelline RA. Acute epiploic appendagitis and its mimics. Radiographics. 2005; 25(6):1521–1534

Case 129

Daniel E. Knapp

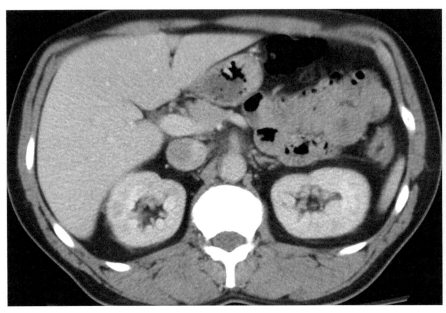

Fig. 129.1 CT axial images of the abdomen with intravenous contrast has fat stranding surrounding superior mesenteric artery (SMA) and subtle wall thickening. (Image courtesy of Rocky C. Saenz.)

■ Clinical History

A 39-year-old female with general abdominal pain (▶Fig. 129.1).

■ Key Finding

Fat stranding surrounding the SMA.

■ Top 3 Differential Diagnoses

- **SMA vasculitis:** General term for a group of processes characterized by inflammation and necrosis of blood vessels. On cross-sectional imaging, findings include peripheral fat stranding, wall thickening, and luminal narrowing. The classification is based on the size of the blood vessel involved. Consideration for large and medium vessel vasculitis (such as SMA) includes Takayasu arteritis, giant cell arteritis, Henoch–Schonlein purpura, and polyarteritis nodosa.
- **Atherosclerosis:** Plaque formation from deposition of lipid, cholesterol, and other substances results in arterial wall thickening, hardening, calcification, and narrowing. Most common in descending aorta, and has predilection for vessel branch points. Risk factors include hypertension, diabetes mellitus, smoking, and hyperlipidemia.
- **Mesenteric artery thromboembolism:** Vascular occlusion due to thromboembolism. The etiology often is from cardiac sources including acute myocardial infarction, atrial fibrillation, arrhythmia, ventricular aneurysm, or valvular disease. The SMA is susceptible because of high flow rate and takeoff angle from aorta.

■ Additional Diagnostic Considerations

Aortic dissection (involving SMA): Abdominal aortic dissection with intimal flap extension into the SMA.

■ Diagnosis

SMA vasculitis, Takayasu.

✓ Pearls

- Acute mesenteric ischemia is a life-threatening emergency with overall mortality of 60 to 80%.
- Can be chronic (intestinal angina) with classic clinical scenario of post-prandial pain beginning shortly after eating and lasting 1 to 2 hours.
- Angiography may be required for definitive diagnosis.
- Closely evaluate to find bowel ischemia in acute cases.

Suggested Readings

Beaulieu RJ, Arnaoutakis KD, Abularrage CJ, Efron DT, Schneider E, Black JH, III. Comparison of open and endovascular treatment of acute mesenteric ischemia. J Vasc Surg. 2014; 59(1):159–164

Heo SH, Kim YW, Woo SY, Park YJ, Park KB, Kim DK. Treatment strategy based on the natural course for patients with spontaneous isolated superior mesenteric artery dissection. J Vasc Surg. 2017; 65(4):1142–1151

Wilkins LR, Stone JR. Chronic mesenteric ischemia. Tech Vasc Interv Radiol. 2015; 18(1):31–37

Case 130

Rocky C. Saenz

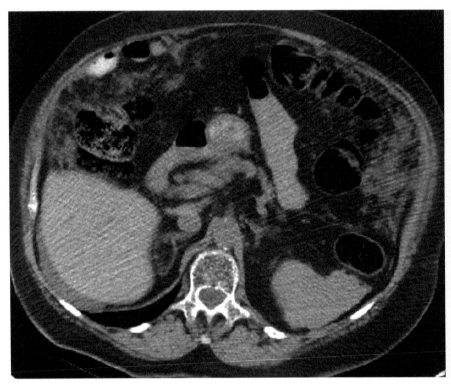

Fig. 130.1 CT of the abdomen with oral contrast shows irregular, nodular foci involving the peritoneum along both paracolic gutters with a small amount of ascites layering adjacent to the liver.

■ Clinical History

A 56-year-old male diabetic with generalized abdominal pain (▶Fig. 130.1).

■ Key Finding

Peritoneal nodular enhancement.

■ Top 3 Differential Diagnoses

- **Peritoneal carcinomatosis:** Peritoneal carcinomatosis is defined as a neoplastic disease involving the peritoneum. On cross-sectional imaging, irregular enhancement of the peritoneum with nodularity is the typical presentation. Peritoneal carcinomatosis classically represents gastrointestinal and ovarian malignancies but can be seen with many other advanced tumors including the appendix, breast, and gallbladder.
- **Peritonitis:** Peritonitis is an infectious or inflammatory process involving the abdomen. On cross-sectional imaging, peritonitis is seen as fine, linear peritoneal enhancement typically involving the periphery of the abdomen. There are many etiologies including perforated abdominal viscus,

appendicitis, inflammatory bowel disease, spontaneous bacterial peritonitis, and pelvic inflammatory disease. When ascites is present, paracentesis may be needed to exclude spontaneous bacterial peritonitis. Treatment is tailored to the etiology of the peritonitis.
- **Pseudomyxoma peritonei:** Pseudomyxoma peritonei refers to the gelatinous ascites secondary to mucinous adenocarcinomas disseminated into the peritoneal cavity. The classic mucinous neoplasms that cause pseudomyxoma peritonei are mucinous adenocarcinoma of the appendix and ovary. On cross-sectional imaging, the liver and spleen demonstrate scalloped contours of low density, which represents the gelatinous implants.

■ Diagnosis

Peritoneal carcinomatosis secondary colon carcinoma.

✓ Pearls

- Nodular peritoneal enhancement should be considered carcinoma until proven otherwise.
- Linear enhancement of the peritoneum is typically an infectious or inflammatory process.

- Pseudomyxoma peritonei is classically associated with mucinous adenocarcinoma.

Suggested Readings

Federle MP, Jeffrey RB, Woodward PJ, Borhani A. Diagnostic Imaging: Abdomen. 2nd ed. Philadelphia, PA: Lippincott Williams & Wilkins; 2009

Filippone A, Cianci R, Delli Pizzi A, et al. CT findings in acute peritonitis: a pattern-based approach. Diagn Interv Radiol. 2015; 21(6):435–440

Levy AD, Shaw JC, Sobin LH. Secondary tumors and tumorlike lesions of the peritoneal cavity: imaging features with pathologic correlation. Radiographics. 2009; 29(2):347–373

Case 131

Kristin Kamienecki

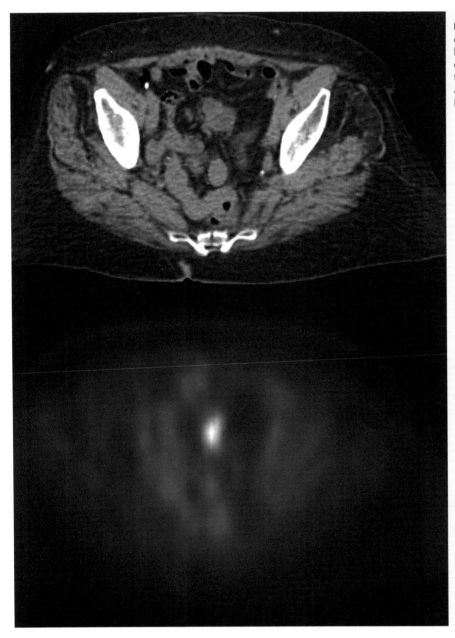

Fig. 131.1 Top image, CT axial image without contrast demonstrates enlarged lower mesenteric lymph nodes. Bottom image, PET (positron emission tomography) axial at the same level as the top image showing FDG (fluorodeoxyglucose) avidity of the lymph nodes. (Image courtesy of Rocky C. Saenz.)

■ **Clinical History**

A 71-year-old female with colon carcinoma (▶Fig. 131.1).

■ Key Finding

Mesenteric lymph nodes.

■ Top 3 Differential Diagnoses

• **Lymphoma:** Classic appearance of mesenteric lymphoma is a lobulated confluent nodal mass that encases the superior mesenteric vessels. This creates the classic "sandwich or hamburger" sign. There usually is associated retroperitoneal and inguinal adenopathy with splenomegaly. Early in the disease, nodes can be small and discrete. Lymph node attenuation typically matches soft tissue with homogenous enhancement.

• **Metastasis:** The most common cause of malignant peritoneal masses is metastatic deposits. Disease spread can be via direct invasion (pancreas, liver, gallbladder, and stomach), ascitic circulation (ovarian, gastrointestinal), hematogenous, or lymphatic routes. Multiple deposits are seen more commonly than a single focus. Diffuse omental involvement can lead to extensive tumor studding (omental caking).

• **Mesenteric adenitis:** Typical presentation is cluster of lymph nodes in the right lower quadrant. The nodes are homogenous in attenuation and classically seen anterior to the right psoas, but may be in the root of the mesentery. Primary mesenteric adenitis is defined as having no identifiable inflammatory cause. Ileal or ileocecal wall thickening may be present. Secondary mesenteric adenitis is characterized by the concomitant intra-abdominal inflammatory process.

■ Additional Diagnostic Considerations

• **Extramedullary hematopoiesis:** Ectopic hematopoiesis occurs outside the bony medulla and is associated with conditions like myelofibrosis, congenital hemolytic anemia, and thalassemia. Mediastinal, retroperitoneal, and pelvic sites of extramedullary hematopoiesis can develop and be mistaken for adenopathy or metastatic disease.

• **Mycobacterium avium-intracellulare:** Consider this diagnosis in the setting of an immunocompromised patient with extensive centrally low attenuation mesenteric and retroperitoneal lymphadenopathy.

■ Diagnosis

Metastatic disease.

✓ Pearls

• Metastatic disease is the most common cause of peritoneal masses.
• Low attenuation adenopathy is a frequent finding in treated lymphoma.

• Lymphomatous involvement of the mesentery is seen in approximately 50% of non-Hodgkin's lymphoma (NHL) cases.

Suggested Readings

Johnson CD, Schmit G. Mayo Clinic Gastrointestinal Imaging Review. Rochester, MN: Mayo Clinic Scientific Press; 2005

Macari M, Hines J, Balthazar E, Megibow A. Mesenteric adenitis: CT diagnosis of primary versus secondary causes, incidence, and clinical significance in pediatric and adult patients. AJR Am J Roentgenol. 2002; 178(4):853–858

Sheth S, Horton KM, Garland MR, Fishman EK. Mesenteric neoplasms: CT appearances of primary and secondary tumors and differential diagnosis. Radiographics. 2003; 23(2):457–473, quiz 535–536

Case 132

Kristin Kamienecki

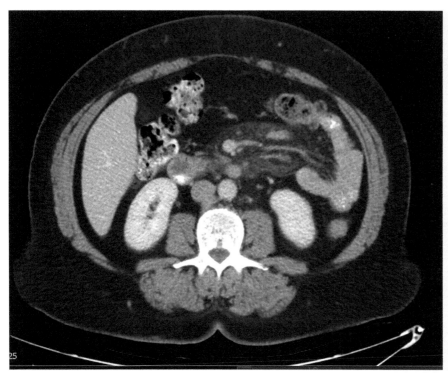

Fig. 132.1 CT axial image with intravenous and oral contrast shows a round area of vague focal increased density around the root of the mesentery consistent with a "misty mesentery." (Image courtesy of Rocky C. Saenz.)

■ Clinical History

A 54-year-old male with occasional left upper quadrant pain (▶Fig. 132.1).

■ Key Finding

Misty mesentery.

■ Top 3 Differential Diagnoses

- **Neoplasm:** This can be the most challenging diagnosis to exclude. Lymphoma is the most common tumor involving the mesentery. It is typically encountered with early stage lymphoma (most commonly non-Hodgkin). More advanced lymphoma is easier to distinguish secondary to the presence of bulky adenopathy. A careful search for the presence of any adenopathy is necessary when misty mesentery is discovered. Treated lymphoma may result in persistent high-attenuation changes of the mesentery even following resolution of lymphadenopathy.
- **Mesenteric panniculitis:** It typically appears on CT as increased attenuation of the mesenteric root just left of midline with adjacent small lymph nodes. This region of increased attenuation may appear mass like and displace bowel loops. This area may exhibit a tumoral pseudocapsule, a peripheral band of soft tissue separating normal mesentery from inflammatory process or demonstrate sparing of the fat surrounding adjacent vessels and nodes, the "fat-ring" or "fat-halo" sign. On MRI, an intermediate T1, slightly higher T2 signal mesenteric mass is seen.
- **Edema:** Mesenteric congestion should be considered if ascites or subcutaneous fluid is identified. A patient history of hypoproteinemia or hepatic/cardiac/renal failure may also be a helpful clue. Vascular disease including portal hypertension or hepatic, portal and mesenteric vein thrombosis are also etiologies. Consider mesenteric edema if the pattern of edema is atypical in location, more focal or contiguous with segmental bowel wall thickening; all findings which could indicate venous thrombosis.

■ Diagnosis

Misty mesentery secondary to treated non-Hodgkin's lymphoma (NHL).

✓ Pearls

- Mass effect on mesenteric vasculature should raise suspicion of primary neoplasm.
- CT appearance of "misty mesentery" should *not* automatically be equated to mesenteric panniculitis.
- Greater than one-third of cirrhotic patients demonstrate "misty mesentery."
- Follow-up imaging may be necessary to find primary cause or to exclude malignancy.

Suggested Readings

Boland G. Gastrointestinal Imaging: The Requisites. 4th ed. Philadelphia, PA: Elsevier/Saunders; 2014

Haaga J. CT and MRI of the Whole Body. 5th ed. Philadelphia, PA: Elsevier; 2009

McLaughlin PD, Filippone A, Maher MM. The "misty mesentery": mesenteric panniculitis and its mimics. AJR Am J Roentgenol. 2013; 200(2):W116–23

Case 133

Elias Antypas

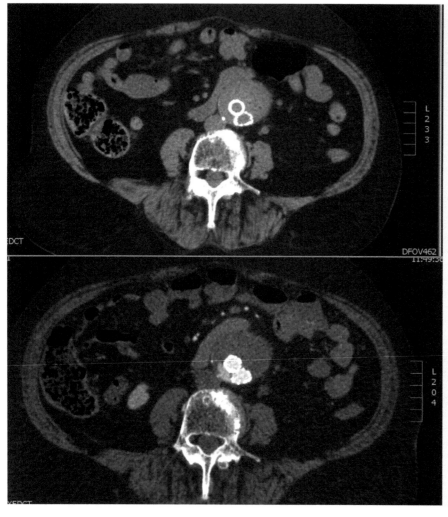

Fig. 133.1 1 CT axial images, top without contrast and bottom with intravenous, show an aortic aneurysm with an endoluminal graft repair. The bottom image has enhancement posterior to the graft. (Image courtesy of Rocky C. Saenz.)

■ Clinical History

A 79-year-old male with a recent aortic aneurysm repair
(►Fig. 133.1).

■ **Key Finding**

Aortic aneurysm endoluminal graft repair with posterior enhancement.

■ **Diagnosis**

Endoleak, Type II

■ **Discussion**

Endoleak of aortic repair: The persistence of blood flow outside an aortic graft within the aneurysm sac following an endoluminal repair. The aneurysm sac typically thromboses and shrinks in diameter when it is excluded from blood flow. Endoleaks are often asymptomatic, but can expand and is at risk of rupture if left untreated. Endoleaks are classified into five types, given as follows:

Type I: This results from the flow around the ends of the endograft and is subdivided into IA (proximal attachment site) and IIA (distal attachment site). These endoleaks require urgent treatment. Attempting additional expansion of the endograft utilizing a large diameter balloon or the use of covered stents at the leaking graft end may help to improve the seal.

Type II: These are the most common type of endoleak accounting for 80% of cases. This results from retrograde arterial flow into the aneurysm sac from patent aortic side branches.

Most common vessels to supply aneurysm are lumbar arteries or the inferior mesenteric artery. Type II leaks are treated with embolization of endoleak nidus.

Type III: These are rare. Type III leaks result from tears in the graft fabric or separation of graft components. This requires intervention as the endograft defect separation will result in reperfusion of the native aneurysm sac with systemic blood resulting in high risk of rupture.

Type IV: Leak through graft fabric as a result of porosity of the graft fabric material.

Type V: There is continued enlargement of the aneurysm sac without an identifiable endoleak, secondary to endotension. This is usually observed, although intervention may be required if sac continues to enlarge despite the lack of endoleak on imaging.

✓ **Pearls**

- CT is the best imaging tool best performed in three phases: unenhanced, arterial, and delayed. Unenhanced studies are helpful because calcification can be mistaken for hemorrhage.
- Type II is the most common type and may resolve spontaneously. Serial CT is done to assess stability.

- Effective treatment of type II leak requires embolization via catheter placed directly into the endoleak nidus. Embolization of only feeding vessels may result in additional recruitment of inflow into the aneurysm sac.

Suggested Readings

Rosen RJ, Green RM. Endoleak management following endovascular aneurysm repair. J Vasc Interv Radiol. 2008; 19(6, Suppl):S37–S43

Yu H, Desai H, Isaacson AJ, Dixon RG, Farber MA, Burke CT. Comparison of type II endoleak embolizations: embolization of endoleak nidus only versus embolization of endoleak nidus and branch vessels. J Vasc Interv Radiol. 2017; 28(2):176–184

Case 134

Kristin Kamienecki

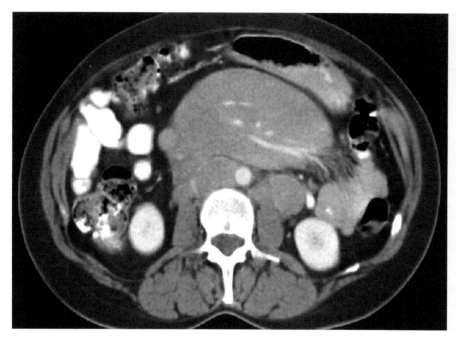

Fig. 134.1 CT axial image with intravenous and oral contrast which shows an oval-shaped lobulated mass encasing the mesenteric vessels and extending into the retroperitoneum. (Image courtesy of Rocky C. Saenz.)

■ Clinical History

A 51-year-old female with abdominal fullness (▶Fig. 134.1).

■ Key Finding

Solid mesenteric mass.

■ Top 3 Differential Diagnoses

- **Metastasis:** It is by far the most common cause of malignant peritoneal mesenteric masses. Peritoneal metastases may occur through direct invasion (typical with pancreas, liver, gallbladder, or stomach). Alternatively, peritoneal metastases may occur by intraperitoneal seeding via ascitic flow (most common sites are the pelvic cul-de-sac, paracolic gutters, and the sigmoid mesocolon). The most common tumors to spread in the peritoneum by seeding are ovarian and gastrointestinal tumors. Deposits may be single or diffuse. Diffuse involvement can invade the omentum leading to subtle studding with nodules or the more overt "caking."
- **Carcinoid:** Most common primary tumor of the small bowel. Tumors are usually small (< 1.5 cm). Growth of these tumors into the mesentery induces an intense fibrotic reaction (sunburst appearance) on CT. Calcification is found in approximately three quarters of cases. The triad of a calcified mesenteric mass, radiating strands, and adjacent bowel wall thickening, or mass is highly suggestive of carcinoid tumor.
- **Lymphoma:** Most commonly seen with non-Hodgkin's lymphoma (NHL), approximately 50% of cases. Classic appearance is a lobulated confluent soft-tissue mass encasing the superior mesenteric vessels, creating the sandwich or hamburger sign. Concomitant retroperitoneal adenopathy, inguinal adenopathy, and splenomegaly often present in cases of mesenteric lymphoma.

■ Additional Diagnostic Considerations

- **Desmoid:** Most commonly incidentally found on CT. Typical as single or sometimes multiple rounded soft-tissue masses within the mesentery, more often multiple in association with Gardner syndrome. Masses may also reside in the retroperitoneum or abdominal wall. They may cause displacement or retraction of bowel loops. Despite benign pathology can invade locally into the adjacent bowel.
- **Abdominal mesothelioma:** Abdominal mesothelioma arises from the serosal lining of the peritoneal cavity and is associated with a history of asbestos exposure. Classic CT findings include ascites and serosal soft-tissue masses, mimicking peritoneal carcinomatosis. Correlation with chest imaging for pleural thickening and calcification is helpful, although peritoneal involvement may occur in the absence of pleural disease.

■ Diagnosis

Lymphoma.

✓ Pearls

- Peritoneal metastasis by far the most common solid peritoneal tumor.
- NHL more commonly associated with mesenteric disease than Hodgkin.
- If mesenteric mass is small and contains calcification consider carcinoid. If the mass is larger, the primary consideration would be sclerosing mesenteritis.

Suggested Readings

Johnson CD, Schmit G. Mayo Clinic Gastrointestinal Imaging Review. Rochester, MN: Mayo Clinic Scientific Press; 2005

Levy AD, Rimola J, Mehrotra AK, Sobin LH. From the archives of the AFIP: benign fibrous tumors and tumorlike lesions of the mesentery: radiologic-pathologic correlation. Radiographics. 2006; 26(1):245–264

Sheth S, Horton, KM, Garland, MR, Fishman, EK. Mesenteric neoplasms: CT appearance of primary and secondary tumors and differential diagnosis. Radiographics. 2003; 23:457–473

Case 135

Elias Antypas

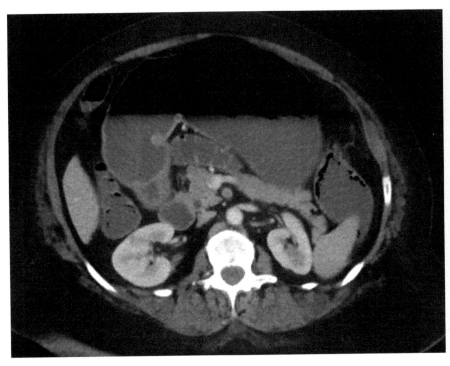

Fig. 135.1 CT axial image with intravenous contrast shows nonopacification of the superior mesenteric artery (SMA). (Image courtesy of Rocky C. Saenz.)

■ Clinical History

A 63-year-old female with generalized pain (▶Fig. 135.1).

■ Key Finding

Nonopacification of the SMA.

■ Top 3 Differential Diagnoses

• **SMA stenosis (atherosclerosis):** Atherosclerotic disease (ASD) is the most common cause of chronic mesenteric ischemia. Atherosclerotic plaque results in narrowing of the ostia and/or lumens of the mesenteric vessels, which are usually circumferential. Poststenotic dilation is commonly present. ASD typically affects the elderly presenting with risk factors such as diabetes, hypertension, and hyperlipidemia.

• **Thromboembolism:** Thrombosis is associated with acute mesenteric ischemia. CT demonstrates a filling defect within the SMA with the remainder of the artery demonstrating a normal appearance. Thrombosis is often associated with bowel infarct with resulting sepsis with a high mortality rate of 70%.

• **Vasculitis:** It is inflammation/necrosis of blood vessels and can affect vessels of all sizes. Abdominal manifestations may be difficult to distinguish from mesenteric ischemia and commonly occur in younger patients. SMA is the most commonly involved vessel with lupus vasculitis.

■ Additional Diagnostic Considerations

Radiation: Radiation-induced vasculopathy can involve the SMA when it is included in the radiation treatment field. Findings may include stenosis and/or pseudoaneurysms of the mesenteric vasculature.

■ Diagnosis

SMA thrombosis.

✓ Pearls

• SMA stenosis secondary to atherosclerosis typically affects elderly with risk factors.

• Filling defect, rather than circumferential narrowing, distinguishes thromboembolism from SMA stenosis.

• Vasculitis should be considered when the CT findings that mimic mesenteric stenosis are observed in a younger patient.

Suggested Readings

Ha HK, Lee SH, Rha SE, et al. Radiologic features of vasculitis involving the gastrointestinal tract. Radiographics. 2000; 20(3):779–794

Hohenwalter EJ. Chronic mesenteric ischemia: diagnosis and treatment. Semin Intervent Radiol. 2009; 26(4):345–351

Lee R, Tung HK, Tung PH, Cheung SC, Chan FL. CT in acute mesenteric ischaemia. Clin Radiol. 2003; 58(4):279–287

Case 136

Chelsea M. Jeranko

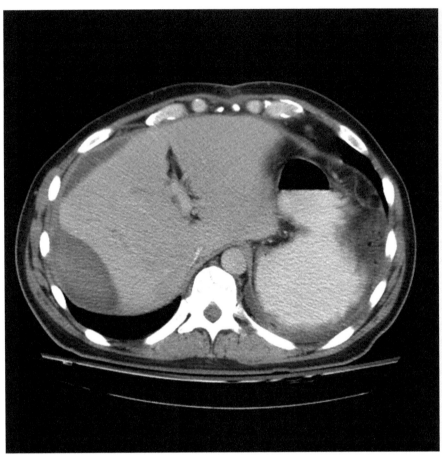

Fig. 136.1 CT of the abdomen with intravenous and oral contrast shows low-attenuation ascites that scallops the margins of the liver.

■ **Clinical History**

A 57-year-old male with abdominal distension (▸Fig. 136.1).

■ Key Finding

Ascites that scallops the margins of the liver.

■ Top 3 Differential Diagnoses

- **Ascites:** Transudative ascites most commonly occurs in the setting of liver disease, heart failure, or renal failure. Ultrasound will demonstrate anechoic, free flowing fluid and it will measure simple fluid by CT attenuation (0–15 Hounsfield units). Exudative ascites has a higher protein content than transudative ascites and therefore can appear complex on the ultrasound and be higher attenuation on CT (15–30 Hounsfield units). Septations, loculation, and peritoneal thickening may be present depending on the etiology of the fluid.

- **Pseudomyxoma peritonei:** Pseudomyxoma peritonei is a descriptive term for mucinous implants throughout the peritoneal cavity. Classification of pseudomyxoma peritonei is debated, as some authors also use the term for mucinous peritoneal dissemination from extra-appendiceal mucin-producing tumors (i.e., colon, ovary, etc.); however, the strict definition encompasses only mucinous dissemination from primary appendiceal neoplasms. The most important diagnostic finding is scalloping of the visceral surfaces of intraperitoneal organs, which can distinguish it from simple ascites. In newly diagnosed cases, close inspection of the appendiceal region should be performed.

- **Peritoneal carcinomatosis:** Metastatic disease to the peritoneal surface most commonly occurs with primary ovarian or gastrointestinal tract tumors. CT and MRI have a low sensitivity for detecting peritoneal metastases less than 1 cm in size. Omental stranding/induration is an early sign of involvement that can progress to discrete nodules that can further coalesce into conglomerate omental masses. Complications include bowel and ureteral obstruction. Peritoneal carcinomatosis with mucinous ascites from an extra-appendiceal mucin-producing tumor can be indistinguishable from pseudomyxoma peritonei and a normal appendix may be a clue as to the diagnosis on CT.

■ Additional Diagnostic Considerations

Peritonitis: Infectious or granulomatous infection may manifest as ascites with loculation due to peritoneal dissemination. The ascites is typically exudative. Bacterial peritonitis can also demonstrate smooth peritoneal thickening and hyperenhancement. Tuberculous peritonitis can be indistinguishable from peritoneal carcinomatosis with complex, loculated ascites and omental thickening. Other manifestations of abdominal tuberculous may be present, such as low-density mesenteric lymphadenopathy or ileocecal wall thickening.

■ Diagnosis

Pseudomyxoma peritonei from appendix adenocarcinoma.

✓ Pearls

- Exudative ascites can appear complex by imaging with septations, loculations, and peritoneal thickening.
- Pseudomyxoma peritonei arises from rupture of an appendiceal mucinous neoplasm.

- The characteristic finding of pseudomyxoma peritonei is scalloping of the liver and spleen surfaces.

Suggested Readings

Diop AD, Fontarensky M, Montoriol PF, Da Ines D. CT imaging of peritoneal carcinomatosis and its mimics. Diagn Interv Imaging. 2014; 95(9):861–872

Levy AD, Shaw JC, Sobin LH. Secondary tumors and tumorlike lesions of the peritoneal cavity: imaging features with pathologic correlation. Radiographics. 2009; 29(2):347–373

Pickhardt PJ, Levy AD, Rohrmann CA, Jr, Kende AI. Primary neoplasms of the appendix: radiologic spectrum of disease with pathologic correlation. Radiographics. 2003; 23(3):645–662

Case 137

Kristin Kamienecki

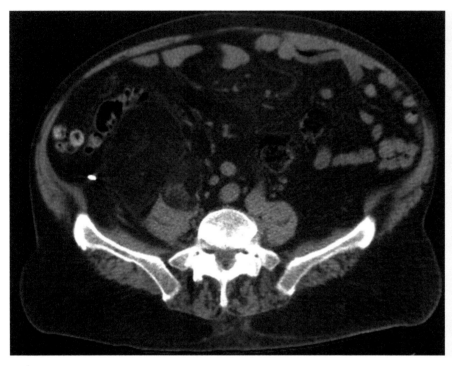

Fig. 137.1 CT axial without contrast in the upper pelvis shows a round fat density lesion in the right lower quadrant with mass effect upon the adjacent bowel and psoas muscle. (Image courtesy of Rocky C. Saenz.)

■ Clinical History

A 66-year-old male with abdominal fullness (▶ Fig. 137.1).

■ **Key Finding**

Fat density mesenteric mass.

■ **Top 3 Differential Diagnoses**

- **Liposarcoma:** Liposarcomas are the most common malignant retroperitoneal soft-tissue tumor in adults. These are more commonly in the retroperitoneum than the mesentery. These are usually large bulky tumors with mass effect. The majority are multiloculated predominately fatty masses with soft-tissue components. Classically, the well-differentiated type has CT and MRI components matching fat with thickened or nodular septa that avidly enhance.

- **Lipoma:** Lipomas may arise anywhere in the body. The classic imaging findings are of macroscopic fat on all radiographic studies. On MRI, the diagnosis can be solidified with loss signal on fat saturation images. Lipomas may have thin fibrous septa without nodular changes.
- **Omental infarction:** Typically appears as a fatty mass with surrounding inflammatory changes of the right lower quadrant omentum. Large areas may show gas within the infarction or fat-fluid levels. Adjacent colon is usually normal.

■ **Additional Diagnostic Considerations**

- **Lipoleiomyoma:** These tumors occur in the uterus and results from smooth muscle degeneration of a leiomyoma. On CT, it presents as a well-marginated, predominantly fat containing uterine mass. Soft-tissue attenuation components are commonly present. MRI imaging features reflect the fatty component as well with T1 hyperintensity with chemical shift artifact. Loss of signal is seen with fat suppression.

- **Epiploic appendagitis:** Torsion of colonic epiploic appendages lead to ischemia and inflammatory changes. Classic imaging findings are focal fat stranding with peripheral rim epicentered away from the colon and absence of or minimal bowel wall thickening. A central hyperattenuating dot may be present representing the thrombosed vascular pedicle.

■ **Diagnosis**

Intra-abdominal lipoma.

✓ **Pearls**

- Liposarcoma is the diagnosis of exclusion when a fatty tumor is seen with nodular enhancement.
- Lipomas should not demonstrate nodular enhancement.

- A fatty lesion with inflammatory changes in the right lower quadrant is most consistent with an omental infarct.

Suggested Readings

Boland G. Gastrointestinal Imaging: The Requisites. 4th ed. Philadelphia, PA: Elsevier/Saunders; 2014
Craig WD, Fanburg-Smith JC, Henry LR, Guerrero R, Barton JH. Fat-containing lesions of the retroperitoneum: radiologic-pathologic correlation. Radiographics. 2009; 29(1):261–290

Pereira JM, Sirlin CB, Pinto PS, Casola G. CT and MR imaging of extrahepatic fatty masses of the abdomen and pelvis: techniques, diagnosis, differential diagnosis, and pitfalls. Radiographics. 2005; 25(1):69–85

Case 138

Elias Antypas

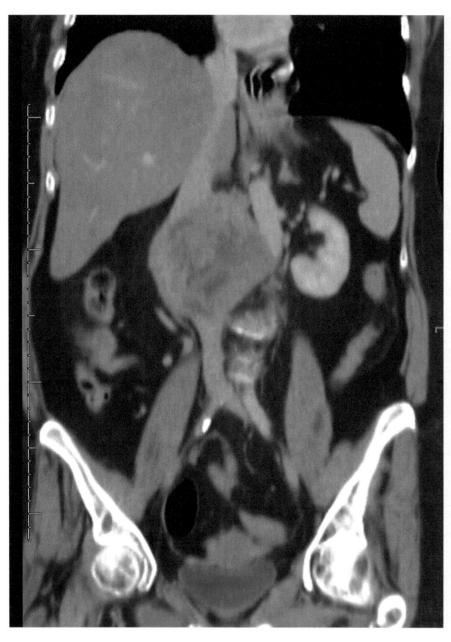

Fig. 138.1 CT coronal image with intravenous shows a large filling defect in the inferior vena cava (IVC) expanding the lumen. (Image courtesy of Rocky C. Saenz.)

■ Clinical History

A 65-year-old female with abdominal pain (▶ Fig. 138.1).

■ Key Finding

Filling defect in the IVC.

■ Top 3 Differential Diagnoses

- **Tumor extension into IVC:** The most common neoplastic etiology is from secondary tumor extension, most commonly from renal cell carcinoma (RCC). Other tumors that are considered include hepatocellular carcinoma (HCC), adrenal cortical carcinoma, and retroperitoneal sarcomas. On CT, these tumors will demonstrate heterogeneous contrast enhancement, expansion of the lumen, and most importantly contiguity of the mass with primary tumor.
- **Venous thrombosis:** Thrombus accounts for the most common cause of a filling defect in the IVC. It is most frequently associated with oral contraceptive use, vasculitis, or

patients with hypercoagulable states. On imaging, it can be difficult to distinguish between tumor and thrombus. Thrombus does not demonstrate enhancement and typically does not expand the lumen.
- **Primary tumor of IVC:** Primary neoplasms of the IVC are exceedingly rare. Leiomyosarcomas are the most common neoplasms arising from large veins. The tumors are more common in women aged 40 to 60 and arise from the smooth muscle cells. Similar to tumor extension, imaging demonstrates enhancement of tumor with expansion of the IVC lumen.

■ Additional Diagnostic Considerations

Pseudothrombus: Admixture of enhanced blood from renal veins with unenhanced blood from the lower body, resulting in a flow-related artifact. Delayed images will resolve apparent filling defect.

■ Diagnosis

IVC leiomyosarcoma.

✓ Pearls

- Malignant IVC involvement most often attributed to tumor extension (RCC) and demonstrates enhancement and vessel expansion.
- Consider venous thrombosis in a patient with hypercoagulable state. Lack of enhancement or venous expansion noted.

- Delayed imaging at 90 to 120 seconds allows more uniform enhancement to exclude admixture of contrast (pseudothrombus) from pathology.

Suggested Readings

Kaufman LB, Yeh BM, Breiman RS, Joe BN, Qayyum A, Coakley FV. Inferior vena cava filling defects on CT and MRI. AJR Am J Roentgenol. 2005; 185(3):717–726

Sheth S, Fishman EK. Imaging of the inferior vena cava with MDCT. AJR Am J Roentgenol. 2007; 189(5):1243–1251

Smillie RP, Shetty M, Boyer AC, Madrazo B, Jafri SZ. Imaging evaluation of the inferior vena cava. Radiographics. 2015; 35(2):578–592

Case 139

Sharon Kreuer

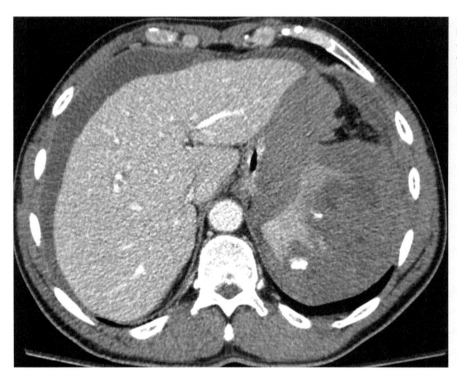

Fig. 139.1 CT axial image with intravenous contrast demonstrates two spherical foci of enhancement in the left upper quadrant in the region of the spleen which are briskly enhancing. Free fluid is noted which is complex in the left upper quadrant. (Image courtesy of Rocky C. Saenz.)

■ Clinical History

A 45-year-old man with pain after car accident (▶Fig. 139.1).

■ Key Finding

Spherical focus of enhancement near the spleen.

■ Top 3 Differential Diagnoses

- **Sentinel clot:** A sentinel clot can be seen in the setting of traumatic or nontraumatic hemoperitoneium. Acute blood products form a hemostatic clot adjacent to the source of hemorrhage and can assist in detecting the site of injury. On CT, a sentinel clot is higher in attenuation than nonclotted blood measuring 45 to 70 HU. Nonclotted blood tends to pool in the dependent aspects of the abdomen and pelvis, including the hepatorenal recess, paracolic gutters, and pelvic cul-de-sac. Dependent, nonclotted hemoperitoneum has attenuation of 30 to 45 HU. Active extravasation can be assessed with the use of intravenous contrast with arterial and venous phase imaging and may require emergent embolization.
- **Pseudoaneurysm/mycotic aneurysm:** A pseudoaneurysm is aneurysmal dilatation that is contained by the adventicial layer of the arterial wall or perivascular soft tissue. Etiologies include iatrogenic and non-iatrogenic trauma and infection. False aneurysms from an infectious source are known as mycotic aneurysms and are commonly caused by bacterial endocarditis. With sonographic imaging, a classic yin-yang flow pattern may be demonstrated. Pseudoaneurysms have a high risk of rupture resulting in hemoperitoneum and are most commonly treated via endovascular embolization or placement of a covered stent.
- **True aneurysm:** A fusiform or saccular dilatation of the artery that involves all three layers. There are a multitude of etiologies including atherosclerosis, hypertension, trauma, and connective tissue disorders. True aneurysms are less prone to rupture than pseudoaneurysm; however, the treatment is similar.

■ Additional Diagnostic Considerations

Arterial venous fistula (AVF): AVF is an abnormal communication between venous and arterial vessels. Some common causes include abdominal trauma, percutaneous intervention, and vessel erosion related to tumor or inflammation. This may involve almost any organ in the abdomen. CT and MRI show early arterial enhancement of venous vessels. Angiography is used to plan and execute treatment by transcatheter or surgical occlusion.

■ Diagnosis

Sentinel clot secondary to a splenic laceration.

✓ Pearls

- Sentinel colt has a higher attenuation than dependent extravasated blood.
- Clot forms as a physiologic hemostatic response and can aid in detection of bleeding source.

- True and false aneurysms are treated similarly, but pseudoaneurysms are more prone to rupture.

Suggested Readings

González, SB, Vilanova Busquets, JC, Figueiras, RG, et al. Imaging arteriovenous fistulas. AJR Am J Roentgenol. 2009; 193:1425–1433

Jesinger RA, Thoreson AA, Lamba R. Abdominal and pelvic aneurysms and pseudoaneurysms: imaging review with clinical, radiologic, and treatment correlation. Radiographics. 2013; 33(3):E71–96

Lubner M, Menias C, Rucker C, et al. Blood in the belly: CT findings of hemoperitoneum. Radiographics. 2007; 27(1):109–125

Case 140

Robert A. Jesinger

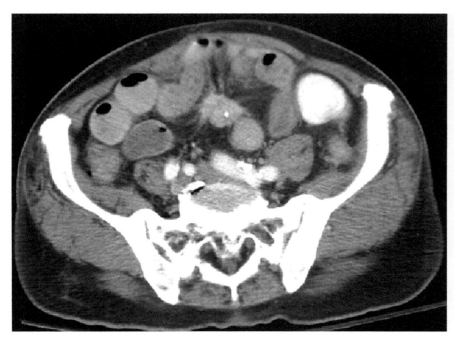

Fig. 140.1 Enhanced axial CT image through the lower abdomen demonstrates a solid enhancing mass in the small bowel mesentery. There is retraction of mesenteric vessels toward the mass suggestive of a desmoplastic reaction. A punctate calcification is noted in the center of the mass. (Image courtesy of Rocky C. Saenz.)

■ Clinical History

A 38-year-old man with chronic abdominal pain (▶Fig. 140.1).

■ Key Finding

Mesenteric mass with calcifications.

■ Top 3 Differential Diagnoses

• **Carcinoid tumor:** Gastrointestinal carcinoid tumor is a slow-growing hypervascular lesion arising from neuroendocrine cells within the bowel. Mesenteric involvement incites a desmoplastic response, resulting in a spiculated mesenteric mass with intense reactive scarring. Calcifications are visible in up to 70% of cases. Mesenteric involvement is typically secondary with the primary neoplasm most commonly within the appendix or ileum. While the primary lesion is often occult, CT or MR enterography or somatostatin receptor scintigraphy are the best modalities to localize the primary mass.

• **Sclerosing mesenteritis:** Most common CT appearance is solitary, ill-defined mass at the root of the small bowel mesentery with marked calcification. Tethering of adjacent bowel loops and vascular encasement is also frequent. Differentiation of retractile mesenteritis from a mesenteric carcinoid metastasis can be impossible.

• **Metastatic disease:** Metastatic disease to the bowel mesentery can occur via direct spread (pancreatic and colon carcinoma), hematogenous dissemination (breast and lung carcinoma), lymphatic spread (lymphoma), or peritoneal seeding (gastric and ovarian carcinoma). Enhanced CT is the modality of choice for assessing number of lesions, margins (round vs. irregular), internal components (soft tissue, fluid, calcification, etc.), enhancement characteristics, as well as identification of the primary source of neoplasm.

■ Additional Diagnostic Considerations

• **Reactive lymphadenopathy:** Reactive lymphadenopathy may present as a mesenteric mass and is typically due to an infectious process within the abdomen. Although virtually any abdominal infection may result in conglomerate lymphadenopathy, *Mycobacterium* (tuberculosis and avium-intracellulare), and *Tropheryma whipplei* (Whipple's disease) are particularly prone to lymph node enlargement. In particular, these infectious agents result in characteristic lymphadenopathy with central low attenuation.

• **Desmoid tumor/fibrosing mesenteritis:** Mesenteric desmoid tumors consist of focal regions of mass-like fibrosis. They are most commonly associated with familial adenomatous polyposis and cranial osteomas (Gardner syndrome). CT reveals a circumscribed or stellate soft-tissue mesenteric mass. Larger lesions may undergo central necrosis, and calcification may be seen posttreatment. A related entity referred to as fibrosing mesenteritis is similar to desmoid tumor both radiographically and pathologically; however, it occurs in the absence of familial adenomatous polyposis and is a diagnosis of exclusion.

■ Diagnosis

Carcinoid tumor.

✓ Pearls

• Reactive adenopathy is commonly seen with gastroenteritis.
• Carcinoid tumor incites a desmoplastic reaction and commonly calcifies.

• Mesenteric adenopathy with central low attenuation is concerning for tuberculosis, Mycobacterium avium-intracellulare, and Whipple's disease.

Suggested Readings

Lattin GE, Jr, O'Brien WT, Duncan MD, Peckham S. Sclerosing mesenteritis. Appl Radiol. 2007; 36(5):40–41

Levy AD, Rimola J, Mehrotra AK, Sobin LH. From the archives of the AFIP: benign fibrous tumors and tumorlike lesions of the mesentery: radiologic-pathologic correlation. Radiographics. 2006; 26(1):245–264

Sheth S, Horton KM, Garland MR, Fishman EK. Mesenteric neoplasms: CT appearances of primary and secondary tumors and differential diagnosis. Radiographics. 2003; 23(2):457–473, quiz 535–536

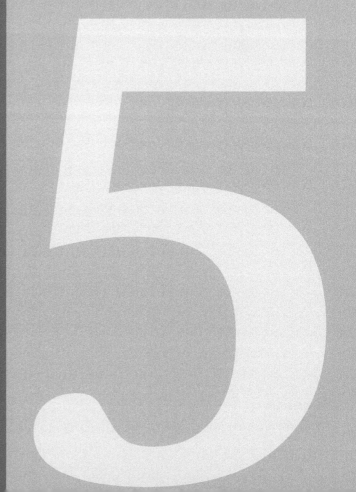

Part 5

Abdominal Wall and Soft Tissues

Case 141

Rocky C. Saenz

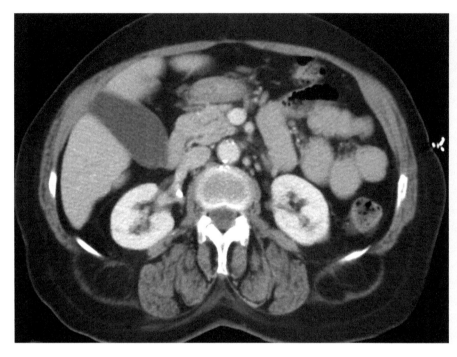

Fig. 141.1 CT axial images of the lower abdomen with intravenous and oral contrast demonstrates retroperitoneal fat herniating though the posterior abdominal walls bilaterally.

■ **Clinical History**

A 50-year-old male with back pain (▶Fig. 141.1).

■ Key Finding

Retroperitoneal fat herniating though the posterior abdominal wall.

■ Top 3 Differential Diagnoses

- **Lumbar hernia**: Lumbar hernia is a hernia through the lumbar triangle. Lumbar hernias can contain essentially any retroperitoneal organ. These are divided into superior and inferior lumbar triangle hernias. Superior hernias are also known as Grynfeltt–Lesshaft and inferior hernias are also called Petit's hernias. The superior hernias are more common. These occur between the quadratus lumborum, 12th rib, and the internal oblique muscle. The boundaries of the inferior hernias consist of the iliac crest, external abdominal oblique muscles, and the margins of the latissimus dorsi muscle. Acute abdominal trauma more commonly results in Petit's hernias. Both superior and inferior hernias may be related to incisions from a recent procedure. Secondary to the large size of lumbar hernias, it is uncommon for associated incarceration and strangulation of herniated bowel.
- **Congenital diaphragmatic hernia**: Congenital diaphragmatic hernias include Bochdalek hernias, which are the most common type of congenital diaphragmatic hernia, and involve the posterior–lateral aspect of the diaphragm and typically present in infancy. Another type of congenital diaphragmatic hernia is a Morgagni hernia, which involves the anterior aspect of the diaphragm and typically presents later in life. Traumatic diaphragmatic hernia typically occurs after trauma and causes abdominal or retroperitoneal structures to herniate into the chest cavity secondary to the negative intrathoracic pressure. There is a high association of intra-abdominal organ injury with traumatic diaphragmatic rupture.
- **Abdominal wall lipoma**: Lipomas are benign fatty tumors that can occur anywhere in the body. These tumors follow fat on all cross-sectional studies. These lesions are typically incidentally found. On MRI, fat saturation sequences are helpful to solidify the diagnosis. Imaging findings of lipomas that suggest liposarcoma include nodules of soft tissue and foci of enhancement.

■ Diagnosis

Superior lumbar hernia, Grynfeltt–Lesshaft.

✓ Pearls

- Grynfeltt–Lesshaft hernias are uncommon to cause bowel strangulation.
- Petit's hernias occur just above the iliac crest.

- Nodular enhancement of a lipoma raises the concern for liposarcoma.

Suggested Readings

Aguirre DA, Santosa AC, Casola G, Sirlin CB. Abdominal wall hernias: imaging features, complications, and diagnostic pitfalls at multi-detector row CT. Radiographics. 2005; 25(6):1501–1520

Federle MP, Jeffrey RB, Woodward PJ, Borhani A. Diagnostic Imaging: Abdomen. 2nd ed. Philadelphia, PA: Lippincott Williams & Wilkins; 2009

Killeen KL, Girard S, DeMeo JH, Shanmuganathan K, Mirvis SE. Using CT to diagnose traumatic lumbar hernia. AJR Am J Roentgenol. 2000; 174(5):1413–1415

Case 142

Elias Antypas

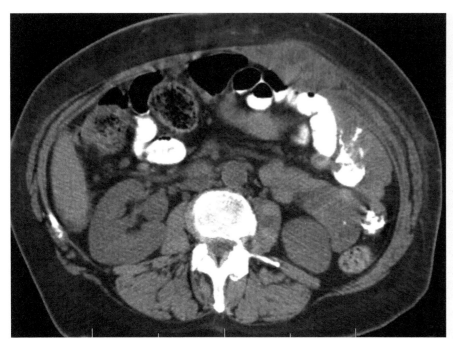

Fig. 142.1 CT axial image with oral contrast shows enlargement of the abdominis rectus along its left side. (Image courtesy of Rocky C. Saenz D.O.)

■ Clinical History

A 74-year-old female taking a new medication with abdominal pain (▶Fig. 142.1).

■ Key Finding

Enlargement of the abdominis rectus.

■ Top 3 Differential Diagnoses

- **Hematoma:** In a patient with history of trauma or anticoagulation use, hematoma is the most common etiology. On noncontrast CT, a hematoma can appear to be isoattenuating to the muscle but can be of higher attenuation with acute bleeding. While there is lack of enhancement on contrast-enhanced CT, focal hyperattenuation within the hematoma can represent active extravasation. Follow-up imaging will show regression. MR appearance is variable due to different appearances of blood products over time.

- **Abscess:** On contrast-enhanced CT, this can be seen as a low-density fluid collection with a peripherally enhancing rim. With MRI, appearance is variable and depends on its internal contents. Typically, it has high T2 signal that becomes more heterogeneous with increasing amounts of necrosis, debris, or gas.
- **Neoplasm:** Usually tumors demonstrate enhancement when compared to precontrasted images. Tumors that may involve the rectus abdominis include, but not limited to, lipoma, desmoid, fibrous tumor, metastasis, or lymphoma.

■ Additional Diagnostic Considerations

- **Endometriosis:** Endometriomas are hemorrhagic cysts, resulting from functioning endometrium outside of the uterus. The abdominal wall is the most common site of extrapelvic involvement. Classic presentation is an abdominal wall mass near a C-section scar in a patient with cyclical pain. On MRI, endometriomas appear hyperintense on T1-weighted image, but demonstrate hypointense signal on T2-weighted image known as "T2 shading."

- **Ventral hernia:** These hernias occur through the linea alba of the abdominal wall and are in the midline. On physical examination, hernias can be confused for soft-tissue masses. On imaging, the diagnosis is obvious when the "mass" is noted to be contiguous with the bowel. CT is useful to evaluate obstruction, incarceration, strangulation, and necrosis.

■ Diagnosis

Rectus abdominis hematoma

✓ Pearls

- Hematoma is the most common cause of a rectus abdominis mass, it is strongly associated with trauma or use of anticoagulation.
- Consider endometrioma in a female with an abdominal wall mass that enlarges with menses.

- An abdominal wall abscess may have a fistulous connection to the bowel (oral contrast may be beneficial in the diagnosis).

Suggested Readings

Gidwaney R, Badler RL, Yam BL, et al. Endometriosis of abdominal and pelvic wall scars: multimodality imaging findings, pathologic correlation, and radiologic mimics. Radiographics. 2012; 32(7):2031–2043

Stein L, Elsayes KM, Wagner-Bartak N. Subcutaneous abdominal wall masses: radiological reasoning. AJR Am J Roentgenol. 2012; 198(2):W146–51

Case 143

Gregory D. Puthoff

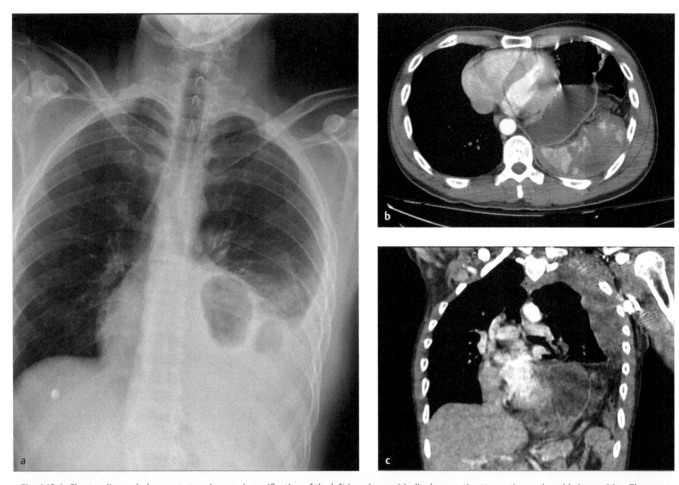

Fig. 143.1 Chest radiograph demonstrates abnormal opacification of the left lung base with diaphragmatic attenuation and ovoid air opacities. The axial and coronal CT images demonstrate intrathoracic stomach and spleen. The spleen demonstrates grade V laceration with surrounding hematoma. Additionally, there is abnormal soft-tissue attenuation material along the lateral left chest wall. (Image courtesy of Rocky C. Saenz D.O.)

■ Clinical History

A 31-year-old male with left upper quadrant pain after a motor vehicle accident (▶ Fig. 143.1).

■ Key Finding

Diaphragmatic attenuation.

■ Top 3 Differential Diagnoses

- **Congenital diaphragmatic hernia**: Congenital diaphragmatic hernias include Bochdalek hernias, which are the most common type of congenital diaphragmatic hernia, and involve the posterior–lateral aspect of the diaphragm and typically present in infancy. Another type of congenital diaphragmatic hernia is a Morgagni hernia, which involves the anterior aspect of the diaphragm and typically presents later in life. Traumatic diaphragmatic hernia typically occurs after trauma and causes abdominal or retroperitoneal structures to herniate into the chest cavity secondary to the negative intrathoracic pressure. There is a high association of intra-abdominal organ injury with traumatic diaphragmatic rupture.
- **Traumatic diaphragmatic hernia**: Traumatic diaphragmatic hernia or diaphragmatic rupture typically occurs after significant abdominal trauma. The abdominal or retroperitoneal structures herniate into the chest cavity secondary to the negative intrathoracic pressure. There is a high association of intra-abdominal organ injury with traumatic diaphragmatic rupture. The most common location is on the left.
- **Hiatal hernia**: It is a type of acquired hernia that occurs when abdominal structures herniate through the esophageal hiatus, typically the stomach. This can be differentiated from other types of diaphragmatic hernias by its central location and involvement of the esophageal hiatus. There are two types of hiatal hernias: sliding and paraesophageal. Sliding is the most common type of hiatal hernia and occurs when the gastroesophageal junction herniates above the esophageal hiatus, whereas the paraesophageal hiatal hernia occurs when the gastroesophageal junction remains within the normal location and a portion of the stomach herniates through the hiatus.

■ Additional Diagnostic Considerations

- **Congenital pulmonary airway malformation (CPAM):** It is a congenital lung lesion that can mimic diaphragmatic hernia on a chest radiograph secondary to its multicystic properties. CPAM is usually diagnosed within the antenatal period and may present with respiratory distress and pulmonary hypoplasia, although it may present into adulthood. Cross-sectional imaging is critical and will demonstrate an intact diaphragm.
- **Pericardial cyst:** Pericardial cysts occur within the cardiophrenic recess and are more common on the right side. Pericardial cysts arise from the pericardium and may mimic a diaphragmatic hernia on a chest radiograph, but are easily differentiated on cross-sectional imaging secondary to the well-defined and uniformly low-attenuated fluid pericardial cyst arising from the pericardium.

■ Diagnosis

Traumatic diaphragmatic hernia/rupture

✓ Pearls

- There is a high association of intra-abdominal organ injury with traumatic diaphragmatic rupture.
- Diaphragmatic injuries/ruptures are most common on the left side.
- Pericardial cysts may mimic a diaphragmatic hernia and are more common on the right side.

Suggested Readings

Biyyam DR, Chapman T, Ferguson MR, Deutsch G, Dighe MK. Congenital lung abnormalities: embryologic features, prenatal diagnosis, and postnatal radiologic-pathologic correlation. Radiographics. 2010; 30(6):1721–1738

Iochum S, Lu, dig T, Walter F, Sebbag H, Grosdidier G, Blum AG. Imaging of diaphragmatic injury: a diagnostic challenge? Radiographics. 2002; 22(Spec No):S103–S116, discussion S116–S118

Pineda V, Andreu J, Cáceres J, Merino X, Varona D, Domínguez-Oronoz R. Lesions of the cardiophrenic space: findings at cross-sectional imaging. Radiographics. 2007; 27(1):19–32

Case 144

Chelsea M. Jeranko

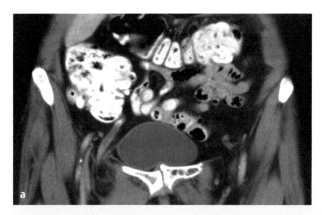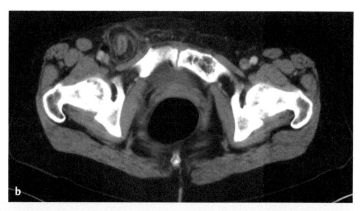

Fig. 144.1 CT coronal and axial images with intravenous and oral contrast. The top coronal image demonstrates the appendix with a proximal appendicolith entering an inguinal hernia defect. The bottom axial image shows the appendix with hyperemic walls, thickening, and peripheral fat stranding. (Image courtesy of Rocky C. Saenz D.O.)

■ Clinical History

A 30-year-old male with right lower quadrant pain (▶ Fig. 144.1).

◼ Key Finding

Appendix with an inguinal hernia.

◼ Top 3 Differential Diagnoses

- **Amyand's hernia**: An inguinal hernia sac can contain essentially any organ within the lower abdomen. When the appendix is found within an inguinal hernia sac, it is termed an Amyand's hernia. Amyand's hernias can be complicated by appendiceal inflammation, incarceration, or strangulation. Incarceration is a clinical diagnosis when the hernia sac cannot be reduced manually. Strangulation occurs due to ischemia, and imaging findings include bowel wall thickening, mesenteric vessel engorgement, fat stranding, and free fluid. Emergent surgical repair is indicated in the setting of a strangulated hernia.

- **Littre's hernia**: A Meckel's diverticulum contained within an inguinal hernia sac is termed a Littre's hernia. This is an uncommon type of hernia; however, it is prone to complications, particularly incarceration and strangulation.
- **Richter's hernia**: A Richter's hernia is protrusion of the antimesenteric bowel wall into an abdominal wall hernia sac. Strangulation is common and can occur in the absence of obstructive symptoms. It occurs most commonly with femoral hernias.

◼ Additional Diagnostic Considerations

Inguinal hernia: Inguinal hernias are the most common type of abdominal wall hernia. They can be direct or indirect, with indirect inguinal hernias being more common. These can be differentiated on imaging based on the relationship of the hernia sac to the inferior epigastric vessels. The neck of an indirect inguinal hernia arises superior and lateral to the inferior epigastric vessels while direct inguinal hernias emerge anterior and medial to the inferior epigastric vessels. Ultrasound has a lower sensitivity for inguinal hernias than CT and can be used as a first-line modality in nonurgent presentations. CT is helpful in identifying the contents of the hernia sac and complications related to the hernia, particularly in patients with acute symptoms.

◼ Diagnosis

Amyand's hernia with appendicitis

✓ Pearls

- An appendix contained within an inguinal hernia sac is termed an Amyand's hernia.
- Richter's and Littre's hernias are rare and prone to incarceration and strangulation.

- Indirect inguinal hernias are the most common type of inguinal hernia; however, direct inguinal hernias are considered more benign.

Suggested Readings

Aguirre DA, Santosa AC, Casola G, Sirlin CB. Abdominal wall hernias: imaging features, complications, and diagnostic pitfalls at multi-detector row CT. Radiographics. 2005; 25(6):1501–1520

Bhosale PR, Patnana M, Viswanathan C, Szklaruk J. The inguinal canal: anatomy and imaging features of common and uncommon masses. Radiographics. 2008; 28(3):819–835, quiz 913

Burkhardt JH, Arshanskiy Y, Munson JL, Scholz FJ. Diagnosis of inguinal region hernias with axial CT: the lateral crescent sign and other key findings. Radiographics. 2011; 31(2):E1–E12

Case 145

Rocky C. Saenz

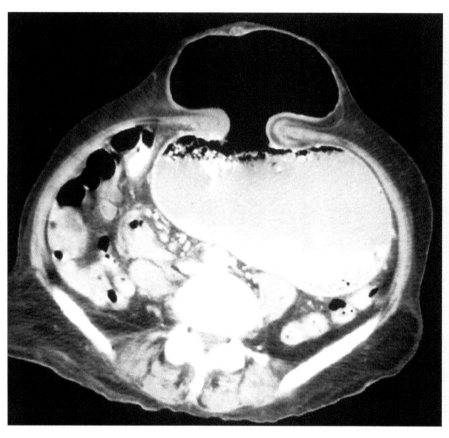

Fig. 145.1 CT axial image with intravenous and oral contrast through the pelvis shows protrusion of the stomach through the center of the abdominal wall. The hernia sac contains a portion of the stomach. (Image courtesy of Rocky C. Saenz D.O.)

■ Clinical History

A 72-year-old male with pelvic pain and bulging (▶Fig. 145.1).

■ Key Finding

Bowel herniating along the midline of the abdominal wall.

■ Top 3 Differential Diagnoses

• **Umbilical hernia**: These hernias occur when abdominal contents protrude through the umbilical ring and are typically in the midline. Umbilical hernias are commonly seen with chronic ascites in cirrhotic patients. These are termed congenital when diagnosed in infancy and considered acquired when developed at a later age. It is particularly important to evaluate the presence of bowel strangulation, which occurs when bowel becomes entrapped in the hernia and becomes ischemic.

• **Spigelian hernia**: These hernias occur through the lateral ventral abdominal wall where the semilunar and semicircular lines intersect at the lateral border of the rectus abdominus (the spigelian aponeurosis). These hernias are inferior to the level of the umbilicus. Typically, spigelian hernias are asymptomatic and present as a palpable mass. This condition may lead to symptoms of bowel incarceration or obstruction.

• **Ventral hernia:** These hernias occur through the linea alba of the abdominal wall and are typically in the midline. CT is useful to evaluate obstruction, incarceration, strangulation, and necrosis. Risk factors include obesity, diabetes, pulmonary disease, and steroid use. Many of these patients, approximately 20%, have multiple hernias.

■ Diagnosis

Ventral hernia

✓ Pearls

• Spigelian hernias occur along the lateral abdominal wall.
• When hernia sacs become enlarged or are symptomatic, surgical reduction is needed.

• Always evaluate herniated bowel for the presence of ischemia and obstruction.

Suggested Readings

Elsayes KM, Staveteig PT, Narra VR, Leyendecker JR, Lewis JS, Jr, Brown JJ. MRI of the peritoneum: spectrum of abnormalities. AJR Am J Roentgenol. 2006; 186(5):1368–1379

Federle MP, Jeffrey RB, Woodward PJ, Borhani A. Diagnostic Imaging: Abdomen. 2nd ed. Philadelphia, PA: Lippincott Williams & Wilkins; 2009

Case 146

Rocky C. Saenz

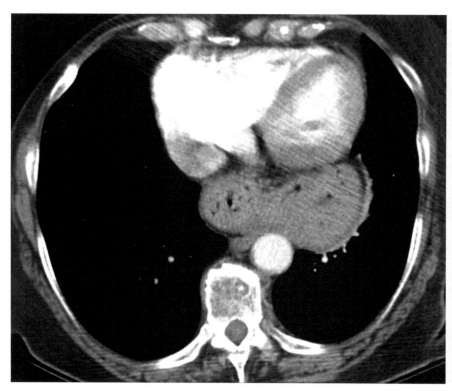

Fig. 146.1 CT chest axial image with intravenous contrast demonstrates a focal soft-tissue density behind the heart.

■ Clinical History

A 49-year-old male with occasional pyrosis (▶Fig. 146.1).

■ **Key Finding**

Retrocardiac soft-tissue density.

■ **Top 3 Differential Diagnoses**

- **Sliding hiatal hernia**: Hiatal hernia is a type of acquired hernia that occurs when abdominal structures herniate through the esophageal hiatus, typically the stomach. There are two types of hiatal hernias: sliding and paraesophageal. Sliding hiatal hernia represents 90% of hiatal hernias. These occur when the gastroesophageal junction herniates above the esophageal hiatus. Classic symptoms include substernal pain, dysphagia, and regurgitation. When the esophageal B ring and gastric folds are seen more than 2 cm above the diaphragm, it can also present as a retrocardiac opacity with an air fluid level on a chest X-ray. They may self-reduce in the upright position and are commonly associated with gastroesophageal reflux. In 5% of the patients, Cameron ulcers are seen in the herniated stomach on an endoscopy. These are usually treated medically to control gastroesophageal reflux disease (GERD).
- **Paraesophageal hiatal hernia**: Paraesophageal hernia is a type of hiatal hernia that occurs when the gastric fundus herniates through the esophageal hiatus with the gastroesophageal junction remaining in the normal position. Usually asymptomatic but can have chest pain, GERD, vomiting, and anemia. Paraesophageal hernias are often treated surgically, as there is an increased risk for gastric volvulus.
- **Congenital diaphragmatic hernia**: Congenital diaphragmatic hernias include Bochdalek hernias, which are the most common type of congenital diaphragmatic hernia, and involve the posterior–lateral aspect of the diaphragm and typically present in infancy. Another type of congenital diaphragmatic hernia is a Morgagni hernia, which involves the anterior aspect of the diaphragm and typically presents later in life. Traumatic diaphragmatic hernia typically occurs after trauma and causes abdominal or retroperitoneal structures to herniate into the chest cavity secondary to the negative intrathoracic pressure. There is a high association of intra-abdominal organ injury with traumatic diaphragmatic rupture.

■ **Additional Diagnostic Considerations**

Phrenic ampulla: The phrenic ampulla is a normal anatomical segment of the distal esophagus located between the esophageal A and B rings. This segment is slightly more distensible than the normal esophagus and can have a bulbous configuration when fully distended, mimicking a sliding hiatal hernia. It is of no clinical significance.

■ **Diagnosis**

Hiatal hernia, sliding

✓ **Pearls**

- Sliding hiatal hernias are the most common type of hernias.
- Bochdalek hernias are the most common type of congenital diaphragmatic hernias.
- Paraesophageal hernias are at risk for volvulus, and therefore they are surgically reduced.

Suggested Readings

Biyyam DR, Chapman T, Ferguson MR, Deutsch G, Dighe MK. Congenital lung abnormalities: embryologic features, prenatal diagnosis, and postnatal radiologic-pathologic correlation. Radiographics. 2010; 30(6):1721–1738

Federle MP, Jeffrey RB, Woodward PJ, Borhani A. Diagnostic Imaging: Abdomen. 2nd ed. Philadelphia, PA: Lippincott Williams & Wilkins; 2009

Huang SY, Levine MS, Rubesin SE, Katzka DA, Laufer I. Large hiatal hernia with floppy fundus: clinical and radiographic findings. AJR Am J Roentgenol. 2007; 188(4):960–964

Case 147

Daniel E. Knapp

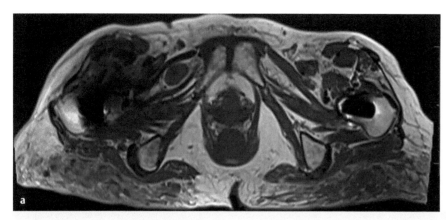 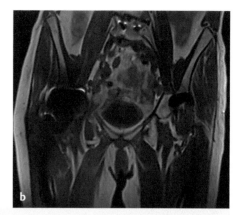

Fig. 147.1 MRI T1-weighted axial and coronal images of the pelvis without contrast. The top axial image demonstrates a loop of small bowel protruding through the right obturator foramen. The bottom coronal image shows similar findings. (Images courtesy of Rocky C. Saenz D.O.)

■ **Clinical History**

A 30-year-old male with right lower quadrant pain (▶ Fig. 147.1).

■ Key Finding

Abdominal or pelvic contents protruding through the obturator foramen.

■ Top 3 Differential Diagnoses

- **Obturator hernia:** Obturator hernias occur when bowel or mesenteric fat protrude through the obturator foramen. Obturator hernia is a rare type of abdominal hernia representing less than 1% of hernias. These are commonly seen in elderly female patients. Obturator hernia is exacerbated by conditions that increase abdominal pressure; chronic obstructive pulmonary disease, constipation, and pregnancy. These hernias can present with bowel obstruction. The obturator foramen is covered by a protective membrane that passes through the obturator nerve, artery, and vein. These hernias extend through this membrane.
- **Inguinal hernia:** Inguinal hernias are the most common type of abdominal hernia (75–80%). Inguinal hernias can be divided into two types: direct and indirect. Direct inguinal hernia contents pass through Hesselbach's triangle formed by the boundaries of inguinal ligament, lateral margin of rectus abdominis, and inferior epigastric artery. The hernia sac is anteromedial to the origin of inferior epigastric artery. Indirect inguinal hernia contents exit through the inguinal canal, having passed through the deep internal inguinal ring. Hernia sac is superolateral to inferior epigastric artery. These can follow spermatic cord and course into the scrotum. Almost any abdominal structure can potentially herniate, some notable structures include small bowel wall (Richter's hernia), inflamed appendix (Amyand's hernia), or Meckel's diverticulum (Littre's hernia). It is particularly important to evaluate the presence of small bowel strangulation that occurs when bowel becomes entrapped in the hernia and becomes ischemic.
- **Femoral hernia:** Femoral hernias occur when contents extend through the femoral rings and into femoral canal, medial to femoral vein and inferior to inferior epigastric vein. These hernias are less common than inguinal hernias and occur with herniation into the femoral canal below the inguinal ligament. Femoral hernias occur more commonly in women and on the right side. Evaluation of femoral vein occlusion secondary to mass effect is important, especially if there is incarcerated bowel within a femoral hernia.

■ Additional Diagnostic Considerations

Sciatic hernia: When hernia contents protrude through the greater or lesser sciatic foramen. This is an extremely rare type of pelvic floor hernia.

■ Diagnosis

Obturator hernia.

✓ Pearls

- As with any case of hernia, radiographic signs of ischemia and obstruction must be evaluated.
- Obturator hernias may present with Howship–Romberg sign. Symptoms include pain in medial aspect of thigh or hip with abduction, extension, and/or internal rotation of the knee, which are caused by irritation of the obturator nerve. Flexion of knee relieves pain in 25 to 50% of cases.
- Inguinal hernias are the most common type of hernia.

Suggested Readings

Aguirre DA, Santosa AC, Casola G, Sirlin CB. Abdominal wall hernias: imaging features, complications, and diagnostic pitfalls at multi-detector row CT. Radiographics. 2005; 25(6):1501–1520

Bhosale PR, Patnana M, Viswanathan C, Szklaruk J. The inguinal canal: anatomy and imaging features of common and uncommon masses. Radiographics. 2008; 28(3):819–835, quiz 913

Pandey R, Maqbool A, Jayachandran N. Obturator hernia: a diagnostic challenge. Hernia. 2009; 13(1):97–99

Case 148

Gregory D. Puthoff

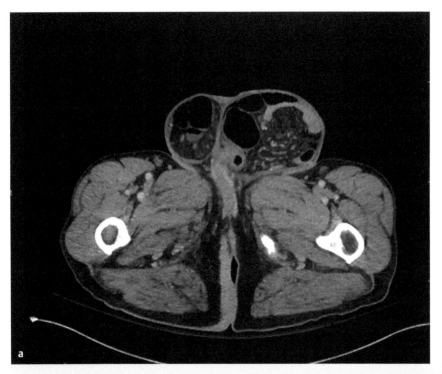
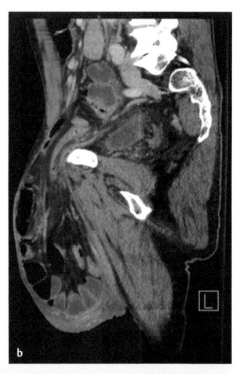

Fig. 148.1 Contrast-enhanced axial CT image through the lower pelvis demonstrates bilateral pelvic inguinal hernias. The hernia sacs both contain loops of nonenlarged bowel.

■ Clinical History

A 52-year-old male with pelvic pain and bulging (▶ Fig. 148.1).

■ Key Finding

Bilateral pelvic hernias.

■ Top 3 Differential Diagnoses

- **Inguinal hernia**: Inguinal hernias can be classified as direct or indirect, depending on whether the herniation occurs through the internal inguinal ring (indirect) or through the weakened abdominal wall musculature (direct). Imaging of inguinal region hernias is important to evaluate the presence of herniation of abdominal structures. Almost any abdominal structure can potentially herniate, some notable structures include small bowel wall (Richter's hernia), inflamed appendix (Amyand's hernia), or Meckel's diverticulum (Littre's hernia). It is particularly important to evaluate the presence of small bowel strangulation that occurs when bowel becomes entrapped in the hernia and becomes ischemic. Entrapped bowel can also become obstructed, resulting in a bowel obstruction, which will present as proximal bowel dilation with air fluid levels that is decompressed distally.

- **Femoral hernia**: Femoral hernias are less common than inguinal hernias and occur with herniation into the femoral canal below the inguinal ligament. Femoral hernias occur more commonly in women and on the right side. Evaluation of femoral vein occlusion secondary to mass effect is important, especially if there is incarcerated bowel within a femoral hernia.
- **Inguinal lipoma:** Spermatic cord lipomas are benign fatty tumors of the spermatic cord, which are typically incidentally found. Evaluation of spermatic cord lipomas will demonstrate well defined fat density lesion centered within the spermatic cord. These fatty tumors should not be contiguous with retroperitoneal fat, which helps differentiate lipomas from normal fat within an inguinal hernia.

■ Additional Diagnostic Considerations

- **Hydrocele/Varicocele**: Scrotal pathology may extend superiorly into the inguinal canal, which may mimic an inguinal hernia. This particularly occurs with scrotal hydroceles and dilated veins from varicoceles. Careful evaluation of the inguinal hernia and scrotal region should be performed, as these conditions can often coexist.

- **Inguinal mass**: Soft-tissue masses can present involving the inguinal region. Masses arising from adjacent inguinal lymph nodes or soft-tissue masses may present as a mass within this region. An inguinal mass will not be continuous with the intra-abdominal cavity.

■ Diagnosis

Bilateral inguinal hernias, indirect.

✓ Pearls

- Indirect inguinal hernias are the most common type of abdominal hernias.
- Femoral hernias are more common in females and may compress the femoral vein.

- Always evaluate herniated bowel for the presence of ischemia and obstruction.

Suggested Readings

Bhosale PR, Patnana M, Viswanathan C, Szklaruk J. The inguinal canal: anatomy and imaging features of common and uncommon masses. Radiographics. 2008; 28(3):819–835, quiz 913

Burkhardt JH, Arshanskiy Y, Munson JL, Scholz FJ. Diagnosis of inguinal region hernias with axial CT: the lateral crescent sign and other key findings. Radiographics. 2011; 31(2):E1–E12

Case 149

Alex R. Martin

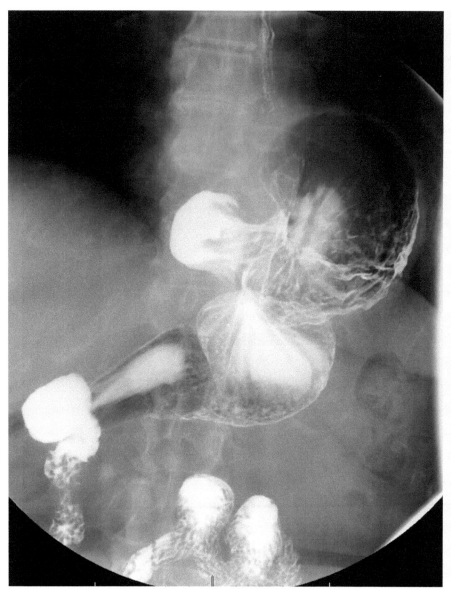

Fig. 149.1 Frontal image from a barium esophagram demonstrates gastric mucosa superior to the diaphragm, the esophagus passes medial to the supradiaphragmatic stomach.

■ Clinical History

A 73-year-old female with dyspepsia (▶Fig. 149.1).

■ **Key Finding**

Stomach herniating above diaphragm.

■ **Top 3 Differential Diagnoses**

• **Sliding hiatal hernia**: There is superior displacement of the gastroesophageal junction and gastric cardia through the esophageal hiatus. When the esophageal B ring and gastric folds are seen more than 2 cm above the diaphragm, it can also present as a retrocardiac opacity with an air fluid level on a chest X-ray. They may self-reduce in the upright position and are commonly associated with gastroesophageal reflux.

• **Paraesophageal hiatal hernia**: There is herniation of the gastric fundus through the esophageal hiatus with the fundus typically located anterior and lateral to the esophagus. The majority have an associated sliding hiatal hernia. Paraesophageal hernias are often treated surgically, as there is an increased risk for gastric volvulus.

• **Epiphrenic diverticulum**: Pulsion diverticulum of the distal esophagus occurs due to increased intraluminal pressure and is associated with esophageal dysmotility. These are false diverticula that are most commonly on the right posterolateral aspect of the esophagus, which can cause dysphagia, regurgitation, and compression of the distal esophagus.

■ **Additional Diagnostic Considerations**

Phrenic ampulla: The phrenic ampulla is a normal anatomical segment of the distal esophagus located between the esophageal A and B rings. This segment is slightly more distensible than the normal esophagus and can have a bulbous configuration when fully distended, mimicking a sliding hiatal hernia. It is of no clinical significance.

■ **Diagnosis**

Paraesophageal hiatal hernia.

✓ **Pearls**

• Sliding hiatal hernias are very common and associated with increased risk of gastroesophageal reflux disease (GERD) and Barrett's esophagus.

• Paraesophageal hernias are associated with an increased risk of gastric volvulus.

• Epiphrenic diverticulum can mimic a sliding hiatal hernia but will not contain gastric folds.

Suggested Readings

Canon CL, Morgan DE, Einstein DM, Herts BR, Hawn MT, Johnson LF. Surgical approach to gastroesophageal reflux disease: what the radiologist needs to know. Radiographics. 2005; 25(6):1485–1499

Chen YM, Ott DJ, Gelfand DW, Munitz HA. Multiphasic examination of the esophagogastric region for strictures, rings, and hiatal hernia: evaluation of the individual techniques. Gastrointest Radiol. 1985; 10(4):311–316

Fasano NC, Levine MS, Rubesin SE, Redfern RO, Lauf, er I. Epiphrenic diverticulum: clinical and radiographic findings in 27 patients. Dysphagia. 2003; 18(1):9–15

Case 150

Stacy J. Ries

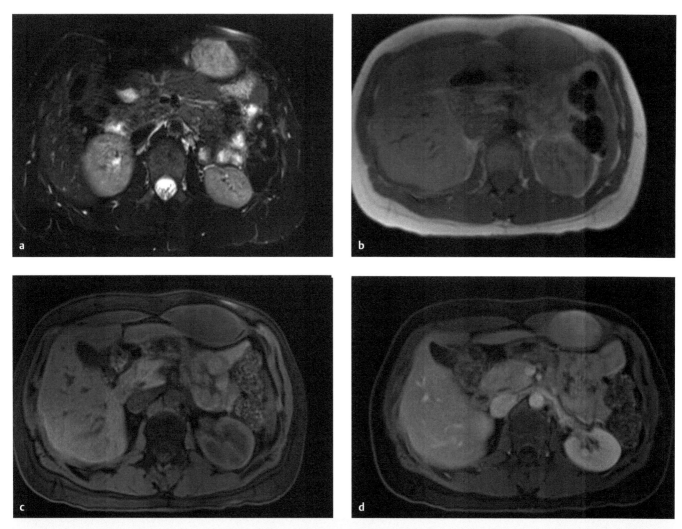

Fig. 150.1 **(a)** MRI demonstrates a predominantly hyperintense, well circumscribed, ovoid, solitary intramuscular mass within the left rectus abdominis on T2-weighted imaging. **(b)** The mass has slight intermediate signal on T1-weighted imaging. **(c)** The T1-weighted precontrast fat saturation image shows slight hypointensity relative to skeletal muscle. **(d)** The mass has homogeneous enhancement on the T1-weighted postcontrast fat saturation image.

■ **Clinical History**

A 28-year-old female complains of left mid abdominal pain (▶ Fig. 150.1).

■ Key Finding

Rectus abdominis intramuscular mass.

■ Top 3 Differential Diagnoses

- **Desmoid tumor**: Desmoid tumors are locally aggressive but are benign tumors and sometimes referred to as aggressive fibromatosis. They can occur spontaneously, in sites of prior trauma or with high estrogen states but are most commonly seen at prior surgical sites. Therefore, these can be seen during pregnancy at the site of prior cesarean scars. They are classified as intra-abdominal, abdominal, or extra-abdominal. On imaging, these tumors are generally homogeneous and isoattenuated to skeletal muscle on the CT. Initially, the tumors are typically T1 hypointense and T2 hyperintense, and later becoming T2 heterogeneous due to increase in collagen deposition. Finally, desmoids will be hypointense on both T1- and T2-weighted images due to an increase in fibrous tissue. Typically, these demonstrate homogeneous enhancement. Some cases are associated with familial adenomatous polyposis or Gardner's syndrome. Definitive treatment is wide local excision, as there is a tendency to recur but not metastasize.
- **Rectus sheath hematoma**: Hematomas may occur in the setting of trauma or be iatrogenic secondary to intervention. These may also occur spontaneously in a patient taking blood thinners or with a coagulopathy. Typical presentation is with acute abdominal pain. There should be lack of internal enhancement on CT and MRI with lack of internal blood flow on the ultrasound. Hematomas may be heterogeneous on CT and MRI, as the blood products degenerate.
- **Rectus sheath abscess:** Abscesses typically demonstrate peripheral rim enhancement and should fit the appropriate clinical setting of fever and leukocytosis. Usually these follow fluid signal on MRI and fluid attenuation on CT. The minority of cases may demonstrate foci of air. When larger than 3 cm, percutaneous drainage may be helpful.

■ Additional Diagnostic Considerations

- **Endometriosis**: Endometrial tissue is directly deposited iatrogenically into areas such as a cesarean section scar at the time of surgery. The history of cyclical pain aids to clinch the diagnosis. In the abdominal wall, endometrial implants will display different imaging characteristics than when in the pelvic cavity. It will be T1 isointense or mildly hyperintense and T2 isointense or slightly hyperintense with avid enhancement. The margins are typically ill-defined and on the CT the mass will typically be isoattenuated.
- **Lymphoma**: Extranodal lymphoma can occur almost anywhere. These are soft masses that conform to surrounding structures and have commonality with the above differentials in that they are typically homogenous on CT, well-circumscribed, and homogeneously enhanced. However, lymphoma is typically T1 and T2 isointense.

■ Diagnosis

Desmoid tumor.

✓ Pearls

- Desmoid tumors are typically homogenous, circumscribed, and at sites of prior scar tissue.
- Hematomas should be avascular on the ultrasound and heterogeneous on the MRI.
- Abscess is the favored diagnosis with a peripheral rim enhancing lesion with air.
- Endometriosis of the abdominal wall should be considered with prior cesarean and cyclical abdominal pain.

Suggested Readings

Dinauer PA, Brixey CJ, Moncur JT, Fanburg-Smith JC, Murphey MD. Pathologic and MR imaging features of benign fibrous soft-tissue tumors in adults. Radiographics. 2007; 27(1):173–187

Federle MP, Jeffrey RB, Woodward PJ, Borhani A. Diagnostic Imaging: Abdomen. 2nd ed. Philadelphia, PA: Lippincott Williams & Wilkins; 2009

Stein L, Elsayes KM, Wagner-Bartak N. Subcutaneous abdominal wall masses: radiological reasoning. AJR Am J Roentgenol. 2012; 198(2):W146–51

Index of Differential Diagnoses

Index of Key Findings

Note: The index is ordered by case number within each part.